Evidence-Based Clinical Practice in Exotic Animal Medicine

Editors

NICOLA DI GIROLAMO
ALEXANDRA L. WINTER

VETERINARY CLINICS OF NORTH AMERICA: EXOTIC ANIMAL PRACTICE

www.vetexotic.theclinics.com

Consulting Editor
JÖRG MAYER

September 2017 • Volume 20 • Number 3

ELSEVIER

1600 John F. Kennedy Boulevard • Suite 1800 • Philadelphia, Pennsylvania, 19103-2899
http://www.vetexotic.theclinics.com

VETERINARY CLINICS OF NORTH AMERICA: EXOTIC ANIMAL PRACTICE Volume 20, Number 3
September 2017 ISSN 1094-9194, ISBN-13: 978-0-323-54576-1

Editor: Colleen Dietzler
Developmental Editor: Meredith Madeira

Veterinary Clinics of North America: Exotic Animal Practice (ISSN 1094-9194) is published in January, May, and September by Elsevier, Inc., 360 Park Avenue South, New York, NY 10010-1710. Subscription prices are $265.00 per year for US individuals, $460.00 per year for US institutions, $100.00 per year for US students and residents, $311.00 per year for Canadian individuals, $554.00 per year for Canadian institutions, $347.00 per year for international individuals, $554.00 per year for international institutions and $165.00 per year for Canadian and foreign students/residents. To receive student/resident rate, orders must be accompanied by name of affiliated institution, date of term, and the *signature* of program/residency coordinator on institution letterhead. Orders will be billed at individual rate until proof of status is received. Foreign air speed delivery is included in all *Clinics* subscription prices. All prices are subject to change without notice. **POSTMASTER:** Send address changes to *Veterinary Clinics of North America: Exotic Animal Practice*, Elsevier Health Sciences Division, Subscription Customer Service, 3251 Riverport Lane, Maryland Heights, MO 63043. **Customer Service: Telephone: 1-800-654-2452** (U.S. and Canada); **1-314-447-8871** (outside U.S. and Canada). **Fax: 1-314-447-8029. E-mail: journalscustomerservice-usa@elsevier.com (for print support); journalsonlinesupport-usa@elsevier.com (for online support)**.

Reprints. For copies of 100 or more of articles in this publication, please contact the Commercial Reprints Department, Elsevier Inc., 360 Park Avenue South, New York, New York 10010-1710. Tel.: 212-633-3874; Fax: 212-633-3820; E-mail: reprints@elsevier.com.

Veterinary Clinics of North America: Exotic Animal Practice is covered in *MEDLINE/PubMed (Index Medicus)*.

Contributors

CONSULTING EDITOR

JÖRG MAYER, Dr med vet, Msc
Diplomate, American Board of Veterinary Practitioners (Exotic Companion Mammals); Diplomate, European College of Zoological Medicine (Small Mammals); Diplomate, American College of Zoological Medicine; Associate Professor of Zoological Medicine, Department of Small Animal Medicine and Surgery, University of Georgia College of Veterinary Medicine, Athens, Georgia, USA

EDITORS

NICOLA DI GIROLAMO, DMV, MSc (EBHC), PhD
Diplomate, European College of Zoological Medicine (Herpetology); Tai Wai Small Animal and Exotic Hospital, Tai Wai, Shatin, Hong Kong; Founder, EBMVet, Cremona, Italy

ALEXANDRA L. WINTER, BVSc
Diplomate, American College of Veterinary Surgeons; Editor, Journal of the American Veterinary Medical Association, American Veterinary Medical Association, Schaumburg, Illinois, USA

AUTHORS

JULIE A. BALKO, VMD
Veterinary Fellow in Zoo Animal Anesthesia, Analgesia, and Pharmacology, Brookfield Zoo, Chicago Zoological Society, Brookfield, Illinois, USA

JOÃO BRANDÃO, LMV, MS
Assistant Professor and Service-Chief, Zoological Medicine Service, Department of Veterinary Clinical Sciences, Center for Veterinary Health Sciences, Oklahoma State University, Stillwater, Oklahoma, USA

LUCILE CHASSANG, DVM, IPSAV (med zool)
Department of Exotic, Centre Hospitalier Vétérinaire Frégis, Arcueil, France

SATHYA K. CHINNADURAI, DVM, MS
Diplomate, American College of Zoological Medicine; Diplomate, American College of Veterinary Anesthesia and Analgesia; Senior Staff Veterinarian, Brookfield Zoo, Chicago Zoological Society, Brookfield, Illinois, USA

MARCUS CLAUSS, MSc, Dr med vet
Diplomate, European College of Veterinary and Comparative Nutrition; Professor, Clinic for Zoo Animals, Exotic Pets and Wildlife, Vetsuisse Faculty, University of Zurich, Zurich, Switzerland

NICOLA DI GIROLAMO, DMV, MSc (EBHC), PhD
Diplomate, European College of Zoological Medicine (Herpetology); Tai Wai Small Animal and Exotic Hospital, Tai Wai, Shatin, Hong Kong; Founder, EBMVet, Cremona, Italy

MICHELLE A. GIUFFRIDA, VMD, MSCE
Diplomate, American College of Veterinary Surgeons; Assistant Professor, Small Animal Surgery, Department of Surgical and Radiological Sciences, UC Davis School of Veterinary Medicine, Davis, California, USA

DAVID SANCHEZ-MIGALLON GUZMAN, LV, MS
Diplomate, European College of Zoological Medicine (Avian, Small Mammal); Diplomate, American College of Zoological Medicine; Associate Professor of Clinical Zoological Companion Animal Medicine and Surgery, Department of Medicine and Epidemiology, UC Davis School of Veterinary Medicine, Davis, California, USA

JEAN-MICHEL HATT, MSc, Dr med vet
Diplomate, American College of Zoological Medicine; Diplomate, European College of Zoological Medicine (Avian); Professor, Clinic for Zoo Animals, Exotic Pets and Wildlife, Vetsuisse Faculty, University of Zurich, Zurich, Switzerland

KAREL HAUPTMAN, DVM, PhD
Professor, Avian and Exotic Animal Clinic, Faculty of Veterinary Medicine, University of Veterinary and Pharmaceutical Sciences Brno, Brno, Czech Republic

JENNIFER M. HELLIER, BSc (Hons)
Department of Biostatistics, Institute of Psychiatry, Psychology and Neuroscience, King's College London, London, United Kingdom

JOHN HODSOLL, PhD
Department of Biostatistics, Institute of Psychiatry, Psychology and Neuroscience, King's College London, London, United Kingdom

MINH HUYNH, DVM, MRCVS
Diplomate, European College of Zoological Medicine (Avian); Department of Exotic, Centre Hospitalier Vétérinaire Frégis, Arcueil, France

VLADIMIR JEKL, DVM, PhD
Diplomate, European College of Zoological Medicine (Small Mammal); Associate Professor, Avian and Exotic Animal Clinic, Faculty of Veterinary Medicine, University of Veterinary and Pharmaceutical Sciences Brno, Brno, Czech Republic

ZDENEK KNOTEK, DVM, PhD
Diplomate, European College of Zoological Medicine (Herpetology); Professor, Avian and Exotic Animal Clinic, Faculty of Veterinary Medicine, University of Veterinary and Pharmaceutical Sciences Brno, Brno, Czech Republic

SYLVAIN LARRAT, med vet, MSc, DES
Diplomate, American College of Zoological Medicine; Clinique Vétérinaire Benjamin Franklin, Brech/Auray, France

REINT MEURSINGE REYNDERS, DDS, MS (Oral Biology),
MSc (Evidence-Based Health Care), PhD
Department of Oral and Maxillofacial Surgery, Academic Medical Center, University of Amsterdam, Amsterdam, The Netherlands; Private Practice of Orthodontics, Milan, Italy

MARK A. MITCHELL, DVM, MS, PhD
Diplomate, European College of Zoological Medicine (Herpetology); Director and Professor, Department of Veterinary Clinical Sciences, Louisiana State University School of Veterinary Medicine, Baton Rouge, Louisiana, USA

DENNIS OONINCX, BEc, MSc, PhD
Laboratory of Entomology, Plant Sciences Group, Wageningen University, Wageningen, The Netherlands

LAURA L. PAVLECH, DVM, MSLS
Department of Research and Instruction, Hirsh Health Sciences Library, Tufts University, Boston, Massachusetts, USA

SEAN M. PERRY, DVM
Graduate Assistant, Department of Veterinary Clinical Sciences, Louisiana State University School of Veterinary Medicine, Baton Rouge, Louisiana, USA

ELIZABETH G. RYAN, PhD
Department of Biostatistics, Institute of Psychiatry, Psychology and Neuroscience, King's College London, London, United Kingdom

NOÉMIE M. SUMMA, Dr Med Vet, IPSAV
Clinical Instructor of Zoological Medicine, Department of Clinical Sciences, University of Montreal School of Veterinary Medicine, Montreal, Québec, Canada

JEROEN VAN LEEUWEN, MSc, PhD
Biometris, Plant Sciences Group, Wageningen University, Wageningen, The Netherlands

CLAIRE VERGNEAU-GROSSET, med vet, IPSAV, CES
Diplomate, American College of Zoological Medicine; Clinical Instructor, Zoological Medicine Service, Veterinarian, Aquarium du Québec, University of Montreal School of Veterinary Medicine, Saint-Hyacinthe, Québec, Canada

ALEXANDRA L. WINTER, BVSc
Diplomate, American College of Veterinary Surgeons; Editor, Journal of the American Veterinary Medical Association, American Veterinary Medical Association, Schaumburg, Illinois, USA

GRAHAM ZOLLER, DVM, IPSAV (med zool)
Department of Exotic, Centre Hospitalier Vétérinaire Frégis, Arcueil, France

Contents

In the field of exotic animal medicine, there is much work to do, more than in human medicine and in companion animal medicine. The work in this field should be directed toward an evidence-based knowledge accumulation. Sound evidence supporting tests and treatments will ensure better health care for exotic animal patients.

High-quality clinical practice requires veterinarians to stay abreast of new research and integrate relevant findings into patient care. Clinicians can achieve this goal using evidence-based practice (EBP), the stepwise process of integrating best research evidence into existing clinical decision-making processes. This article provides explanations and recommendations for performing key steps of the EBP process, with a focus on issues the exotic animal practitioner might encounter. Key areas of discussion include the development of focused PICO questions, types of literature and search strategies, and basic clinical epidemiology principles, including chance error, bias, confounding, and generalizability.

Rabbit medicine has been continuously evolving over time with increasing popularity and demand. Tremendous advances have been made in rabbit medicine over the past 5 years, including the use of imaging tools for otitis and dental disease management, the development of laboratory testing for encephalitozoonosis, or determination of prognosis in rabbits. Recent pharmacokinetic studies have been published, providing additional information on commonly used antibiotics and motility-enhancer drugs, as well as benzimidazole toxicosis. This article presents a review of evidence-based advances for liver lobe torsions, thymoma, and dental disease in rabbits and controversial and new future promising areas in rabbit medicine.

This literature review covers approximately 35 years of veterinary medicine. This article develops the current state of knowledge in pet ferret medicine regarding the most common diseases according to evidence-based data and gives insight into further axis of research. Literature review was conducted through identification of keywords (title + ferret) with Web-based database searching. To appreciate the methodological quality and the level of evidence of each article included in the review, full-text versions were reviewed and questions addressed in the articles were formulated. Analysis of the articles' content was performed by the authors, and relevant clinical information was extracted.

objective, and reproducible. Case reports and case series are limited in their scope and application. Cross-sectional studies, likewise, cannot provide answers to specific variable testing with a temporal application. It is essential for the reptile specialty to expand into case-control studies, cohort studies, and experimental/intervention studies. Unfortunately, much of the reptile literature remains limited to descriptive studies. This article reviews current evidence-based topics in reptile medicine and shares how everyone practicing in the field can contribute to improving this specialty.

Evidence-Based Rabbit Housing and Nutrition   871

Marcus Clauss and Jean-Michel Hatt

Because most research on rabbit husbandry, welfare, and nutrition was performed on production animals, evidence for best practices in pet rabbits is scarce, and guidelines must be based on transfer of results, deduction, and common sense. Rabbits benefit from being kept with at least one conspecific; from large enclosures and multistory hutches; from drinking water offered ad libitum in open dish drinker systems; and from receiving hay ad libitum, with restricted amounts of fresh grass, herbs, or green leafy vegetables, and a high-fiber complete diet. Offering hay ad libitum bears several advantages and should be considered a matter of course.

Evidence-Based Reptile Housing and Nutrition   885

Dennis Oonincx and Jeroen van Leeuwen

The provision of a good light source is important for reptiles. For instance, ultraviolet light is used in social interactions and used for vitamin D synthesis. With respect to housing, most reptilians are best kept pairwise or individually. Environmental enrichment can be effective but depends on the form and the species to which it is applied. Temperature gradients around preferred body temperatures allow accurate thermoregulation, which is essential for reptiles. Natural distributions indicate suitable ambient temperatures, but microclimatic conditions are at least as important. Because the nutrient requirements of reptiles are largely unknown, facilitating self-selection from various dietary items is preferable.

Advancements in Evidence-Based Analgesia in Exotic Animals   899

Julie A. Balko and Sathya K. Chinnadurai

The importance of appropriate recognition, assessment, and treatment of pain in all veterinary species, including exotic animals, cannot be overstated. Although the assessment of pain perception in nondomestic species is still in its infancy, this does not preclude appropriate analgesic management in these species. Although analgesic drug selection is often based on data extrapolated from similar species, as the pharmacokinetics and pharmacodynamics of many drugs can vary greatly between species, an evidence-based approach to analgesic therapy should be used whenever possible. This article provides an overview of recent advances in evidence-based analgesic management in companion exotic animals.

> Anesthesia and sedation of pet nondomestic species are often necessary for both invasive and noninvasive procedures. Even minimally invasive procedures can be stressful for small prey species that are not domesticated or acclimated to human contact and restraint. Recent advancements in evidence-based practice will continue to improve the field based on scientifically sound best practices and rely less on anecdotal recommendations. This article focuses on new scientific literature that has been published in the past 5 years. For ease of reading, the authors divide the article to highlight advances in anesthetic pharmacology and discoveries in anesthetic physiology and monitoring.

> An essential component of evidence-based practice is finding the best available evidence to answer a clinical question. Finding evidence is difficult for veterinarians in general, and exotic animal clinicians in particular, owing to the lack of studies that provide a high level of clinically relevant evidence and limited access to resources. Knowing where and how to search for evidence can facilitate evidence-based practice.

> Clinical research attempts to answer questions about patient populations by studying small samples of patients drawn from those populations. Statistics are used to describe the data collected in a study and to make inferences about the larger populations. Practitioners of evidence-based practice need a basic understanding of these principles to critically appraise the results of research studies. The main paradigm for statistical inference in medicine is called hypothesis testing, which involves generating a null hypothesis and examining the strength of evidence against it.

> Correlation and regression assess the association between 2 or more variables. This article reviews the core knowledge needed to understand these analyses, moving from visual analysis in scatter plots through correlation, simple and multiple linear regression, and logistic regression. Correlation estimates the strength and direction of a relationship between 2 variables. Regression can be considered more general and quantifies the numerical relationships between an outcome and 1 or multiple variables in terms of a best-fit line, allowing predictions to be made. Each technique is discussed with examples and the statistical assumptions underlying their correct application.

> Developing and conducting systematic reviews and meta-analyses is a complex process that requires many judgments and the input from a

wide variety of stakeholders. This article presents an introduction on how to develop, conduct, and report these research studies. Veterinary clinicians should seek systematic reviews to address their research questions. Criteria for including meta-analyses in a systematic review are presented. However, before applying the findings of systematic reviews and meta-analyses to a particular patient, clinicians should weigh a variety of issues. The quality of the review is particularly important.

Reporting the results of primary research is a key step in knowledge creation. Many well-conducted studies are rejected by journal editors, criticized by peers, or unsuitable for systematic reviewers because of poor reporting. This article summarizes the most important methodological items to report when writing an original research article.

VETERINARY CLINICS OF NORTH AMERICA: EXOTIC ANIMAL PRACTICE

FORTHCOMING ISSUES

January 2018
Exotic Animal Neurology
Susan Orosz, *Editor*

May 2018
Therapeutics
Yvonne R.A. van Zeeland, *Editor*

RECENT ISSUES

May 2017
Reproductive Medicine
Vladimir Jekl, *Editor*

January 2017
Exotic Animal Oncology
David Guzman, *Editor*

September 2016
Disorders of the Oral Cavity
Vittorio Capello, *Editor*

ISSUE OF RELATED INTEREST

Veterinary Clinics of North America: Small Animal Practice
September 2017, (Vol. 47, Issue 5)
Topics in Cardiology
Joao S. Orvalho, *Editor*

THE CLINICS ARE NOW AVAILABLE ONLINE!
Access your subscription at:
www.theclinics.com

Preface

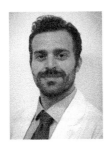 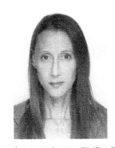

Nicola Di Girolamo, DMV, MSc (EBHC),   Alexandra L. Winter, BVSc, DACVS
PhD, DECZM (Herpetology)
Editors

When we first set out to create an issue focused on the application of principles of evidence-based medicine (EBM) for busy exotic animal practitioners, we assumed that this was likely an impossible task. EBM is not a classic medical "specialty"; rather this describes an approach to the delivery of patient care. Furthermore, we hoped to provide content in a readily understandable format for immediate application in day-to-day clinical practice, that would be useful for trainees (interns, residents, fellows, graduate students) as well as practicing clinicians.

With this task in mind, we have organized the content into two broad sections. The first includes articles describing current advances in exotic animal medicine divided by species. Two chapters dedicated to the current status of methods of analgesia and anesthesia in exotic species are also included. Accompanying this clinical information, a separate section is dedicated to addressing various core principles underlying the practice of EBM. These include basic and more advanced statistics, and an introduction to systematic reviews. We felt that chapters on how to search the literature and how to write a research article would be particularly useful for recent graduates, interns, and residents.

Evidence-based medicine is defined as the integration of the best available research, with clinical experience and patient (and owner) values, when addressing any clinical scenario; notice that the patient is always at the core of evidence-based practice. As veterinarians, we face particularly unique challenges in our efforts to search for the best available evidence; as such, these challenges may be exacerbated for clinicians working with exotic species. The diversity of the species treated, the variety of the treatments provided, and the poor quality of current scientific resources are just some of the challenges that we face daily. Nonetheless, we hope that readers will find the information presented in this issue of value in their everyday practice. We are grateful for the outstanding contributions of all of the authors. It has been an incredibly rewarding collaborative experience to work on putting this issue of *Veterinary Clinics of North America: Exotic Animal Practice* together and it would not have been possible without the extraordinary work of the editorial team at Elsevier, to whom we express our thanks.

Vet Clin Exot Anim 20 (2017) xiii–xiv
http://dx.doi.org/10.1016/j.cvex.2017.06.001
1094-9194/17/© 2017 Published by Elsevier Inc.

vetexotic.theclinics.com

Nicola Di Girolamo, DMV, MSc (EBHC), PhD, DECZM (Herpetology)
Tai Wai Small Animal & Exotic Hospital
75 Chik Shun Street
Tai Wai, Shatin, Hong Kong

EBMVet
Via Sigismondo
Trecchi 20, Cremona, Italy

Alexandra L. Winter, BVSc, DACVS
American Veterinary Medical Association
1931 N. Meacham Road
Suite 100, Schaumburg
IL 60173, USA

E-mail addresses:
nicoladiggi@gmail.com (N. Di Girolamo)
awinter@avma.org (A.L. Winter)

Why Should We Direct Our Efforts Toward Evidence-Based Knowledge Creation?

Nicola Di Girolamo, DMV, MSc (EBHC), PhD, DECZM (Herpetology)[a,b,*],
Alexandra L. Winter, BVSc, DACVS[c]

KEYWORDS

- Exotic animal medicine • Evidence-based medicine • Clinical epidemiology
- History of evidence-based medicine

KEY POINTS

- In the field of exotic animal medicine, there is much greater need for novel research, compared with human and companion animal medicine.
- Work in this field should be directed toward evidence-based knowledge accumulation.
- Sound evidence supporting tests and treatments will ensure better health care for exotic animal patients.

In 1958, an edition of a popular book on how to care for infants, *Baby and Child Care*, a best-seller from world-renowned pediatrician Dr Benjamin Spock, was published with the novel advice, "it is preferable to accustom a baby to sleeping on his stomach." The cover of the book depicted an infant lying on his belly, and this was a recurrent motif in the book. Hospitals and parents throughout the world followed this suggestion, resulting in millions of babies sleeping in a prone position. Subsequently, the number of infants dying of sudden infant death syndrome (SIDS) dramatically increased.[1] Observational studies demonstrated the association between prone sleeping and SIDS, but only in the 1980s did the message that prone sleeping was harmful spread to health care professionals and lay people. In the United States, between 1992 and 1996, the prevalence of infants placed in the prone sleep position declined by 66% and the rate of SIDS declined by 38%.[2]

The authors have nothing to disclose.
[a] Tai Wai Small Animal & Exotic Hospital, 75 Chik Shun Street, Tai Wai, Shatin, Hong Kong;
[b] EBMVet, Via Sigismondo Trecchi 20, Cremona, Italy; [c] American Veterinary Medical Association, 1931 N. Meacham Road, Suite 100, Schaumburg, IL 60173, USA
* Corresponding author. EBMVet, Via Sigismondo Trecchi 20, Cremona, Italy.
E-mail address: nicoladiggi@gmail.com

Vet Clin Exot Anim 20 (2017) 733–735
http://dx.doi.org/10.1016/j.cvex.2017.04.011
1094-9194/17/© 2017 Elsevier Inc. All rights reserved.

In the late 1980s, it was common to treat human patients who suffered myocardial infarction with antiarrhythmic drugs. Cardiologists supported this approach, because these antiarrhythmic drugs effectively suppressed arrhythmias.[3] What was not clear at the time was that patients taking such antiarrhythmic drugs had a dramatically higher risk of mortality compared with patients who took placebos.[4] Prescription of these drugs in clinically asymptomatic patients led to a countless number of deaths.

In the early 1990s, there was some evidence that in dogs with experimentally induced endotoxemia, administration of an inhibitor of nitric oxide formation improved cardiovascular function.[5] When first tested in humans, the drug actually had positive hemodynamic effects.[6] In a randomized controlled trial, however, including approximately 800 patients with septic shock, the administration of the nitric oxide synthase inhibitor was associated with a 10% increase in mortality rate.[7]

Until the early 2000s, short-term administration of corticosteroids to human patients with head injury was a common practice. The physiologic reasoning behind this was straightforward and included the potential to decrease inflammation. Aggregate mortality results from 13 small randomized trials of steroid treatment of head injury published before 1997 found a 2% lower mortality in patients treated with steroids.[8] However, because of small sample sizes of the trials, the pooled results suggested no real benefit of steroid treatment. In 2004, early results of the CRASH (Corticosteroid Randomization After Significant Head Injury) trial were published. This large randomized controlled trial included more than 10,000 patients with head injury, who were randomized to receive treatment with either short-term corticosteroids or placebo. The results demonstrated that the group of patients allocated to corticosteroid treatment had a 3% higher risk of death.[9]

These are just a few examples of patient harm that the practice of evidence-based medicine can avoid. One example shows how much expert opinions can be wrong. Prone sleeping was recommended in books between 1943 and 1988, and evidence available from 1970 proved this was harmful.[10] Another example demonstrates that physiologic reasoning cannot substitute for clinical testing. Opinions are opinions not evidence, and physiologic systems, while important, are unpredictable. Several examples presented illustrate the importance of objective (hard) outcomes. Often, improvement in study variables (eg, ECG parameters, serum biochemical tests results, cytological markers), are not followed by improvements in patient-important outcomes, for example, survival time and quality of life. No treatment should be implemented in clinical practice if improvement in patient-important outcomes has not been demonstrated.

Much continued work is required to develop a high-quality evidence base in the field of exotic animal medicine. This is imperative to ensure that clinicians can best serve the needs of their patients, owners and deliver optimal health care.

REFERENCES

1. de Jonge GA, Engelberts AC, Koomen-Liefting AJ, et al. Cot death and prone sleeping position in The Netherlands. BMJ 1989;298(6675):722.

2. Willinger M, Hoffman HJ, Wu KT, et al. Factors associated with the transition to nonprone sleep positions of infants in the United States: the National Infant Sleep Position Study. JAMA 1998;280(4):329–35.

3. Cardiac Arrhythmia Pilot Study (CAPS) Investigators. Effects of encainide, flecainide, imipramine and moricizine on ventricular arrhythmias during the year after acute myocardial infarction: the CAPS. Am J Cardiol 1988;61:501–9.

4. Echt DS, Liebson PR, Mitchell LB, et al. Mortality and morbidity in patients receiving encainide, flecainide, or placebo. The cardiac arrhythmia suppression trial. N Engl J Med 1991;324(12):781–8.
5. Kilbourn RG, Cromeens DM, Chelly FD, et al. NG-methyl-L-arginine, an inhibitor of nitric oxide formation, acts synergistically with dobutamine to improve cardiovascular performance in endotoxemic dogs. Crit Care Med 1994;22(11):1835–40.
6. Watson D, Grover R, Anzueto A, et al. Cardiovascular effects of the nitric oxide synthase inhibitor NG-methyl-L-arginine hydrochloride (546C88) in patients with septic shock: results of a randomized, double-blind, placebo-controlled multicenter study (study no. 144-002). Crit Care Med 2004;32(1):13–20.
7. López A, Lorente JA, Steingrub J, et al. Multiple-center, randomized, placebo-controlled, double-blind study of the nitric oxide synthase inhibitor 546C88: effect on survival in patients with septic shock. Crit Care Med 2004;32(1):21–30.
8. Alderson P, Roberts I. Corticosteroids in acute traumatic brain injury: systematic review of randomised controlled trials. BMJ 1997;314:1855–9.
9. Roberts I, Yates D, Sandercock P, et al. Effect of intravenous corticosteroids on death within 14 days in 10008 adults with clinically significant head injury (MRC CRASH trial): randomised placebo-controlled trial. Lancet 2004; 364(9442):1321–8.
10. Gilbert R, Salanti G, Harden M, et al. Infant sleeping position and the sudden infant death syndrome: systematic review of observational studies and historical review of recommendations from 1940 to 2002. Int J Epidemiol 2005;34(4):874–87.

Practical Application of Evidence-Based Practice

Michelle A. Giuffrida, VMD, MSCE, DACVS

KEYWORDS

- Evidence-based practice • Evidence-based medicine • Clinical epidemiology

KEY POINTS

- Evidence-based practice (EBP) is the integration of clinical expertise, client values and preferences, and best research evidence into the decision-making process for clinical care.
- Practical application of EBP involves asking well-focused questions, searching the literature for relevant research evidence, critically appraising the evidence, and applying findings to patient care.
- A high-quality evidence base is lacking in many areas of veterinary medicine. Practitioners must develop new skills to efficiently identify relevant evidence and examine its internal and external validity.
- Basic understanding of PICO question format, literature search strategies, and clinical epidemiology principles (chance, bias, confounding, and generalizability) are valuable to veterinary EBP practitioners.

Veterinarians desire to provide best-quality medicine to patients, and to counsel clients wisely during the medical decision-making process. Pet owners value our experiences and skills, but they also depend on us to provide care that reflects contemporary knowledge and standards of care. High-quality clinical practice requires veterinarians to be aware of new research and continually integrate relevant findings into patient care. Evidence-based practice (EBP) provides us with a practical framework to achieve this.

EBP is based on the principles of clinical epidemiology, the branch of medicine concerned with conducting, appraising, and applying research studies that focus on patients' medical care and disease outcomes.[1] A contemporary definition of EBP is the integration of clinical expertise, client (or patient) values and preferences, and best research evidence into the decision-making process for clinical care.[2] Clinical expertise is the veterinarian's knowledge base, skills, and personal experiences. Clients'

Disclosure Statement: The author has nothing to disclose.
Small Animal Surgery, Department of Surgical and Radiological Sciences, Davis School of Veterinary Medicine, University of California, One Shields Avenue, Davis, CA 95616, USA
E-mail address: magiuffrida@ucdavis.edu

Vet Clin Exot Anim 20 (2017) 737–748
http://dx.doi.org/10.1016/j.cvex.2017.04.001
1094-9194/17/Published by Elsevier Inc.

values and preferences include their reasons for pet ownership, past experiences, financial resources, emotional attachment, and general medical knowledge. Best research evidence refers to research findings that are relevant to the individual and clinical scenario, and ideally based on sound scientific methodology.

A practical application of EBP involves the following steps:

- Asking a well-formulated question based on a real clinical case or problem
- Acquiring relevant research and information
- Appraising the strength and relevance of the evidence
- Applying the findings to the actual clinical scenario

For most clinicians, successful application of EBP will require developing new clinical epidemiology skills, specifically those related to appraising and interpreting research evidence.[3] This article gives particular attention to the appraisal step of EBP, with a focus on understanding and applying basic epidemiologic principles.

ASKING A QUESTION

The EBP process begins by assessing the patient and articulating a question or problem of interest. Not every patient problem requires a formal application of EBP. In many scenarios, effective diagnostic tests or treatments are established, prognosis for disease is known, or perhaps the client has no interest in moving forward. Relevant EBP questions arise when confronted with the following:

- Unfamiliar species
- Unusual clinical signs or test results
- Rare disease processes
- Common conditions for which there are multiple tests or treatments
- Conflicting recommendations and opinions

Once you have identified the clinical problem, the next step is to formulate a concise, specific, answerable question. A recommended approach is to build questions using PICO, a mnemonic that provides a structured, easy-to-remember formula for creating EBP questions (**Table 1**). A focused and specific question will facilitate the next step in the process, which is to develop a list of publications that are relevant to your clinical problem.

ACQUIRING INFORMATION

Research literature can be categorized into 3 main forms:

- Primary literature: original scientific articles that describe conduct and results of experimental and observational research
  - Aims to answer specific questions or test hypotheses
  - Original scientific journal articles peer-reviewed by experts
  - Difficulties and limitations: large volume; findings of different studies may conflict; rigor and validity of research varies; some topics are studied more than others
- Secondary literature: interpretation, analysis, and summary of primary sources
  - Aims to synthesize existing knowledge on a particular topic, using scientific (systematic) or nonscientific (narrative) methods
  - Textbooks, systematic reviews and meta-analyses, narrative review articles, knowledge summaries, editorials; often peer-reviewed or peer-edited by experts

Table 1
Guidelines for creating focused evidence-based practice questions using a PICO approach

PICO Component	PICO Component Explanation	Therapy Questions	Diagnostic Test Questions	Risk or Prognostic Factor Questions
Patient	The defining characteristics of the patient or problem	Example: species, condition, disease stage, clinical sign	Example: species, condition, disease stage, treatment	Example: species, condition, disease stage, treatment
Intervention	The treatment, exposure, test, prognostic factor, or characteristic you want to understand	Example: medication type, dose, or regimen; surgical procedure, implant, or technique; diet; environment; order of combination treatments	Example: examination finding, blood test, clinical sign, imaging result, biopsy test or technique, survey response	Example: exposure to a toxin, environment, medication or treatment; species, signalment, body weight, stage; concurrent disease or clinical sign
Comparison	The main alternative to the intervention that you are considering	Example: no treatment; a different form of treatment; a different dose, brand, regimen, or order of treatment	Example: a different sign, finding, or test; often an existing test that is considered the gold standard	Example: not having the exposure, characteristic, disease, or sign
Outcome	The result you would like to prevent, cause, or measure	Example: cure or remission rate; test or imaging result; speed of recovery; side effects or complications	Example: identify presence or absence of disease	Example: development or progression of disease, clinical signs, complications, or other events

Example therapy question: In *guinea pigs with conjunctivitis*, do *oral* versus *topical* antibiotics result in a *faster resolution of signs*?

Example diagnostic test question: In *ferrets presenting with weakness and weight loss*, how accurate is a *single fasting glucose measurement* compared with *insulin-glucose ratio* for *ruling out insulinoma*?

Example risk factor question: In *pet aquatic turtles*, is *water temperature* $\geq 80°F$ versus *less than 80°F* a risk factor for *developing shell rot*?

- ○ Difficulties and limitations: authors and editors can introduce personal biases in interpretations and choices of source material; affected by availability and weaknesses of primary literature
- • Gray literature: material that is not available through traditional systems of publication and distribution
  - ○ Aims vary from dissemination of preliminary scientific data to communicating trade information and opinion
  - ○ Conference proceedings, posters, and abstracts; academic theses, lecture notes, and presentations; industry and government reports and fact sheets; and online blogs, newsletters, advice columns, and community forums

○ Difficulties and limitations: rarely undergoes formal peer-review; often contains nonscientific data, unsubstantiated claims, and opinions and experiences from subject matter experts, novices, or even lay people

Primary literature and systematic reviews and meta-analyses are considered to provide the most up-to-date knowledge for dynamic areas of veterinary medicine, such as diagnostic testing and therapy.[4] A systematic review involves a comprehensive search for relevant evidence, followed by critical appraisal conducted according to specific scientific criteria[5]; in contrast, a narrative review or knowledge summary selects and appraises source material according to more subjective and intuitive methods that are at greater risk of bias.[6] Knowledge summaries are intended to be time-saving evidence-based distillations of current research and could become increasingly valuable to EBP veterinarians if the number, scope, and rigor of available summaries improves. Textbooks and narrative review articles are appropriate sources for stable knowledge that does not tend to change, such as anatomy and basic principles, mechanisms, and characteristics of disease.[4] Gray literature is often nonscientific and is usually avoided during EBP, except as a source of anecdote and opinion in situations in which no scientific evidence exists.

A comprehensive literature search requires access to academic citation databases or citation search engines.

- Citation databases selectively catalog citations according to a predefined list of journals, publishers, or subject areas.[7] Veterinary primary and secondary literature is largely indexed in CAB Abstracts and Medline (PubMed) databases.[8] PubMed can be searched for free, whereas CAB requires a subscription.
- Citation search engines such as Google Scholar and Microsoft Academic Search are also free to use and comb the Internet for information that appears to be a citation.[7]

Compared with citation databases, search engines are more likely to return non-scholarly results and gray literature in addition to traditional academic citations.[9] Veterinary online subscription services such as VIN (Veterinary Information Network)[10] also provide access to curated selections of citations, conference proceedings, and self-generated gray literature; because these services provide only selective access to information, they generally should not be relied on for effective EBP. Regardless of which search strategy is used, most full-text articles can be accessed only via subscription or pay-per-use services, although some are available through open-source publishing agreements.

To identify potentially relevant research evidence, enter key words from your PICO question into the search engine or database. A good strategy is to start with the patient population (type of animal and problem) and intervention of interest. It is often necessary to try several iterations of search terms before relevant results are obtained. Some potentially helpful search tips include the following:

- Examine the reference lists of relevant articles or book articles
- Try different ways of searching the species or animal type; birds and reptiles are often identified in article titles using both common names and binomial nomenclature (genus and species) or other zoologic taxa (eg, subspecies or family)
- Include the word "veterinary" in searches of small mammals and exotic species

In the author's experience, the latter recommendation is helpful to narrow the search focus, given the prevalence of preclinical animal research. Search strategies should initially focus on finding evidence that derives from actual clinical patients, rather than colony-housed animals used to study mechanisms of disease and treatment.

As you examine the search output, flag for a more in-depth examination of any articles that seem relevant. In veterinary medicine, and particularly in exotic animal medicine, it is unfortunately common to find no articles that directly address your specific question. For this reason, it is often necessary to retain articles that are partially relevant, even though you might ultimately discard the research as unhelpful during the appraisal process.

APPRAISING THE EVIDENCE

Being able to understand and critically appraise research studies is at the heart of EBP. Practitioners of EBP commonly triage studies using schemes that rank evidence based on the rigor of the study methods, and how consistent results are across similar studies. **Table 2** presents an overview of the different types of evidence and their relative quality. The highest-quality clinical evidence is typically considered to come from high-level syntheses of multiple studies that address specific scenarios and questions.[11] However, this form of evidence generally does not yet exist in veterinary medicine. Rather, most published evidence in veterinary medicine derives from individual studies, many of which are concentrated in the lower echelons of evidence hierarchies.[3] Although available veterinary evidence often provides a relatively low strength of recommendation relative to what is possible, we can still examine and consider it during our EBP process. To do this, we need to understand the basic goals of clinical research and be able to identify major threats to study validity as they might manifest in common veterinary studies, such as case series and cohort studies.

Clinical Research Basics

If we know what causes a disease or complication, we can develop ways to predict, avoid, or treat it; if we know how a medication or surgery affects different patients or disease processes, we are better equipped to recommend treatment appropriately. The main purpose of clinical research is to explore these causal associations between patient exposures and outcomes.

- Exposures are treatments, tests, environmental factors, patient characteristics, diseases; anything that might be the "cause" in a cause-effect relationship.
- Outcomes are the "effect" part of the relationship, typically the development, improvement, or worsening of diseases, side effects, or events.
- Associations are the estimated relationships between exposures and outcomes.

Obviously, we want to know whether true or real associations exist, but in reality well-intentioned research can sometimes result in false or misleading estimates of association. As practitioners, we can also misuse research by extrapolating results to patients or situations to which they do not really apply. The best evidence has both internal and external validity.

- Internal validity means the associations or other results that the study generates are correct, and are not attributable to some rival explanation. The 3 major threats to internal validity are chance, bias, and confounding.
- External validity means the results are generalizable to real-world populations.
- A study's vulnerability to threats against internal and external validity determines its place in the EBP evidence hierarchy.

It is important to realize that study design hierarchies are merely broad guidelines; for example, a randomized controlled trial is in theory a high-quality design but a real trial could nevertheless lack internal or external validity and generate low-quality

Table 2
Broad overview of characteristics, quality, and strength of recommendation of various sources of evidence

	Evidence type	Characteristic features	In veterinary medicine
Highest — Syntheses of multiple individual studies	Summaries and systems	High-level, continuously updated evidence-based syntheses of specific problems; computerized decision-making support systems	Not currently available
	Synopses of systematic reviews and meta-analyses	Summaries of information found in systematic reviews	Not currently available, likely due to lack of systematic reviews
	Systematic reviews and meta-analyses	Comprehensive summaries of evidence surrounding specific research questions	Uncommon; most individual studies are excluded for failure to meet design and reporting criteria
	Synopses of individual studies	Critical appraisals of 1 or more high-quality studies; usually limited to recent works rather than all knowledge to date; published in specialty journals of evidence-based summaries	Uncommon; knowledge summaries that appraise current research are a version of this; variable quality due to inconsistent appraisal criteria and expertise
Individual studies	Randomized controlled trials	Prospective cohort study in which subjects are assigned to exposure by the investigators and observed over time for outcomes of interest; high internal validity when rigorously designed and conducted	Somewhat common; variable quality due to deficiencies in design, conduct, and reporting
	Cohort studies	Prospective or retrospective design in which subjects are grouped based on exposure status and observed over time for outcomes of interest	Common; can be mislabeled as case series; single-arm and nonrandomized clinical trials are cohort studies
	Case control studies	Retrospective design in which subjects are grouped based on outcome status and exposure histories are compared to determine risk factors for the outcome	Uncommon; retrospective cohort studies can be mislabeled as case control studies
	Case series	Retrospective design in which subjects with a particular outcome are selected and described	Common
	Clinical case reports	Detailed reports of individual subject experiences; typically new or unusual tests, presentations, diseases, or therapies	Common
Lowest	Preclinical studies, expert opinions	Cadaver, in vitro studies; nontarget species; laboratory animals; induced disease models; biomechanical models; editorials and opinions	Common

Evidence Quality and Strength of Recommendation

Quality and strength of recommendation relate to internal validity, generalizability, and consistency of evidence.

evidence. Until there is a consistently high-quality body of veterinary clinical evidence, we should examine individual studies for internal and external validity, rather than assume these properties exist simply because of the design.

Chance

- The chance effect refers to arriving at false conclusions by random error
- The chance effect diminishes as the sample size gets larger
- Statistical analysis is used to determine the number of animals needed to minimize the chance effect, and to investigate whether specific results could be observed due to chance alone

Most clinical research involves studying a finite number of patients who are drawn from and presumed to represent the underlying population of interest. For example, a researcher interested in rabbit limb amputations would study a sample of representative cases and extrapolate the results to the general population of amputees. However, even if the cases are truly a random sample of all amputees, they might fail to accurately represent the larger population due to chance alone. The chance effect (also called random error or random variation) diminishes as the sample size gets larger. This makes intuitive sense; we would naturally be more worried that a study involving only 3 rabbits could miss important outcomes or focus on idiosyncrasies compared with a study of 300 rabbits. When the study objective is to compare groups of animals, investigators should calculate in advance how many animals they will need to study to reasonably exclude the chance effect; this is known as a sample size or power calculation and can be performed for both prospective and retrospective studies. If a sufficient number of animals is included based on this type of calculation, it provides a measure of protection against arriving at conclusions based on chance alone. Much of the statistical analysis reported in veterinary clinical research articles is used to examine the likelihood that a given result could be observed due to chance alone. A small P value or a narrow confidence interval can be reassuring signs that the results are probably not due to random error. However, even when analysis demonstrates a low likelihood that a given result would be observed purely by chance, the finding could still be incorrect due to bias or confounding. Imagine flipping a coin and getting heads 99 on of 100 consecutive flips; the chance of this happening is exceptionally small with a fair coin, but the result could reasonably occur if the coin were unbalanced.

Bias

- Bias is a research conduct error that causes an incorrect estimate of association.
- Bias is typically introduced during selection of study subjects and data collection.
- Bias cannot be corrected with statistics or larger sample size.

Bias refers to systematic error in how the research was performed that results in mistaken estimates of association. Bias is essentially a mistake of the researcher, but it cannot always be avoided. When appraising the literature it can be difficult to know whether results are biased, because documenting it depends on knowing the "true" associations, which are generally unknown and the reason for doing the research in the first place! However, we can assess the *potential* for bias by looking at how a study was designed and conducted. If a study is performed using methods that are known to introduce bias, then it is reasonable to assume the results could be incorrect and we should view them with healthy skepticism. On the other hand, if a study is performed with rigorous attention to minimizing bias, then we can be more confident that the resulting estimates will be correct. As discussed previously, this is the basic premise of the evidence hierarchies. There are 2 main types of bias to be aware of: selection bias and information (misclassification) bias.

Selection bias

Selection bias occurs when the study sample is drawn from the population in a nonrandom way, such that it does not accurately represent the underlying population. There are many ways to introduce selection bias. Using retrospective medical record review to identify cases for a study is apt to introduce selection bias, because in real life, patients with the same condition are not randomly assigned to receive diagnostic tests and treatments. For example, owners and veterinarians might be less likely to choose and recommend intensive treatments for older, sicker animals, in which case medical records will be biased toward the treatment experiences of animals with better initial prognoses. Prospective studies are also at risk of bias, such as by selectively enrolling certain types of patients or comparing outcomes between groups of animals whose owners chose the treatment plan. Selection bias also can occur due to different follow-up between groups of study subjects. Longer follow-up is often available for animals whose owners choose more involved, intensive, or experimental treatments, whereas animals that are treated conservatively and do not require close veterinarian contact are more likely to be lost to follow-up. Another example of selection bias is nonresponse bias, wherein subjects respond to a survey or enroll in a research study who are systematically different from those who do not respond or enroll.

Information bias

Information bias occurs when information about study exposures and outcomes is incorrect, typically due to how the data are collected. This type of bias is also referred to as misclassification bias, because it often involves incorrect classification of some subjects' treatment or outcome status. Information bias can occur if some animals were not given the full course of treatment or received additional unreported medications that could have affected outcome; if tests or outcomes are incorrectly or inconsistently measured; or if information is selectively recorded for different patients. Selective recording of information is common in the author's experience, particularly in medical records; for example, certain clinical signs could be recorded in detail when attributed to medication but otherwise ignored. In prospective studies, it is typically recommended to blind anyone who is making outcome assessments (such as owners or investigators), because they might interpret or record information differently if they know which study group an animal is in. Recall bias is also a form of information bias and can occur when people are asked to remember whether their pets were exposed to certain environments or medications, or whether certain outcomes occurred. People whose pets experienced memorable outcomes could be more likely to remember previous exposures, particularly if they are aware of a potential causal link to the outcome.

Bias is not diminished with larger sample size, and it cannot be corrected for with statistics. Bias can obscure a real association or create a spurious one, and it can cause overestimation or underestimation of the magnitude of relationships. Because all research is at some risk of bias, and most clinical veterinary studies use designs that are particularly prone, bias should be considered among alternative explanations for most research findings. Ideally, researchers should address the potential for bias in their results, and discuss how bias, if present, might be expected to impact the magnitude or direction of associations. In reality, the potential for bias often does not receive a great deal of attention in article discussion sections, so the responsibility for considering it largely falls on us as readers and appraisers of the literature.

Confounding

- Confounding refers to a third factor that obscures the true association between an exposure and outcome.
- Confounding is likely to occur when comparing groups of patients that are not balanced with respect to baseline characteristics and prognostic factors.
- Confounding can be mitigated by randomization, matching, and statistical adjustment.

Confounding is present when the observed relationship between an exposure and outcome is actually due wholly or in part to the presence of some extraneous variable. A confounding variable is related to both the exposure and the outcome, but does not lie on the causal pathway between them. For example, imagine a study that observes captive bearded dragons fed 1 of 2 different commercial diets according to owner preference. At the end of 6 months, researchers determine that lizards fed diet X have a much lower incidence of metabolic bone disease, and conclude that diet X is protective against disease. However, it turns out that owners who chose diet X were also much more likely to follow other husbandry practices known to reduce the risk of metabolic bone disease. Confounding is present if the lower rate of metabolic bone disease is partly or completely due to these nondiet husbandry practices; for all we know, the diets could be equivalent. It is easy to see how confounding is problematic, because it can lead us to misunderstand important relationships or make improper changes in practice. Unfortunately, identifying confounding is not always as easy as in this example.

Compared with selection bias, which is an error in how subjects are sampled from the population, confounding is not an error but a real phenomenon that we need to account for. This can be achieved either through study design or statistical analysis. Investigators can control confounding by assigning animals to groups that are balanced with respect to potential confounders, using randomization or matching strategies. Randomization is preferred when possible because it will balance both known and unknown confounders, whereas matching can generally only balance on confounders we are aware of. Alternatively, mathematical modeling can produce adjusted estimates of results that account for confounding; examples of these methods include stratification and Mantel-Haenszel estimation, multivariable regression, and propensity scoring. Most veterinary studies use designs that do not naturally balance potential confounders, such as case series, cohort studies, and nonrandomized trials. Furthermore, in the author's experience, veterinary studies often do not attempt to control for confounding mathematically, or have such small sample sizes that statistical adjustment is not feasible. When evaluating comparative therapeutic studies (eg, studies that compare 2 different treatments or doses, or compare treatment with no treatment), it is helpful to think of confounders as prognostic factors; if the treatment groups are not balanced with respect to known or anticipated prognostic factors, such as age, disease severity, and adjunctive therapies, then confounding could exist and distort the results. Many commonly used statistical tests, such as the Fisher exact test, χ^2 test, t test, Wilcoxon rank sum test (Mann-Whitney U test), simple regression, and log-rank test, simply compare averages or proportions between groups and cannot adjust for confounding. These methods are not incorrect, nor do they necessarily lead to incorrect results, but, if the groups of animals being compared are not balanced and one of these methods alone is used to identify important associations, it is reasonable to consider whether confounding could be a factor.

Generalizability

Generalizability refers to whether research results can be applied to real-world patients and circumstances.

External validity of the study pertains to whether its results can be generalized to other populations, settings, and times. Even if a study generates valid research findings, the results are not necessarily true for animals outside the source population. Imagine a study demonstrating that a new medication effectively controls hyperadrenocorticism in a sample of ferrets with treatment-naïve unilateral disease; the results might be correct, but we cannot assume the medication would have the same effect in ferrets that have failed prior treatments or have bilateral disease, or in other species. Generalizability of both population characteristics and the exposures themselves should be considered. Studies might not be highly generalizable if they are based on limited populations selected for convenience (eg, only the animals that were treated at a given practice), or if attempts to limit bias and confounding result in very narrow or unrealistically homogeneous study populations, such as through strict inclusion and exclusion criteria. If the environment, equipment, practitioner skill level, or other conditions in the study are different from your practice, recognize that the results might not apply; an imaging study could be highly accurate when performed under special conditions and interpreted by a radiologist, but the same test could perform poorly in another setting.

Boxes 1 and 2 provide lists of questions that veterinarians might consider when working through the appraisal of individual studies, or comparing evidence across studies.

APPLYING THE FINDINGS TO THE PATIENT

During the appraisal process, we try to understand cause and effect by looking at groups of patients, but ultimately, we need to make recommendations and

---

Box 1
Practical questions for appraising an individual research study

- How likely is this evidence to be true?
  - Did the study include a large enough number of animals?
  - Is there potential for selection bias in how subjects were chosen for the study?
  - Is there potential for information bias in how data were collected?
  - Does the study account for potential confounding?

- What are the results?
  - What associations (cause-effect relationships) are being investigated?
  - Was an appropriate and balanced comparison made?
  - Were all clinically important outcomes (benefits and harms) considered?
  - Are the conclusions supported by results, considering any limitations?

- Does this evidence generalize to my clinical problem?
  - Does it involve actual clinical patients (vs laboratory animals, cadaver specimens, and so forth)?
  - Are the animals similar to my patients in terms of signalment, disease severity, prognostic factors?
  - Can I provide the test or treatment as described in the study?
  - Are the likely benefits worth the potential harms?

> **Box 2**
> **Practical questions for synthesizing information from multiple studies**
>
> - Is there a systematic review, meta-analysis, or evidence-based knowledge summary related to my question?
> - Do the studies include information from a large enough number of animals?
> - Are the populations similar across studies and similar to my patient?
> - Is the potential for error and confounding similar across studies?
> - Are the conclusions generally consistent across studies?

decisions for our specific patient or problem. It is difficult to predict what might happen for any individual animal, but we can use research evidence to understand the spectrum of options and outcomes, reconcile the data with our own experiences and knowledge, and present the possibilities to pet owners. Balancing the different factors (the patient's state, the client's goals, the veterinarian's experience, and the available evidence) typically requires sorting through trade-offs,[2] and even more critically, doing so in a way that is useful to our clients. Determining the role clients wish to play in decision-making and providing the information they need to make an informed choice is a growing responsibility of clinical expertise.[2]

When evidence is identified that is both valid and relevant, clinicians also can use it to implement discussions with team members or to create clinical protocols; EBP can be particularly impactful when the process of appraisal and action is shared and includes the perspectives and experiences of the whole clinical team.[12] Even if the overall evidence is sparse, low quality, or does not truly generalize to your particular patient, the EBP process still helps ensure that new and potentially valuable information has not been missed, and that critical patient care decisions incorporate the best available knowledge.

SUMMARY

High-quality clinical practice requires veterinarians to stay abreast of new research and integrate relevant findings into patient care. Clinicians can achieve this goal using the stepwise EBP method of integrating best research evidence into existing clinical decision-making processes. Practitioners must have access to current citations and full-text publications to fully implement EBP in the information age. Although a high-quality evidence base is lacking in many areas of veterinary medicine, clinicians can use basic clinical epidemiology skills to appraise and integrate available research evidence into clinical practice.

REFERENCES

1. Sackett DL. Clinical epidemiology: what, who, and whither? J Clin Epidemiol 2002;55:1161–6.
2. Haynes RB, Devereaux PJ, Guyatt GH. Clinical expertise in the era of evidence-based medicine and patient choice. Evid Based Med 2002;38(7):36–8.
3. Vandeweerd JM, Kirschvink N, Clegg P, et al. Is evidence-based medicine so evident in veterinary research and practice? History, obstacles, and perspectives. Vet J 2012;191:28–34.

4. McKibbon KA, Marks S. Searching for the best evidence. Part 1: where to look. Evid Based Nurs 1998;1(3):68–70.

5. Cook DJ, Mulrow CD, Haynes RB. Systematic reviews: synthesis of the best evidence for clinical decisions. Ann Intern Med 1997;126(5):376–80.

6. Evans R, editor. The veterinary evidence handbook for writing knowledge summaries, version 7. RCVS Knowledge; 2016. Available at: www.veterinaryevidence.org. Accessed November 22, 2016.

7. Haddaway NM, Collins AM, Coughlin D, et al. The role of Google Scholar in evidence reviews and its applicability to grey literature searching. PLoS One 2015;10(9):e1038237.

8. Grindlay DJC, Brennan ML, Dean RS. Searching the veterinary literature: a comparison of the coverage of veterinary journals by nine bibliographic databases. J Vet Med Educ 2012;39(4):404–12.

9. Shultz M. Comparing test searches in PubMed and Google Scholar. J Med Libr Assoc 2007;95(4):442–53.

10. Veterinary Information Network, Inc, 2016. Available at: www.vin.com. Accessed November 22, 2016.

11. Haynes RB. Of studies, syntheses, synopses, summaries, and systems: the "5S" model evolution of information services for evidence-based healthcare decisions. Evid Based Med 2006;11:162–4.

12. Rosenberg W, Donald A. Evidence-based medicine: an approach to clinical problem solving. BMJ 1995;310(6987):1122–6.

Evidence-Based Advances in Rabbit Medicine

Noémie M. Summa, Dr Med Vet, IPSAV[a], João Brandão, LMV, MS[b],*

KEYWORDS

- Rabbit • *Oryctolagus cuniculus* • Diagnosis • Prognosis • Therapeutics • Thymoma
- Dental disease • Liver lobe torsion

KEY POINTS

- Diagnostic imaging for the assessment of the tympanic bullae and otitis has been recently investigated and provides helpful information for practitioners.
- Laboratory testing has been evaluated for the diagnosis of common diseases in rabbits, such as encephalitozoonosis.
- Liver torsion seems to be more commonly reported than previously thought in rabbits, with typical clinical presentations that can help veterinarians in their diagnosis.
- New therapeutic alternatives to thoracotomy for thymoma management in rabbits have been developed, with significantly improved survival time.
- Dental disease is a common pathology in rabbits, and new research has been published to better understand the relationship between diet and dental abnormalities, as well as to develop normal reference ranges of tooth characteristic in rabbits.

INTRODUCTION

Rabbit medicine has significantly evolved over the past few decades due to the increase in popularity and owners' demand. When rabbits began to gain popularity, clinicians had a need to use their empirical knowledge and personal experience alone due to limited validated research. Nowadays, with the increase in available scientific information, clinicians do not need to rely on their own personal experience alone, and instead should take advantage of published information. Evidence-based veterinary medicine is a process used to guide clinical decision making, thereby allowing veterinarians to find, appraise, and integrate current best evidence with individual clinical expertise, client wishes, and patient needs.[1] Much research regarding rabbits can

---

Disclosure Statement: The authors have nothing to disclose.
[a] Department of Clinical Sciences, School of Veterinary Medicine, University of Montreal, 3200, rue Sicotte, PO 5000, Saint-Hyacinthe, Quebec J2S 2M2, Canada; [b] Department of Veterinary Clinical Sciences, Center for Veterinary Health Sciences, Oklahoma State University, 2065 West Farm Road, Stillwater, OK 74078, USA
* Corresponding author.
E-mail address: jbrandao@okstate.edu

be found in exotic and laboratory animal–specific journals, as well as in more generic publications. Although the interest in rabbit research by journals is refreshing and beneficial to the veterinary community as a whole, it may make it difficult to keep up with the most up-to-date information. This review explores recent publications regarding rabbit medicine and offers a short review of the significant information from each (**Table 1**).

EVIDENCE-BASED ADVANCES IN DIAGNOSIS
Otitis

Diagnostic imaging for the assessment of the tympanic bullae and otitis has been recently investigated. Radiograph sensitivity has been investigated in a recent prospective study in an experimental setting, in which 40 of 80 tympanic bullae (n = 40 rabbit cadavers) were randomly allocated to be filled with soft tissue material.[2] Each specimen was radiographed in dorsoventral, 40° rostroventral-caudodorsal, and left and right 40° lateroventral-laterodorsal. Radiographs were compared with gross findings by 2 blinded board-certified radiologists. Accuracy was between 77% and 80%, with no statistical difference in sensitivity or specificity between the 3 radiographic projections and the 2 observers. Computed tomography (CT) allows cross-sectional evaluation of the entire head and is reported to be more sensitive than, and as specific as, radiography for diagnosis of middle ear disease in dogs.[3] CT results were consistent with otitis in 57% rabbits with clinical signs of ear disease and in 27% of rabbits without clinical signs. The use of ultrasound for the assessment of the tympanic bullae has also been described in dogs,[4] cats,[5] and cows.[6] The normal ultrasonographic appearance of rabbit tympanic bullae has been described in rabbit cadavers.[7] A nonclinical retrospective study compared the efficacy of ultrasound, radiography, and CT for the identification of fluid in the rabbit bullae.[8] To mimic naturally occurring otitis, 40 of 80 bullae (n = 40 rabbit cadavers) were randomly injected with a water-based lubricant jelly and subsequently imaged with the 3 techniques. Independent examinations were performed by a board-certified radiologist with previous experience imaging tympanic bullae in other species, and a veterinary undergraduate student following a short introductory session using rabbits. Two blinded board-certified radiologists independently interpreted the radiographs and CT, and bullae were classified as empty or fluid filled. Once all the procedures were complete, skulls were frozen and sectioned. CT and sectioning results always agreed, resulting in 100% sensitivity and specificity. Sensitivity and specificity for radiographs was 78.4% and 82.5%, respectively. Sensitivity and specificity for ultrasonography was 97.5% and 97.5%, respectively. The information from this study is useful and promising, as ultrasonography is cheaper and potentially more readily available diagnostic test than CT. However, the use of this methodology for the assessment of clinical cases is lacking.

Laboratory Testing

A retrospective study analyzed blood smears of 482 rabbits presented to a university hospital over a 20-year period.[9] Fragmentation and acanthocytosis were more severe in rabbits with inflammatory disease and malignant neoplasia compared with healthy rabbits. Echinocytosis was significantly associated with renal failure, azotemia, and acid-base/electrolyte abnormalities. The information provided by this study may help maximize the information obtained through hematology in rabbits.

Encephalitozoonosis, a condition caused by the microsporidian *Encephalitozoon cuniculi*, is a relevant disease in pet rabbits. Currently, microsporidia are considered atypical fungi without mitochondria, and all microspora have been reclassified as

Table 1
Grading system presenting the overall quality evidence of the main articles presented in this study

Reference No.	Type of Evidence	Grade	Intervention X	Outcome
Hammond et al,[2] 2010	Prospective blind study: experimental animals	3	Investigate the accuracy of radiographic detection of fluid in the rabbit tympanic bulla for 3 different radiographic projections	No significant difference in sensitivity or specificity among the 3 projections when compared with the gross findings
De Matos et al,[3] 2015	Retrospective study: case series	2	Compare computed tomography (CT) abnormalities of the middle ear in clinical and subclinical rabbits, to determine the prevalence of otitis media, to determine predisposing factors	Subclinical otitis media is frequent, and those with bulla lysis should be closely monitored; lop-eared and rabbits with otitis externa had a higher risk of developing otitis media
King et al,[7] 2007	Prospective study: experimental animals	2	To determine if the tympanic bulla (TB) and associated structures could be evaluated with ultrasound in the rabbit	Lateral approach allowed visualization of the external ear canal to the level of the external acoustic meatus, TB could be visualized only from the ventral approach
King et al,[8] 2012	Prospective blind study: experimental animals	3	To compare ultrasonography, radiography, and CT for the identification of fluid within the TB of rabbit cadavers	CT was the most accurate diagnostic method, but ultrasound produced better results than radiography
Christopher et al,[9] 2014	Retrospective study: case series	2	To investigate the prevalence and type of poikilocytosis in pet rabbits and its association with physiologic factors, clinical disease, and laboratory abnormalities	Poikilocytosis is commonly found in this population, and correlation with some disease processes has been suggested
Cray et al,[12] 2013	Prospective clinical study	2	To evaluate the application of acute phase protein assays for C-reactive protein (CRP), haptoglobin (HP), and serum amyloid A (SAA) in the diagnosis of Encephalitozoon cuniculi	Significant increase in CRP levels, but not HP and SAA, was observed in the diseased group
Cray et al,[13] 2015	Prospective clinical study	2	To evaluate the utility of measuring immunoglobulin (Ig)M, IgG, and CRP levels in rabbits with suspected E cuniculi	Higher titers of IgM and IgG and elevated CRP levels were observed in the diseased group
Di Giuseppe et al,[14] 2016	Prospective clinical study	1	To assess the correlation between γ-globulins and IgM and IgG in E cuniculi–suspected rabbits	Significant quantitative correlation between percentage of γ-globulins and positive IgM and IgG was established in symptomatic rabbits

(continued on next page)

Table 1
(continued)

Reference No.	Type of Evidence	Grade	Intervention X	Outcome
Leipig et al,[15] 2013	Prospective clinical study	2	To evaluated the diagnostic value of histologic spore detection vs immunohistochemistry (IHC), and polymerase chain reaction (PCR) postmortem diagnosis of *E cuniculi*	IHC was more sensitive than histologic spore detection, and PCR proved to be the most sensitive overall
Harvey et al,[22] 2012	Prospective clinical study	2	To measure the level of agreement between forelimb Doppler-measured arterial blood pressure (ABP) vs auricular systolic ABP in isoflurane-anaesthetized rabbits	Doppler is acceptable for monitoring ABP in isoflurane-anaesthetized rabbits and is useful for detection of hypotension
Barter & Epstein,[23] 2014	Prospective experimental study	2	To assess agreement between carotid arterial pressure and auricular arterial, thoracic limb Doppler or thoracic limb oscillometric blood pressure measurements	Limits of agreement for all measurements were large but less so for mean arterial pressure than systolic arterial pressure
Marín et al,[25] 2013	Prospective study: experimental animals	3	To determine disposition kinetics of single dose of marbofloxacin (2 mg/kg) after intravenous (IV), intramuscular (IM), and subcutaneous (SC) administration was determined in rabbits	Kinetic parameters and absence of adverse reactions suggest that marbofloxacin is likely to be effective in rabbits
Carpenter et al,[26] 2009	Prospective study: experimental animals	3	To determine the pharmacokinetics of daily oral marbofloxacin (5 mg/kg) to rabbits during a 10-d period	Marbofloxacin appeared to be absorbed well and tolerated by rabbits
Watson et al,[27] 2015	Prospective study: experimental animals	2	To evaluate the pharmacokinetics and bioavailability of oral and IV orbifloxacin (10 and 20 mg/kg) in rabbits	Further studies are necessary to determine the protein-binding activity of orbifloxacin in rabbits before dosages are recommended
De Vito et al,[28] 2015	Prospective study: experimental animals	3	To compare the pharmacokinetics of metoclopramide after intra-arterial, IM, SC, and perrectal (PR) administrations to normal rabbits	IM and SC administrations may be useful in treating gastrointestinal disorders in rabbits when vascular access is not available, but PR is likely to be unreliable
Graham et al,[29] 2014	Retrospective study: case series	1	To evaluate both clinical and histologic anomalies associated with suspected benzimidazole toxicosis in rabbits	Benzimidazoles should be used judiciously and owners should be informed about potential side effects

Study	Study Design	Level	Objective	Findings
Abu-Akkada & Oda,[31] 2016	Retrospective study: case series	1	To assess whether cardiopulmonary resuscitation (CPR) was effective in rabbits with cardiopulmonary arrest	Prognosis of CPR is similar to other species, tight-fitting facemasks can provide effective respiratory support during CPR, and conventional CPR techniques appear effective in rabbits
Sieg et al,[32] 2012	Observational prospective study	1	To evaluate the use of a portable glucometer in healthy and diseased rabbits, and assess potential prognostic value	Blood glucose can be used to assess the severity of disease and help to differentiate between gut stasis and intestinal obstruction in anorexic rabbits
Buckley et al,[33] 2011	Observational prospective cross-sectional study	3	To evaluate performance of a human and veterinary portable glucometer vs a veterinary benchtop analyzer for measuring blood glucose, and to evaluate the effect of sample characteristics on their performance	Human portable blood glucose monitor (PBGM) is acceptable when benchtops are not available; veterinary PBGM overestimated blood glucose concentration, had decreased accuracy at low hematocrits and at high blood glucose concentrations
Harcourt-Brown & Harcourt-Brown,[34] 2012	Prospective study: experimental animals	1	To assess the feasibility of a commercial continuous interstitial glucose monitoring (CIGM) system in the rabbit, and describe the longitudinal glucose curve	The use of the commercially CIGM was feasible and longitudinal glucose data were determined
Bonvehi et al,[37] 2014	Retrospective study: case series	1	To determine the prevalence and types of hyponatremia, and its relationship with hyperglycemia and mortality in ill pet rabbits	Hyponatremia is common and associated with increase mortality risk; calculation of plasmatic tonicity is necessary for differentiation of types of hyponatremia
Langlois et al,[38] 2014	Prospective clinical trial	1	To determine whole blood and serum concentrations of L-lactate and serum concentrations of D-lactate in healthy rabbits and compare 3 methods of analysis for L-lactate measurement	Serum concentrations of D-lactate in healthy rabbits are in the range of those of other mammals; L-lactate values in healthy rabbits are higher compared with other mammals; units had good correlation
Ardiaca et al,[39] 2016	Prospective clinical trial	1	To establish a reference interval for venous plasmatic L-lactate concentration (PLLC) in pet rabbits and to assess its diagnostic and prognostic significance in ill pet rabbits	Morbidity and mortality are associated with sustained low PLLC in pet rabbits, whereas a good prognosis is associated with an increase in PLLC

(continued on next page)

Table 1
(continued)

Reference No.	Type of Evidence	Grade	Intervention X	Outcome
Di Girolamo et al,[40] 2016	Prospective cohort study	2	To determine whether rectal temperature at hospital admission, independently or in conjunction with other parameters, was associated with all-cause mortality in client-owned rabbits	Rectal temperature was major predictor of death in the present patient cohort
Graham et al,[41] 2014	Retrospective study: case series	2	To determine the clinical signs, diagnostic test results, treatment protocols, and outcomes of rabbits treated for liver lobe in one institution over 5 y	Nonspecific clinical signs (anorexia, lethargy, and decreased defecation) along with anemia and high serum hepatic enzyme activities supports suspicion for liver lobe torsion
Andres et al,[49] 2012	Retrospective study: case series	2	To determine the median survival time (MST) and prognostic factors associated with radiation therapy for the treatment of thymomas in rabbits	MST was good and body weight below 1.57 kg had the worst prognosis
Dolera et al,[50] 2015	Prospective observational study	2	To determine the MST and prognostic factors associated with stereotactic volumetric modulated arc radiotherapy for the treatment of thymomas in rabbits	MST was good and revealed complete responses using the Response Evaluation Criteria in Solid Tumors criteria
Schumacher,[52] 2011	Prospective study: experimental animals	3	To assess the impact of 4 rabbit diets on length and curvature of cheek teeth and eruption and attrition rates of incisors	Presence of increased tooth length, curvature, and interdental spaces indicated early dental pathology in rabbits fed muesli
Meredith et al,[53] 2015	Prospective study: experimental animals	2	To evaluate the use of fluorochromes xylenol orange and calcein green to measure growth rates of rabbit teeth and compared with manual measurements	Application of fluorochrome staining can be used to measure tooth growth
Wyss et al,[54] 2016	Prospective study: experimental animals	2	To determine the effect of 4 different pelleted diets of increasing abrasiveness on incisor and premolar growth and wear, and incisor and cheek tooth length	Diet form (whole vs pelleted) does not necessarily affect cheek teeth, and irrespective of the strong effect of external abrasives, internal abrasives have the potential to induce wear

Reference	Study type	Level	Objective	Findings
Jekl & Redrobe,[56] 2013	Prospective study: case series	1	Skull radiographic and CT images were compared with postmortem assessment in clinical cases	CT images provided more details about the extent of the dental pathology than radiographs
Van Caelenberg et al,[57] 2011	Prospective study: case series	1	Comparison of diagnostic consistency and diagnostic accuracy between survey radiography and CT in rabbits with dental disease	Radiography should not be considered a diagnostic imaging modality of lesser value, but instead complementary to CT
Keating et al,[62] 2012	Prospective observational study	2	To assess the physiologic and behavioral effects of ear tattooing on rabbits, evaluate the analgesic efficacy of topical local anesthetic cream, and to develop a pain scale based on facial expression changes	Ear tattooing causes transient and potentially severe pain in rabbits, which is minimized by application of local anesthetic cream; pain scale was suggested
Leach et al,[63] 2011	Retrospective study: video recording	2	Determine the perception of pain in rabbits by different observers with different levels of experience	Observers focused on the face, which is unlikely to be effective when using behavioral indicators of pain because they involve other body areas
Benato et al,[68] 2014	Observational prospective study	1	To determine the effect of probiotics on fecal levels of 4 important candidate gastrointestinal bacteria in pet rabbits	Inclusion of dietary probiotic supplementation using Enterococcus faecium NCIMB 30183 can increase fecal levels of certain bacterial flora of healthy adult rabbits
Reusch et al,[73] 2009	Clinical trial	1	To calculate reference range for the urinary protein:creatinine ratio (UPC) in healthy and diseased rabbits	No significant variation in the UPC due to the body weight, breed, sex, neutered status, or husbandry of the rabbits
Mancinelli et al,[75] 2012	Clinical trial	1	To determine γ-glutamyl-transferase (GGT) activity and GGT index in the urine of clinically healthy domestic rabbits	Urine GGT activity and the GGT index did not differ significantly between sexes but statistically significant difference was found in the GGT index with neutered status

fungus.[10,11] A study evaluated the application of acute-phase protein assays for C-reactive protein (CRP), haptoglobin (HP), and serum amyloid A (SAA) in the diagnosis of E cuniculi infection in pet rabbits.[12] A nearly 10-fold mean increase in CRP levels was observed in the diseased group, but no significant difference in HP or SAA levels was reported. Another study evaluated the utility of measuring immunoglobulin IgM, IgG, and CRP levels in E cuniculi–suspected cases.[13] When comparing healthy with suspected cases, higher titers of IgM and IgG and elevated CRP levels were observed in the diseased group. The use of combinations of these tests decreased the sensitivity of the diagnostic panel but increased the specificity, which resulted in a positive predictive value ranging from 92% to 100%. Another study suggests that total serum protein was not effective in predicting an antibody response, in contrast to γ-globulin ranges from serum electrophoresis, which could predict whether the patient was positive for IgM and/or IgG.[14] Diagnosis of E cuniculi may require postmortem examination. Samples from 81 rabbits (brain, heart, lungs, intestines, liver, and kidneys) were morphologically examined for lesions attributed to E cuniculi, as well as for the presence of spores and E cuniculi antigen, and 55 rabbits were tested for E cuniculi DNA.[15] Immunohistochemistry was more sensitive (42%, 16/38) than histologic spore detection, and real-time polymerase chain reaction (PCR) proved to be the most sensitive (30/35, 86% of the examined rabbits with E cuniculi infection). For definitive diagnosis, standard histology of the predilection sites and a specific etiologic assay, preferably real-time PCR, should be performed. Microsporidia, including E cuniculi, are increasingly recognized as causing opportunistic infections in immunocompromised humans.[16] Although human disease is unlikely, E cuniculi is a zoonotic organism and people exposed to infected rabbits may be at risk.[17,18] Using indirect fluorescent antibody test, E cuniculi antibodies were identified in 34 of 44 non–human immunodeficiency virus immunocompromised patients and 5 of 44 immunocompetent individuals in Egypt.[19] In China, seroprevalence of E cuniculi detected using enzyme-linked immunosorbent assay in healthy humans was 9.76% (29/300). In this study, prevalence rates varied between regions. Besides rabbits, E cuniculi is commonly found in rodents, dogs, other canids, and primates.[20] Pasteurized cow's milk may be a potential source of infection in humans, as spores in cow milk remained infective to mice following pasteurization treatments at 72°C for 15 seconds or 85°C for 5 seconds.[21]

Blood Pressure

Blood pressure is a common diagnostic test performed for assessment of cardiac function and to monitor anesthesia in rabbits. A prospective clinical study measured the agreement between Doppler-measured arterial blood pressure (ABP) in the forelimb, and directly measured auricular systolic and mean ABP in isoflurane-anesthetized rabbits.[22] Good agreement was found between direct and Doppler systolic ABP. The mean between-method difference comparing direct and Doppler measurements was +1 ± 8 mmHg, and the difference was consistent over the measured pressure range (directly measured systolic arterial blood pressure [SAP] range: 44 to 99 mmHg; directly measured mean arterial blood pressure [MAP] range: 33 to 83 mmHg). Doppler measurements less than 80 mmHg were a reliable indicator of arterial hypotension. Another prospective study assessing the agreement between carotid arterial pressure and auricular arterial, thoracic limb Doppler, or thoracic limb oscillometric blood pressure showed that limits of agreement for all measurements were large but less so for MAP than SAP.[23] Variation in bias with SAP should be considered when using these measurements clinically.

EVIDENCE-BASE ADVANCES IN THERAPEUTICS
Antibacterial Drugs

Marbofloxacin is a fluoroquinolone with concentration-dependent bactericidal activity against gram-negative bacteria, some gram-positive bacteria, and *Mycoplasma* spp. In a previous study, marbofloxacin was the most effective agent against bacterial strains isolated from upper respiratory tract diseases in rabbits, compared with enrofloxacin, danofloxacin, oxytetracycline, or doxycycline.[24] Pharmacokinetics of marbofloxacin after intravenous (IV), intramuscular (IM), and subcutaneous (SC) administration was determined in 6 New Zealand white rabbits at a single dose of 2 mg/kg.[25] Half-life time ($t_{1/2}$) following IV administration was 1.42 hours, and volume of distribution at steady state was 1.99 L/kg, suggesting a wide distribution and a good tissue penetration. Maximum plasma concentrations (Cmax) following IM and SC administration were 2.04 ± 0.32 and 1.64 ± 0.15 mg/L, at 0.33 ± 0.16 hours and 0.50 ± 0.18 hours, respectively. The absolute bioavailabilities after IM and SC administration were high at approximately 123% and 114%, with $t_{1/2}$ of 7.72 and 6.65 hours, and short maximum concentration peak (Tmax) at 0.33 and 0.5 hours, respectively. The Cmax/minimum inhibitory concentration (MIC) ratios for both routes of administration were in favor of a high protection against resistance emergence, based on MIC values reported against *Pasteurella multocida*. Similar findings were observed in a previous study with repeated per os (PO) administrations of 5 mg/kg of marbofloxacin every 24 hours in rabbits.[26] Pharmacokinetics of orbifloxacin, another concentration-dependent bactericidal fluoroquinolone, was also recently investigated after a single dose of 10 or 20 mg/kg, PO and IV, in 6 New Zealand white rabbits.[27] Mean ± SD Cmax of orbifloxacin following 10 and 20 mg/kg dose was 1.66 ± 0.51 μg/mL and 3.00 ± 0.97 μg/mL, at 2.0 and 3.3 hours, respectively. The mean ± SD $t_{1/2}$ was 7.3 ± 1.1 hours and 8.6 ± 0.55 hours for 10 mg/kg and 20 mg/kg dose, respectively. Mean bioavailability was 46.5% to 52.5%, similar to horses, and lower than dogs and quails. As protein-binding capacity of orbifloxacin was not evaluated in this study, a dose for rabbits could not be recommended.

Digestive Motility

Metoclopramide is a benzamide originally used as an antiemetic with prokinetic effect in monogastric and polygastric species. Metoclopramide acts as an antagonist of dopamine-2 (D2) and serotonin (5-HT3) receptors in rabbits, and speeds gastric emptying, relaxes the pyloric sphincter, and promotes aboral movement of stomach chyme in humans.[28] This drug is often used in rabbits with gastrointestinal stasis to stimulate digestive transit. Pharmacokinetics of metoclopramide was evaluated at 2 mg/kg intra-arterial (IA), IM, and SC, and 4 mg/kg perrectal (PR) doses in 6 healthy New Zealand rabbits. No neurologic adverse effects reported in other species were observed in this study. Absorption of metoclopramide after IM and SC administration was reliable, with a short Tmax of less than 10 minutes, fast elimination, and high bioavailability of 96% and 112%, respectively, similar to IA injection. PR route had erratic absorption and should not be used. IM and SC administrations of metoclopramide could be a useful alternative when IA and IV injection are not available. However, as metoclopramide is a lipophilic drug, SC absorption might be altered in overweight rabbits and the injection might cause SC and IM irritation due to its acidic pH (2.5–6.5). Currently, there is no reliable clinical evidence of the effectiveness and of the safety of this drug in rabbits.

Toxicosis

Benzimidazoles, such as albendazole or fenbendazole, act by binding invertebrate tubulin, affecting cellular mitosis and inhibiting the polymerization of the parasite cytoskeleton. Benzimidazoles are reported to have in vitro efficacy against *E cuniculi*.[29] These drugs are supposed to have a greater affinity for the parasitic tubulin compared with the similar mammalian structure; however, toxicosis has been reported in several species, with acute and chronic degenerative changes in rapidly dividing cells, such as bone marrow (aplastic anemia), intestinal mucosa, and genital organs. In a retrospective study including 13 rabbits of suspected benzimidazole toxicosis from 2 pathology institutions, common clinical signs included sudden lethargy, gastrointestinal stasis, petechiation, pale mucous membranes, hemorrhage, elevated body temperature, and sudden unexpected death.[29] Earliest onset of disease was 14 days after starting treatment; however, clinical signs were evident most of the time only after 30 days of treatment. Most common blood abnormalities included anemia, leukopenia, thrombocytopenia, and elevated hepatic enzymes. Weekly complete blood count should be considered during treatment and digestive support ± blood transfusion should be provided in suspected cases of toxicosis. Many rabbits in this study were exposed to higher doses than recommended or prolonged treatment duration of albendazole (30–41 mg/kg PO every 12–24 hours for 14–42 days) and fenbendazole (225 mg/kg PO every 24 hours for 30 days). Underlying causes, such as hepatic disorders or greater absorption following drug-induced intestinal inflammation or necrosis, might play a role. However, some rabbits developed suspected toxicosis at published dosages for albendazole, fendazole, and oxibendazole. Recommended doses for benzimidazoles in rabbits for the treatment of encephalitozoonosis vary over time and, according to the investigators, with albendazole at 7.4 to 20 mg/kg PO every 24 hours for 3 to 14 days, fenbendazole at 20 mg/kg PO every 24 hours for 28 days, and oxibendazole at 30 mg/kg PO every 24 hours for 7 to 14 days, then 15 mg/kg PO every 24 hours for 30 to 60 days.[30] Suspicion of benzimidazole toxicosis was associated with poor prognosis, as only 1 rabbit survived. Some veterinarians usually treat pet rabbits that are asymptomatic but are positive for *E cuniculi* based on laboratory results. The safety and effectiveness of treatment of asymptomatic rabbits needs to be properly demonstrated by epidemiologic research before implementing this treatment in clinical practice. Furthermore, a study has evaluated the efficacy of fenbendazole (20 mg/kg PO) before and after experimental infection of immunosuppressed rabbits with *E cuniculi*.[31] Fenbendazole was administered as prophylactic therapy for 7 successive days before infection or as a treatment for 4 weeks initiated on the 28th day after challenge. The study concluded that fenbendazole was effective to some extent in protecting some rabbits; however, when administered as a therapeutic treatment, no significant effects were observed. No clinical signs or mortality were reported during the study. In a nonrandomized case series, the effectiveness of benzimidazoles for treatment of *E cuniculi* was investigated.[32] Standard treatment consisted of oxytetracycline (from 2000 to 2003; n = 50), or fenbendazole and oxytetracycline (from 2004 to 2008; n = 45), and the rabbits were randomly assigned to treatment groups with or without dexamethasone. Each therapeutic regimen was given for 10 days, along with fluids, B vitamins, and nutritional support added as needed. Inclusion of fenbendazole in the treatment protocol was associated with increased survival rates on day 10 (*P* = .043), better neurologic scores (*P* = .008), and improved long-term survival (*P* = .025) based on the results of univariate analyses. Dexamethasone showed no effect on neurologic score or on short-term or long-term survival. As stated by the investigators, conclusions of such type of study may be biased by several factors, including improvement with supportive care alone.

EVIDENCE-BASED ADVANCES IN PROGNOSIS
Resuscitation

A retrospective study has assessed if cardiopulmonary resuscitation (CPR) was effective for cardiopulmonary arrest in pet rabbits.[33] Ten arrests occurred during or within 24 hours of anesthesia, and 5 were unassociated with anesthesia. Two rabbits were intubated before CPR, 3 during CPR. Facemasks were used in 7 animals, tracheostomy in 1, and the method of ventilation was unknown in 2 rabbits. Other treatments performed included the administration of pharmaceuticals. In 7 of 15 rabbits, return to spontaneous ventilation occurred, of which 1 was discharged, whereas the others died either shortly after resuscitation (2/7) or within 2 to 26 hours (4/7). The prognosis associated with CPR in rabbits is similar to that reported in other species. Tight-fitting facemasks can provide effective respiratory support during CPR when intubation is not feasible.

Glucose

Glucose is essential for the normal cell function. In one study, a significant relationship between blood glucose, food intake, and signs of stress, and severity of clinical disease was found.[34] Severe hyperglycemia (>360 mg/dL) was associated with conditions with poor prognosis and confirmed intestinal obstruction, whereas rabbits with confirmed gastrointestinal ileus had lower values (153 mg/dL). It is important to consider that in this study, the glucose measurement was performed using a single human portable blood glucose meter (PBGM) and results were not compared with a laboratory unit, some of the normal animals may have been suffering from undiagnosed conditions, the results of normoglycemic animals included animals that were showing signs of stress, and some animals were sedated and different types of sedation protocols were used. Nevertheless, this study shows potential clinical application and highlights the value of glucose assessment in rabbits.

Blood glucose is commonly measured using laboratory machines or PBGM. Accuracy of both human and veterinary PBGM has been compared with a veterinary benchtop analyzer.[35] Human PBGM underestimated blood glucose concentration, decreased accuracy at high hematocrits, and had the lowest total error, whereas veterinary PBGMs overestimated blood glucose concentration, had decreased accuracy at low hematocrits, and at high blood glucose concentrations had the highest total error. The addition of approximately 10 mg/dL to the results obtained with the human PBGM would provide the more reliable result. The use of commercial continuous interstitial glucose monitoring has been shown to be feasible in rabbits.[36] The results confirmed normal physiologic glucose concentration to be between 100 and 200 mg/dL, similar to phlebotomy. Glucose concentrations did not substantially change during the day or postprandially, but substantial elevation was observed during surgery (up to 280 mg/dL), which decreased to normal levels 2 to 3 hours postsurgery. One animal died after 5 hours of severe hyperglycemia (>400 mg/dL). Prevalence and types of hyponatremia, and its relationship with hyperglycemia and mortality in ill pet rabbits also has been reported.[37] The results indicate that hyponatremia and hyperglycemia are common in ill pet rabbits. Severe hyponatremia increases the risk of mortality and plasmatic sodium levels decrease with hyperglycemia, therefore simultaneous measurement of sodium and glucose should be performed.

Lactate

Whole blood L-lactate measured using a portable analyzer and a blood gas analyzer were compared with high-performance liquid chromatography analysis.[38] L-lactate values were higher when compared with other mammals, and good correlation was found between the portable and blood gas analyzers. L-lactate and its association with morbidity and mortality at 14 days have been reported. A better prognosis was associated with an increase of 3.3 mmol/L within 48 hours after arrival.[39] The results showed that, contrary to other species, morbidity and mortality is associated with sustained low L-lactate, whereas a good prognosis is associated with an increase in concentration.

Temperature

Rectal temperature on intake has been shown to provide a prognosis factor in terms of overall survival.[40] Rabbits with hypothermia at admission had a risk of death before or within 1 week after hospital discharge 3 times higher than rabbits without hypothermia. For each 1.8°F (1°C) decrease in admission rectal temperature, the odds of death were doubled.

EVIDENCE-BASED ADVANCES IN COMMON DISORDERS
Liver Lobe Torsion

Liver lobe torsion is a rare condition of unknown cause reported in several species, including dogs, horses, pigs, otters, rats, mice, and rabbits.[41,42] In a retrospective study over 5 years in a referral institution, a case series of 16 liver lobe torsions in rabbits were described, suggesting that liver lobe torsions may be more common in this species than previously believed.[41] Affected rabbit age ranged from 1.5 to 9.0 years, with no sex predilection. Lop breeds, specifically mini lops, were overrepresented. Most common clinical signs included anorexia, lethargy, and decreased fecal production. Abdominal pain was observed in 12 of 16 rabbits. A mass effect or palpable liver edge in the cranial abdomen was palpable in only 3 of 16 rabbits. Asymptomatic liver torsions also have been described in the past, as an incidental finding in rabbits during necropsy.[43] Most common blood abnormalities included anemia and elevated levels of alanine aminotransferase, alkaline phosphatase, and aspartate aminotransferase. Blood urea nitrogen and creatinine were also commonly elevated in this study, which was not observed in other previous reports.[44] Subjectively prolonged clotting time in rabbits with liver lobe torsion was in favor of poor prognosis.[41] Abdominal radiographs were performed in 12 rabbits and were suggestive of liver disease in 3 cases. Abnormal ultrasonography with Doppler was diagnostic in 14 of 14 rabbits, with lack of or decrease in blood flow in all affected liver lobes. Other common ultrasonographic findings included hepatomegaly or an abnormally large liver lobe, rounded lobar margins, mixed liver parenchymal echogenicity, and hyperechoic perihepatic mesentery. Abdominal effusion may or may not be detected in rabbits with liver torsion[41,43,44]; however, it appears to be a common finding in dogs and horses.[45–47] In dogs, abdominal effusion is suspected to result from the increase in hydrostatic pressure associated with hepatic vein obstruction.[45] Two rabbits had more than 1 torsed liver lobe.[41] The caudate lobe was affected in 10 of 16 rabbits, followed by the right lateral lobe in 5 of 16 rabbits, the left lateral lobe in 2 of 6 rabbits, and the right medial lobe in 1 of 6 rabbit. As in other reports,[44] the caudate lobe was the most common affected hepatic lobe (63%), theoretically because of its narrow attachment to the dorsal hilar region of the liver.[41,44] Explorative laparotomy and liver lobectomy were performed in 9 of 16 rabbits with 100% survival and minimal postoperative complications, whereas supportive care alone was provided for 7 of 16 rabbits, with 3 successful outcomes.[41] These 3 rabbits had recurrent episodes of digestive stasis for 1 month to several years after hospital discharge. Histologic examination was performed in 7 of 9 rabbits and was consistent with acute or, more interestingly, chronic liver lobe torsion. Underlying causes in these cases could not be determined. Current theories include laxity secondary to trauma or congenital absence of hepatic supporting ligaments, bacterial or parasitic hepatitis, or episodes of gastrointestinal stasis resulting in gastric dilation and stretching of the left triangular ligament, as hypothesized in dogs.[41,42,44] This study highlights that liver lobe torsion should be suspected in rabbits presented with nonspecific signs of gastrointestinal stasis, anemia, and high serum hepatic enzyme activities.[41]

Thymoma

Thymoma is commonly reported in rabbits, with ages ranging from 3 to 10 years (median, 6.1 year).[48] Most common clinical signs include dyspnea, bilateral exophthalmos, and anorexia.[48–50] Some rabbits are asymptomatic.[49,50] Reported suspected paraneoplastic syndromes in rabbits with thymoma include anemia and dermatosis.[48–50] Diagnosis is generally based on radiographs, thoracic ultrasound with fine-needle aspiration (FNA), and/or CT scan with FNA.[48–50] The mediastinal mass can appear cystic or noncystic.[43] FNA is reported to be diagnostic in most cases.[50] Historically, surgical management via thoracotomy has been associated with high perioperative mortalities.[48] The use of radiotherapy (RT) for the treatment of thymoma has been investigated in 2 recent case series.[49,50]

In 1 case series of 19 rabbits with megavoltage RT, 6 rabbits were treated with intensity-modulated radiotherapy (IMRT) of 42 to 48 Gy, and 13 rabbits with hypofractionated RT of 24 to 32 Gy.[49] Hypofractionated protocols include fewer RT sessions compared with IMRT, with a higher dose at each session, thus decreased number of anesthesia and cost for the owner. However, risks of radiation-induced side effects are higher than with IMRT. Megavoltage RT was effective for management of thymoma in these rabbits, with resolution of clinical signs within 4 to 42 days after starting RT and decreased thymoma volume from 30.0% to 86.6%. Median survival time (MST) was 313 days. When excluding 3 rabbits with acute death during RT, MST reached 727 days. These 3 deaths occurred within the first 2 weeks of RT, on the same day as an RT session. Type of radiation protocol was not significantly associated with survival time. Interestingly, rabbits weighing less than 1.57 kg had an MST of 312 days, whereas rabbits weighing more than 1.57 kg had an MST of 727 days. Three rabbits developed complications secondary to RT: 1 rabbit died secondary to radiation-induced cardiac failure at 1240 days post-IMRT, 1 rabbit had radiation-induced pneumonitis 3 months post-hypofractioned RT, and 1 rabbit had suspected radiation-induced mild to severe hair loss. Three rabbits died secondary to thymoma recurrence. One rabbit had 2 RTs 2 years apart, after recurrence of clinical sings. Two rabbits had follow-up serial radiographs, showing decrease and static but incomplete resolution of the mediastinal mass. One rabbit with follow-up CT 11 months after RT had an increase thymoma compared to the last RT session, but still smaller than on presentation.

Another recent study described 15 rabbits with thymoma treated with a total of 40 Gy during 6 sessions over 11 days with volumetric modulated arc radiotherapy (VMAT).[50] Compared with classic RT, VMAT allows dose escalation, hypofractionated protocols with decreased number of anesthesia events, and protocol adaptation during RT via an on-board CT as the thymoma volume decreases, which decreases risk of radiation-induced side effects. No rabbit received anti-inflammatory therapy in this study. Clinical improvement was achieved after the first RT in all rabbits, with more than 30% reduction of the thymoma volume. No death occurred during RT and complete response with elimination of all enhancing tumor volume was achieved in all cases at their final follow-up CT. None of the rabbits progressed once achieving a complete response during the 2-year follow-up period. Anemia resolved in 3 of 4 rabbits by 3 months after completion of treatment. No acute or late radiation toxicity was reported. MST was not reached, with a lower value for the 95% confidence interval of 777 days, whereas survival time in another publication[48] for 2 rabbits with medical management was only respectively 150 days and 270 days in 2 rabbits medically managed with cyst aspiration alone or cyst aspiration and with prednisolone administration. Currently, the evidence that supports radiotherapy is low to very low.[51] There is strong need of a randomized comparison of medical versus radiotherapeutic treatment of thymomas, as well as to determine the natural course of thymomas in untreated rabbits.

Dental Disease

Dental disease is considered as one of the most common disorders in pet rabbits, with up to 60% to 65% of young rabbits showing dental abnormalities, such as hooks, points, periodontal disease, or abnormal grading of molar and premolar abnormalities (**Fig. 1**).[52] Rabbit teeth grow and erupt continuously.[53] Tooth average crown length and periodontal probing depth seems to vary minimally among rabbits, whereas eruption rate can vary widely among individuals.[52,53] Reference ranges of tooth characteristics in rabbits without dental disease have been published (**Table 2**).[52–55] Tooth wear can decrease secondary to pain, congenital abnormalities, neoplasia, trauma, or inappropriate diet, which can increase tooth length and result in dental abnormalities.[52,53] Two studies compared the effects of pelleted diets with different degrees of

Mandibular cheek tooth	Exposed crown	Reserved crown	Root
Normal	- ~ 10° angle laterally - no sharp points	- no curvature - no elongation	- pointed
Grade I	- greater angle laterally - elongated - small sharp points	- no curvature - no or slight elongation apically	- pointed
Grade II	- even greater angle - elongated - curved - hooks/sharp points evident	- curved - elongated apically	- shortened - deformation possible
Grade III	- Grade II with all changes more prominently displayed	- Grade II with all changes more prominently displayed	- normal shape not evident

Fig. 1. Criteria for grading cheek teeth in rabbits. (*From* Schumacher M. Measurement of clinical crown length of incisor and premolar teeth in clinically healthy rabbits. J Vet Dent 2011;28(2):93; with permission.)

Table 2
Reference ranges of clinical crown length and periodontal probing depth of cheek and incisor teeth in rabbits with no clinical signs of dental disease

Tooth	Incisors		Molars (M) and Premolars (PM)				References
	Maxillary	Mandibular	Maxillary PM2	Mandibular PM3	Mandibular PM4		
Average crown length, mm	6.1 ± 0.9	6.4 ± 0.6	1.5 ± 0.4	3.1 ± 0.4	2.6 ± 0.4		Schwartz et al,[45] 2006
Periodontal probing depth, mm	2.2 ± 0.4	5.1 ± 0.8	0.5–1.0				Schwartz et al,[45] 2006
Eruption rate, mm/wk	1.9–2.0	2.2–2.4[47,48]	1.4–3.2 0.93 + 0.18 on hay diet 2.14 + 0.28 on grass/rice hulls/sand pelleted diet				Tennent-Brown et al,[47] 2012; Künzel et al,[48] 2012

abrasiveness and a whole grass hay–only diet on tooth eruption and attrition rate in domestic rabbits. Tooth growth was strongly related to tooth wear but differed correspondingly between diets and tooth positions.[54,55] As an interesting fact, tooth growth slowed down within its physiologic range in response to reduced attrition and wear.[55] In another study, the effects of 4 different diets (Timothy hay only; extruded diet with hay; muesli with hay; and muesli only) on length and curvature of cheek teeth via radiographs and eruption and attrition rates of incisors was evaluated in Dutch rabbits (n = 32).[53] Regardless of the diet, eruption rate of the incisors was similar to attrition rate, as described in another study.[56] However, incisor eruption and attrition rates were higher for the hay-only group compared with both groups fed muesli. After 9 months, a greater degree of curvature of the lower first cheek teeth was present in the muesli-only group compared with rabbits eating hay only or extruded diet with hay. After 17 months, rabbits fed muesli only and muesli with hay had longer lower first cheek teeth and larger interdental spaces between the first 2 M than rabbits fed extruded diet and hay, and hay only. Three rabbits fed muesli only developed evidence of dental disease by 17 months. Low intake of forage, but not calcium and phosphorus imbalance, appeared to be implicated in the development of dental disease based on this study. However, the effect of calcium and phosphorus on the onset of dental disease is still controversial among investigators.[56]

Advanced imaging is commonly used for dental assessment, and 2 recent studies compared CT with survey radiography. In a study with 4 pet rabbits with dental pathology, radiographs and CT provided similar findings that correlated with postmortem; however, CT images provided more detail of the lesions.[57] In another study, survey radiology (5 views; laterolateral, either left-to-right or right-to-left view, oblique view left 15° ventral-right dorsal, oblique view right 15° ventral-left dorsal, ventrodorsal, rostrocaudal) was compared with CT in 30 rabbits with dental disease by 2 non–board-certified radiologists.[58] CT accuracy was superior in 24 patients (80%) in diagnosis and prognosis, and in 17 patients (56.6%) for guiding extraoral dental and surgical treatment. Radiography provided superior accuracy in 5 patients (16.6%) for guiding intraoral dental treatment. The results of this study suggested that radiography should not be considered a diagnostic imaging modality of lesser value, but instead complementary to CT. Normal and diseased rabbit skull anatomy has also been described using cone-beam CT and micro-CT.[59–61]

CURRENT CONTROVERSIES AND CLINICAL TOPICS REQUIRING ADDITIONAL EVIDENCE
Pain Assessment

Pain assessment can be challenging in rabbits, and scoring systems have been developed to assess pain and its severity.[62–64] In a crossover study, New Zealand rabbits (n = 8) were evaluated for their facial expressions via a Rabbit Grimace Scale (**Fig. 2**), and physiologic and behavioral reactions following actual or sham ear tattooing, with or without application of topical local anesthetic (EMLA cream).[62] Tattooing without EMLA cream resulted in greater facial expression scores of pain, as well as significantly greater struggling behavior, vocalization, higher peak heart rate, and SAP and MAP compared with all other treatments. The investigators concluded that the Rabbit Grimace Scale appeared reliable and accurate for the assessment of acute pain in rabbits, similar to the grimace scale developed in mice[65] and rats.[66] In another study, video recordings of rabbits experiencing different degrees of postoperative pain were assessed by rabbit-experienced and inexperienced observers (n = 151).[63] The ethogram of pain behavior from another study[67] was used in this study (**Table 3**). Regardless of the experience or the gender of observers, observing

Orbital Tightening

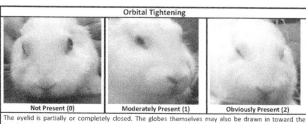

| Not Present (0) | Moderately Present (1) | Obviously Present (2) |

The eyelid is partially or completely closed. The globes themselves may also be drawn in toward the head so that they protrude less. If the eye closure reduces the visibility of the eye by more than half, it would be scored as '2' or 'obviously present'.

Cheek Flattening

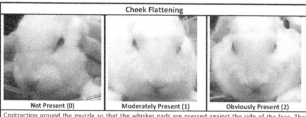

| Not Present (0) | Moderately Present (1) | Obviously Present (2) |

Contraction around the muzzle so that the whisker pads are pressed against the side of the face. The side contour of the face and nose is angular and the rounded appearance of the cheeks to either side of the nose is lost.

Nose Shape

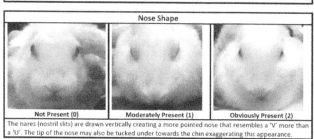

| Not Present (0) | Moderately Present (1) | Obviously Present (2) |

The nares (nostril slits) are drawn vertically creating a more pointed nose that resembles a 'V' more than a 'U'. The tip of the nose may also be tucked under towards the chin exaggerating this appearance.

Whisker Position

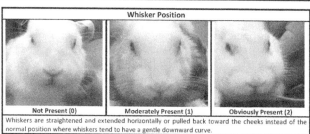

| Not Present (0) | Moderately Present (1) | Obviously Present (2) |

Whiskers are straightened and extended horizontally or pulled back toward the cheeks instead of the normal position where whiskers tend to have a gentle downward curve.

Ear Position

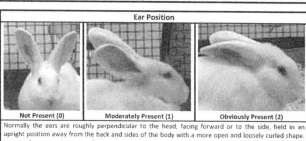

| Not Present (0) | Moderately Present (1) | Obviously Present (2) |

Normally the ears are roughly perpendicular to the head, facing forward or to the side, held in an upright position away from the back and sides of the body with a more open and loosely curled shape. In pain the ears rotate away from normal position to face towards the hindquarters, tend to move backward and be held closer to the back or sides of the body and have a more tightly folded or curled shape (i.e. more like a tube).

Fig. 2. Grimace Scale in rabbits. (*From* Keating SC, Thomas AA, Flecknell PA, et al. Evaluation of EMLA cream for preventing pain during tattooing of rabbits: changes in physiological, behavioural and facial expression responses. PLoS One 2012;7:e44437; with permission.)

Table 3
Ethogram of pain behavior used to determine pain severity in rabbits after ovario-hysterectomy

Behavior	Description
Twitch	Rapid movement of fur and back
Flinch	Body jerks upward for no apparent reason
Wince	Rapid movement of the backward in a rocking motion accompanied by eye dosing and swallowing action
Stagger	Partial loss of balance
Fall	Complete loss of balance when moving
Press	Abdomen pushed toward floor, usually before walking
Arch	Fur arching of the back upward
Writhe	Contraction of the oblique flank muscles
Shuffle	Walking at a very slow pace
Quiver	Slow rhythmic side-to-side movement

Adapted from Leach MC, Coulter CA, Richardson CA, et al. Are we looking in the wrong place? Implications for behavioural-based pain assessment in rabbits (*Oryctolagus cuniculi*) and beyond? PLoS One 2011;6:e1334; with permission.

the face led to poor pain evaluation, whereas observing the back and hindquarters was correlated with correct assessments.[63] However, no Grimace Scale seemed to have been provided to the observers. In conclusion, attention should be paid to the head via the Rabbit Grimace Scale, body posture, and behavior when assessing pain in rabbits.

Probiotics

Rabbits are hindgut fermenters and rely heavily on cecal flora for digestion. Any imbalance of cecal flora can have detrimental effects.[68] Although the rabbit cecum contains 400 different species of bacteria, 25 species are the most abundant.[68] In adult rabbits, strict anaerobes are the most prevalent bacteria, of which *Bacteroides* spp is the most important. The use of probiotics in rabbits is a highly controversial topic, as bacteria need to be resistant to low rabbit gastric pH and be able to colonize the digestive tract.[69] Two probiotics (*Saccharomyces cerevisiae* NCYC Sc47 and *Enterococcus faecium* NCIMB 30183) were given orally for 2 weeks in healthy rabbits. Administration of one of the probiotics (*E faecium* NCIMB 30183) was associated with a significant increase in fecal levels of *E faecium*.[68] However, probiotic treatment did not affect fecal levels of *Bacteroides* species, *Fibrobacter succinogenes* or *Clostridium spiroforme*, body weight, or fecal weight and diameter. Further research is needed to evaluate the health benefits of this probiotic.

NEW IDEAS

Although rabbits are commonly kept exotic small mammal pets and have long been used in medical research, naturally occurring and induced thyroid dysfunction is rarely reported. Hyperthyroidism in 2 pet rabbits has been reported in a non–peer-review format.[70] Although normal values of thyroid scintigraphy by means of IV technetium-99m pertechnetate, and normal circulating concentration of free and total thyroid hormones have been reported as proceedings, further studies assessing its clinical application are needed.[71,72] Indeed, the previously mentioned hyperthyroidism cases in pet rabbits were strongly supported by the results of scintigraphy; however, the serum levels of circulating thyroid hormones were not clearly elevated. Nevertheless, thyroid dysfunction may not be considered in clinical cases due to low prevalence, lack of case reports, and limited validated diagnostic tests.

Renal disease in a common condition in rabbits; however, diagnosis can be challenging. Renal assessment is commonly performed using blood chemistry and urinalysis. The calculated reference ranges for urinary protein:creatinine ratio (UPC) of *E cuniculi*–seronegative rabbits is reported to range from 0.11 to 0.4.[73] Another study supported these findings; in 84.8% rabbits with renal disease, the UPC was greater than 0.4.[74] UPC may be a useful tool for the assessment of renal function. Another potentially useful tool is urinary γ-glutamyl-transferase (GGT).[75] The GGT and the GGT index reference intervals in fresh urine samples of healthy and sick rabbits were found to be 2.7 to 96.5 IU/L and 0.043 to 1.034, respectively. An emerging renal marker in dogs and cats is symmetric dimethylarginine (SDMA). SDMA is a renal biomarker that is primarily excreted by the kidneys and accumulates in patients with kidney failure.[76] SDMA also has been shown to be an earlier indicator of kidney disease in dogs and cats.[76,77] Although the use of this marker in rabbits has not been shown to have diagnostic value, normal tissue and blood values have been reported in rabbits.[78] Future studies assessing its clinical application and potential predictive value for renal disease are needed.

As previously mentioned, *E cuniculi* has been recently reclassified as a fungal organism. It is interesting that the most common treatment for this condition is benzimidazoles, particularly fenbendazole and albendazole, primarily used as anthelmintic agents, which would make sense based on the previous classification as a parasite. These drugs also have been shown to inhibit in vitro growth of some fungi, for example, *Cryptococcus neoformans*.[79] A few case reports of ocular disease caused by microsporidian organisms in humans, including *E cuniculi*, were treated purposely or coincidentally with antifungals like itraconazole.[80–82] Nevertheless, albendazole is still considered the most common treatment for *E cuniculi* in humans.[83–85] In vitro susceptibility of 1 *E cuniculi*–positive rabbit to itraconazole has been shown to be poor[86]; however, new research assessing the in vitro and/or in vivo effect of newer generations of triazoles may provide interesting results.

REFERENCES

1. Gibbons PM, Mayer J. Evidence in exotic animal practice: a "how-to guide". J Exot Pet Med 2009;18:174–80.

2. Hammond G, Sullivan M, Posthumus J, et al. Assessment of three radiographic projections for detection of fluid in the rabbit tympanic bulla. Vet Radiol Ultrasound 2010;51:48–51.

3. De Matos R, Ruby J, Van Hatten RA, et al. Computed tomographic features of clinical and subclinical middle ear disease in domestic rabbits (*Oryctolagus cuniculus*): 88 cases (2007–2014). J Am Vet Med Assoc 2015;246:336–43.

4. Dickie A, Doust R, Cromarty L, et al. Ultrasound imaging of the canine tympanic bulla. Res Vet Sci 2003;75:121–6.

5. King A, Weinrauch S, Doust R, et al. Comparison of ultrasonography, radiography and a single computed tomography slice for fluid identification within the feline tympanic bulla. Vet J 2007;173:638–44.

6. Bernier Gosselin V, Babkine M, Gains M, et al. Validation of an ultrasound imaging technique of the tympanic bullae for the diagnosis of otitis media in calves. J Vet Intern Med 2014;28:1594–601.

7. King A, Hall J, Cranfield F, et al. Anatomy and ultrasonographic appearance of the tympanic bulla and associated structures in the rabbit. Vet J 2007;173:512–21.

8. King A, Posthumus J, Hammond G, et al. Comparison of ultrasonography, radiography and a single computed tomography slice for the identification of fluid within the tympanic bulla of rabbit cadavers. Vet J 2012;193:493–7.

9. Christopher MM, Hawkins MG, Burton AG. Poikilocytosis in rabbits: prevalence, type, and association with disease. PLoS One 2014;9:e112455.

10. Vergneau-Grosset C, Larrat S. Microsporidiosis in vertebrate companion exotic animals. J Fungi 2015;2:3.

11. Thomarat F, Vivares CP, Gouy M. Phylogenetic analysis of the complete genome sequence of Encephalitozoon cuniculi supports the fungal origin of microsporidia and reveals a high frequency of fast-evolving genes. J Mol Evol 2004;59:780–91.

12. Cray C, Rodriguez M, Fernandez Y. Acute phase protein levels in rabbits with suspected Encephalitozoon cuniculi infection. J Exot Pet Med 2013;22:280–6.

13. Cray C, McKenny S, Perritt E, et al. Utility of IgM titers with IgG and C-reactive protein quantitation in the diagnosis of suspected Encephalitozoon cuniculi infection in rabbits. J Exot Pet Med 2015;24:356–60.

14. Di Giuseppe M, Romano P, Gelli D, et al. Correlation between γ-globulins and Encephalitozoon cuniculi immunoglobulins in suspected infected rabbits. Comp Clin Path 2016;25:1237–9.

15. Leipig M, Matiasek K, Rinder H, et al. Value of histopathology, immunohistochemistry, and real-time polymerase chain reaction in the confirmatory diagnosis of Encephalitozoon cuniculi infection in rabbits. J Vet Diagn Invest 2013;25:16–26.

16. Didier E, Vossbrinck C, Baker M, et al. Identification and characterization of three Encephalitozoon cuniculi strains. Parasitology 1995;111:411–21.

17. Carhan A, Ozkan O, Ozkaya E. The first identification of Encephalitozoon cuniculi infection in an animal care worker in Turkey. Iran J Parasitol 2015;10:280.

18. Yaoqian P, Shuai W, Xingyou L, et al. Seroprevalence of Encephalitozoon cuniculi in humans and rabbits in China. Iran J Parasitol 2015;10:290.

19. Abu-Akkada SS, El Kerdany EDH, Rasha Fadly M, et al. Encephalitozoon cuniculi infection among immunocompromised and immunocompetent humans in Egypt. Iran J Parasitol 2015;10:561.

20. Snowden K, Logan K, Didier E. Encephalitozoon cuniculi strain III is a cause of encephalitozoonosis in both humans and dogs. J Infect Dis 1999;180:2086–8.

21. Kváč M, Tomanová V, Samková E, et al. Encephalitozoon cuniculi in raw cow's milk remains infectious after pasteurization. Foodborne Pathog Dis 2016;13:77–9.

22. Harvey L, Knowles T, Murison PJ. Comparison of direct and Doppler arterial blood pressure measurements in rabbits during isoflurane anaesthesia. Vet Anaesth Analg 2012;39:174–84.

23. Barter LS, Epstein SE. Comparison of Doppler, oscillometric, auricular and carotid arterial blood pressure measurements in isoflurane anesthetized New Zealand white rabbits. Vet Anaesth Analg 2014;41:393–7.

24. Rougier S, Galland D, Boucher S, et al. Epidemiology and susceptibility of pathogenic bacteria responsible for upper respiratory tract infections in pet rabbits. Vet Microbiol 2006;115:192–8.

25. Marín P, Álamo L, Escudero E, et al. Pharmacokinetics of marbofloxacin in rabbit after intravenous, intramuscular, and subcutaneous administration. Res Vet Sci 2013;94:698–700.

26. Carpenter JW, Pollock CG, Koch DE, et al. Single- and multiple-dose pharmacokinetics of marbofloxacin after oral administration to rabbits. Am J Vet Res 2009; 70:522–6.

27. Watson MK, Wittenburg LA, Bui CT, et al. Pharmacokinetics and bioavailability of orbifloxacin oral suspension in New Zealand White rabbits (*Oryctolagus cuniculus*). Am J Vet Res 2015;76:946–51.

28. De Vito V, Kim T-W, Rota S, et al. Pharmacokinetics of metoclopramide after Intra-ARTERIAL, intramuscular, subcutaneous, and perrectal administration in rabbits. J Exot Pet Med 2015;24:361–6.

29. Graham JE, Garner MM, Reavill DR. Benzimidazole toxicosis in rabbits: 13 cases (2003 to 2011). J Exot Pet Med 2014;23:188–95.

30. Fiorello C, Divers S. Rabbits. In: Carpenter J, editor. Exotic animal formulary. 4th edition. St Louis (MO): Elsevier/Saunders; 2013. p. 517–57.

31. Abu-Akkada S, Oda S. Prevention and treatment of *Encephalitozoon cuniculi* infection in immunosuppressed rabbits with fenbendazole. Iran J Vet Res 2016;17:98.

32. Sieg J, Hein J, Jass A, et al. Clinical evaluation of therapeutic success in rabbits with suspected encephalitozoonosis. Vet Parasitol 2012;187:328–32.

33. Buckley GJ, DeCubellis J, Sharp CR, et al. Cardiopulmonary resuscitation in hospitalized rabbits: 15 cases. J Exot Pet Med 2011;20:46–50.

34. Harcourt-Brown F, Harcourt-Brown S. Clinical value of blood glucose measurement in pet rabbits. Vet Rec 2012;170:674.

35. Selleri P, Di Girolamo N, Novari G. Performance of two portable meters and a benchtop analyzer for blood glucose concentration measurement in rabbits. J Am Vet Med Assoc 2014;245:87–98.

36. Mayer J, Schnellbacher R, Rich E, et al. Use of a commercial continuous interstitial glucose monitor in rabbits (*Oryctolagus cuniculus*). J Exot Pet Med 2016;25:220–5.

37. Bonvehi C, Ardiaca M, Barrera S, et al. Prevalence and types of hyponatraemia, its relationship with hyperglycaemia and mortality in ill pet rabbits. Vet Rec 2014; 174:554.

38. Langlois I, Planché A, Boysen S, et al. Blood concentrations of d- and l-lactate in healthy rabbits. J Small Anim Pract 2014;55:451–6.

39. Ardiaca M, Dias S, Montesinos A, et al. Plasmatic l-lactate in pet rabbits: association with morbidity and mortality at 14 days. Vet Clin Pathol 2016;45:116–23.

40. Di Girolamo N, Toth G, Selleri P. Prognostic value of rectal temperature at hospital admission in client-owned rabbits. J Am Vet Med Assoc 2016;248:288–97.

41. Graham JE, Orcutt CJ, Casale SA, et al. Liver lobe torsion in rabbits: 16 cases (2007 to 2012). J Exot Pet Med 2014;23:258–65.

42. Basseches J. Liver lobe torsion in pet rabbits. Vet Clin North Am Exot Anim Pract 2014;17:195.

43. Weisbroth S. Torsion of the caudate lobe of the liver in the domestic rabbit (*Oryctolagus*). Vet Pathol 1975;12:13–5.

44. Stanke NJ, Graham JE, Orcutt CJ, et al. Successful outcome of hepatectomy as treatment for liver lobe torsion in four domestic rabbits. J Am Vet Med Assoc 2011;238:1176–83.

45. Schwartz SGH, Mitchell SL, Keating JH, et al. Liver lobe torsion in dogs: 13 cases (1995–2004). J Am Vet Med Assoc 2006;228:242–7.

46. Bhandal J, Kuzma A, Starrak G. Spontaneous left medial liver lobe torsion and left lateral lobe infarction in a rottweiler. Can Vet J 2008;49:1002.

47. Tennent-Brown BS, Mudge MC, Hardy J, et al. Liver lobe torsion in six horses. J Am Vet Med Assoc 2012;241:615–20.

48. Künzel F, Hittmair KM, Hassan J, et al. Thymomas in rabbits: clinical evaluation, diagnosis, and treatment. J Am Vet Med Assoc 2012;48:97–104.

49. Andres K, Kent M, Siedlecki C, et al. The use of megavoltage radiation therapy in the treatment of thymomas in rabbits: 19 cases. Vet Comp Oncol 2012;10:82–94.

50. Dolera M, Malfassi L, Mazza G, et al. Feasibility for using hypofractionated stereotactic volumetric modulated arc radiotherapy (VMAT) with adaptive planning for treatment of thymoma in rabbits: 15 cases. Vet Radiol Ultrasound 2015;57: 313–20.

51. GRADE Working Group. Grading quality of evidence and strength of recommendations. BMJ 2004;328:1490–4.

52. Schumacher M. Measurement of clinical crown length of incisor and premolar teeth in clinically healthy rabbits. J Vet Dent 2011;28:90–5.

53. Meredith A, Prebble J, Shaw D. Impact of diet on incisor growth and attrition and the development of dental disease in pet rabbits. J Small Anim Pract 2015;56: 377–82.

54. Wyss F, Müller J, Clauss M, et al. Measuring rabbit (Oryctolagus cuniculus) tooth growth and eruption by fluorescence markers and bur marks. J Vet Dent 2016;33: 39–46.

55. Müller J, Clauss M, Codron D, et al. Growth and wear of incisor and cheek teeth in domestic rabbits (Oryctolagus cuniculus) fed diets of different abrasiveness. J Exp Zool A Ecol Genet Physiol 2014;321:283–98.

56. Jekl V, Redrobe S. Rabbit dental disease and calcium metabolism–the science behind divided opinions. J Small Anim Pract 2013;54:481–90.

57. Van Caelenberg A, De Rycke L, Hermans K, et al. Comparison of radiography and CT to identify changes in the skulls of four rabbits with dental disease. J Vet Dent 2011;28:172–81.

58. Capello V, Cauduro A. Comparison of diagnostic consistency and diagnostic accuracy between survey radiography and computed tomography of the skull in 30 rabbits with dental disease. J Exot Pet Med 2016;25:115–27.

59. Riggs G, Arzi B, Cissell DD, et al. Clinical application of cone-beam computed tomography of the rabbit head: part 1–normal dentition. Front Vet Sci 2016;3:93.

60. Sasai H, Iwai H, Fujita D, et al. The use of micro-computed tomography in the diagnosis of dental and oral disease in rabbits. BMC Vet Res 2014;10:209.

61. De Rycke LM, Boone MN, Van Caelenberg AI, et al. Micro-computed tomography of the head and dentition in cadavers of clinically normal rabbits. Am J Vet Res 2012;73:227–32.

62. Keating SC, Thomas AA, Flecknell PA, et al. Evaluation of EMLA cream for preventing pain during tattooing of rabbits: changes in physiological, behavioural and facial expression responses. PLoS One 2012;7:e44437.

63. Leach MC, Coulter CA, Richardson CA, et al. Are we looking in the wrong place? Implications for behavioural-based pain assessment in rabbits (Oryctolagus cuniculi) and beyond? PLoS One 2011;6:e13347.

64. Hampshire V, Robertson S. Using the facial grimace scale to evaluate rabbit wellness in post-procedural monitoring. Lab Anim 2015;44:259–60.

65. Langford DJ, Bailey AL, Chanda ML, et al. Coding of facial expressions of pain in the laboratory mouse. Nat Med 2010;7:447–9.

66. Sotocinal SG, Sorge RE, Zaloum A, et al. The Rat Grimace Scale: a partially automated method for quantifying pain in the laboratory rat via facial expressions. Mol Pain 2011;7:55.

67. Leach MC, Allweiler S, Richardson C, et al. Behavioural effects of ovariohysterectomy and oral administration of meloxicam in laboratory housed rabbits. Res Vet Sci 2009;87:336–47.

68. Benato L, Hastie P, O'Shaughnessy P, et al. Effects of probiotic Enterococcus faecium and Saccharomyces cerevisiae on the faecal microflora of pet rabbits. J Small Anim Pract 2014;55:442–6.

69. Myers D. Probiotics. J Exot Pet Med 2007;16:195–7.
70. Brandão J, Higbie C, Rick M, et al. Naturally occurring idiopathic hyperthyroidism in two pet rabbits. ExoticsCon 2015 Proceedings. San Antonio (TX), August 29 – September 2, 2015. p. 341–2.
71. Brandão J, Ellison M, Beaufrere H, et al. Quareporttive 99M-Technetium pertechnetate thyroid scintigraphy in euthyroid New Zealand white rabbits (Oryctolagus cuniculus). Proceedings of the American College of Veterinary Radiology Conference. St Louis (MO): American College of Veterinary Radiology. October 21–24, 2014. p. 62.
72. Brandão J, Rick M, Tully TN. Measurement of serum free and total thyroxine and triiodothyronine concentrations in rabbits. Exoticscon 2016 Proceedings. August 27– September 1, 2016. p. 485–6.
73. Reusch B, Murray J, Papasouliotis K, et al. Urinary protein: creatinine ratio in rabbits in relation to their serological status to Encephalitozoon cuniculi. Vet Rec 2009;164:293–5.
74. Selleri P, Bongiovanni L, Isani G, et al. Protein to creatinine ratio in pet rabbits with suspect or histologically confirmed renal disease. ExoticsCon 2015 Proceedings. August 29 – September 2, 2015. p. 333.
75. Mancinelli E, Shaw D, Meredith A. γ-Glutamyl-transferase (GGT) activity in the urine of clinically healthy domestic rabbits (Oryctolagus cuniculus). Vet Rec 2012;171:475–8.
76. Hall J, Yerramilli M, Obare E, et al. Serum concentrations of symmetric dimethylarginine and creatinine in dogs with naturally occurring chronic kidney disease. J Vet Intern Med 2016;30:794–802.
77. Hall J, Yerramilli M, Obare E, et al. Comparison of serum concentrations of symmetric dimethylarginine and creatinine as kidney function biomarkers in cats with chronic kidney disease. J Vet Intern Med 2014;28:1676–83.
78. McDermott J. Studies on the catabolism of Ng-methylarginine, Ng, Ng-dimethylarginine and Ng, Ng-dimethylarginine in the rabbit. Biochem J 1976; 154:179–84.
79. Cruz M, Bartlett M, Edlind T. In vitro susceptibility of the opportunistic fungus Cryptococcus neoformans to anthelmintic benzimidazoles. Antimicrob Agents Chemother 1994;38:378–80.
80. Yee RW, Tio FO, Martinez JA, et al. Resolution of microsporidial epithelial keratopathy in a patient with AIDS. Ophthalmology 1991;98:196–201.
81. Sridhar M, Sharma S. Microsporidial keratoconjunctivitis in a HIV-seronegative patient treated with debridement and oral itraconazole. Am J Ophthalmol 2003; 136:745–6.
82. Rossi P, Urbani C, Donelli G, et al. Resolution of microsporidial sinusitis and keratoconjunctivitis by itraconazole treatment. Am J Ophthalmol 1999;127:210–2.
83. Fournier S, Liguory O, Sarfati C, et al. Disseminated infection due to Encephalitozoon cuniculi in a patient with AIDS: case report and review. HIV Med 2000; 1:155–61.
84. Didier ES, Maddry JA, Brindley PJ, et al. Therapeutic strategies for human microsporidia infections. Expert Rev Anti Infect Ther 2005;3:419–34.
85. Ridoux O, Drancourt M. In vitro susceptibilities of the microsporidia Encephalitozoon cuniculi, Encephalitozoon hellem, and Encephalitozoon intestinalis to albendazole and its sulfoxide and sulfone metabolites. Antimicrob Agents Chemother 1998;42:3301–3.
86. Franssen F, Lumeij J, Van Knapen F. Susceptibility of Encephalitozoon cuniculi to several drugs in vitro. Antimicrob Agents Chemother 1995;39:1265–8.

Evidence-Based Advances in Ferret Medicine

Minh Huynh, DVM, MRCVS, DECZM (Avian)*, Lucile Chassang, DVM, IPSAV (med zool), Graham Zoller, DVM, IPSAV (med zool)

KEYWORDS

- Ferret • Adrenal gland disease • Insulinoma • Lymphoma • Reference

KEY POINTS

- Ferret medicine is still a young discipline with a limited level of evidence.
- Randomized trials are still uncommon in ferret literature due to economic and ethical reasons.
- Clinical research could be stimulated through individual methodology and statistics but also through the creation of international working groups in order to progress in a more efficient medicine for ferret patients.

INTRODUCTION

Ferrets were domesticated about 2000 years ago. They were used primarily for hunting purposes and then as laboratory models, especially for influenza. Pet ferrets became popular worldwide in the early 1980s; ferret medicine started to grow from that time, with the first case report of estrogen-related aplastic anemia in a female ferret in 1981.[1] This literature review covers about 35 years of publications related to ferret medicine. The content of relevant articles was scrutinized by the authors, and pertinent clinical information was extracted. Whenever possible, several sources were confronted and compared.

CLINICAL EXAMINATION

Ferret clinical examination has the same requirements as other small mammals. Objective assessments include recording of the heart rate, respiratory rate, and rectal temperature (**Table 1**).

Heart rates reported in textbooks range from 160 to 250 beats per minute (bpm).[6,7] Data were extracted from articles focusing on the echocardiography and

Disclosure Statement: The authors have nothing to disclose.
Exotic Department, Centre Hospitalier Vétérinaire Frégis, 43 Avenue Aristide Briand, Arcueil 94110, France
* Corresponding author.
E-mail address: nacologie@gmail.com

Vet Clin Exot Anim 20 (2017) 773–803
http://dx.doi.org/10.1016/j.cvex.2017.04.009

Table 1
Summary of articles found through the literature review regarding normal heart rate of ferrets

Article Type	Number of Articles
Cross-sectional study	2[2,3]
Prospective descriptive observational study	1[4]
Unrandomized crossover trial	1[5]
Narrative review	3
No access	3

electrocardiogram in ferrets. Because of the very active nature of ferrets, most of the studies were performed under anesthesia. Only one study (ranked with low level of evidence) reported about conscious examination.[3] In such an article, the heart rate varied between 210 and 405 bpm.[2] Those records can be biased by several factors, including electrode implantation or handling, which may enhance stress or cause mild pain and, thus, increase the heart rate.

The same study demonstrated that females had significantly higher heart rates than males (300 ± 58 bpm vs 260 ± 34 bpm), and this was correlated to the body weight.[2] Another study reported a higher heart rate in ferrets younger than 6 months.[5] Normal heart rates recorded under anesthesia in most studies ranged from 200 to 300 bpm.[3–5,8]

Normal respiratory rates were rarely reported. One narrative review reported a rate between 33 and 36 breaths per minute.[9]

Body temperature was investigated with an implantable microchip and rectal thermometry.[10] Normal temperature ranged from 99.0°F to 102.6°F (100.7°F mean; 37.2°C–38.9°C mean 37.8°C). Influence of reproductive status has been investigated in male ferrets whereby temperature was constant during the day but lower at night (38°C ± 0.3°C vs 37.3°C during mating season, 36.6°C during inactive period).[11]

CLINICAL PATHOLOGY

Recommendations provided by the American Society for Veterinary Clinical Pathology are used for a definite species.[12]

For the hematology topic, the authors found 11 articles. It was difficult to compare various methodologies because cohort studies could hardly be compared with narrative reviews, which usually mix various sources to produce data. The effect of sex, age, breed, and method of sampling (under anesthesia or not) as well as method of analysis (manual method vs automated method) were reported.[13–15] Although most values were comparable, marginal values should be interpreted with caution. The clinician should try, whenever possible, to obtain an individual reference value with a standardized sampling method and analysis (**Tables 2 and 3**).

Biochemistry was investigated in 8 articles. The same limitations from the hematology articles could be applied to biochemistry, although typically only 2 variables (sex and age) were studied (**Tables 4 and 5**).

A special effort in the literature can be noticed regarding glucose measurement, which is probably because hypoglycemia is one of the most common presentations in ferret emergencies. Glucose levels are usually measured using portable glucometer because of convenience, cost and because they limit glycolysis (consumption of glucose by the erythrocytes). However, there may be significant variation between

Table 2
Summary of articles found through the literature review regarding normal hematology of ferrets

Article Type	Number of Articles
Crossover trial	1[15]
Before and after trial	1[13]
Repeated cross-sectional study	2[14,16]
Prospective descriptive observational study	2[17,18]
Narrative review	3
No access	2

the different commercial devices. Some guidelines about quality assurance have been published by the ASVCP.[22] Standardization of blood glucose measurement has been a subject of controversy in human medicine.[23] Two studies in ferrets compared various portable devices with a laboratory analyzer.[24,25] Underestimation of the glucose blood value by the portable glucometers was observed, resulting in low specificity (50%) for detecting hypoglycemia. This finding means that half of the ferrets that became hypoglycemic with the portable blood glucometers are actually normoglycemic. Use of portable glucometers is, therefore, not acceptable; a laboratory analyzer should be used instead.

Coagulation

Three prospective descriptive studies were found.[26–28] Variation of coagulation parameters depending on the methods used (fibrometer vs automated coagulation analyzer) is described.[26]

Urinalysis

Three different sources were found, but only one focused on normal values of urinalysis (**Table 6**).[29]

Cerebrospinal Fluid

One study reported the composition of normal cerebrospinal fluid in ferrets (**Table 7**).[30]

Ophthalmic Data

Five different studies with a comparable study design described normal measurement in ferret ophthalmology.[31,32] Intraocular pressure (IOP) was best evaluated with rebound tonometry because the eye is small and repeatability was higher as compared with applanation tonometry.[31] IOP was reported to be higher in males than in females (**Table 8**).[31]

DIAGNOSTIC IMAGING
Radiograph

Radiographs are used primarily to diagnose cardiothoracic abnormalities. All studies found were prospective descriptive studies corresponding to a very low degree of evidence. Three studies focused on cardiac size measurement using a vertebral heart score.[33–35] Only one study actually validated the methodology including ferrets affected by dilated cardiomyopathy.[35] However, dilated cardiomyopathy was a relatively rare echocardiographic finding in one retrospective study.[36] The authors found

Table 3
Hematologic reference value

	Heinz et al,[17] 2012	Smith et al,[19] 2015			Carpenter,[20] 2013		Siperstein,[21] 2008			
Study design	Prospective observational study	Narrative review			Narrative review		Narrative review			
Blood sampling method	Vena saphena lateralis	—			—		—			
Material	EDTA									
Population	111 clinically healthy ferrets	*Female*	*Male*	*2–3 mo*	*Female*	*Male*	*Albino male*	*Albino female*	*Fitch male*	*Fitch female*
Packed cell volume (L/L)	0.6 (0.4–0.7)	33.6–49.8	35.6–55.0	27.0–38.5	34.6–55.0	33.6–61.0	44–61	42–55	36–50	47–51
Hemoglobin (mmol/L)	11.1 (8.6–13.6)	12.0–18.2	12.9–17.4	9.6–13.8	11.9–17.4	12.0–18.5	16.3–18.2	14.8–18.20	7.7–15.4	2.5–8.6
Erythrocytes ($\times 10^{12}$/L)	10.5 (7.4–13.0)	6.5–13.2	6.7–9.34	4.8–7.8	6.77–9.76	7.1–13.2	7.3–12.2	6.8–9.8	—	—
Mean corpuscular volume (fL)	54.3 (49.6–60.6)	44.1–52.5	44.4–53.7	47.8–57.6	44.4–53.7	42.6–52.5	—	—	—	—
Mean corpuscular hemoglobin concentration (mmol/L)	19.3 (17.8–20.9)	33.7–42.2	33.2–35.3	34.7–37.0	33.2–42.2 g/dL	30.3–34.9 g/dL	—	—	—	—
Mean corpuscular hemoglobin (fmol/L)	1.1 (1.0–1.2)	16.5–19.7	16.4–19.4	17.5–22.8	16.4–19.4 pg	13.7–19.7 pg	—	—	—	—
White blood cells ($\times 10^{9}$/L)	7.2 (3.0–16.7)	4.4–15.4	2.5–18.2	5.3–12.6	2.5–18.2	4.4–19.1	4.4–19.1	4.0–18.2	7.7–15.4	2.5–8.6
Band neutrophilic granulocytes (%)	0.0 (0.0–1.2)	—	—	—	0.0–4.2	0.0–2.2	—	—	0.0–2.2	0.0–4.2
Band neutrophilic granulocytes ($\times 10^{9}$/L)	0.0 (0.0–0.1)	—	—	—	—	—	—	—	—	—

Segmented neutrophilic granulocytes (%)	43 (17.2–81.9)	24–76	43–78	46.1–76.6	—	11–82	43–84	24–78	12–41
Segmented neutrophilic granulocytes ($\times 10^9$/L)	3.0 (0.9–7.4)	—	—	—	—	—	—	—	—
Lymphocytes (%)	53.0 (12.6–80.6)	12.0–66.6	42.2–68.2	12–95	12–73	12–54	12–50	28–69	25–95
Lymphocytes ($\times 10^9$/L)	3.4 (0.6–10.5)	—	—	—	—	—	—	—	—
Monocytes (%)	2.0 (0.0–6.5)	1.0–6.3	0.7–4.7	1–8	0–9	0–9	2–8	3.4–6.8	1.7–6.3
Monocytes ($\times 10^9$/L)	0.2 (0.0–0.5)	—	—	—	—	—	—	—	—
Eosinophil granulocytes (%)	2.0 (0.0–5.7)	0.0–8.5	2.1–6.9	0–9	0.0–8.5	0–7	0–5	0–7	1–9
Eosinophil granulocytes ($\times 10^9$/L)	0.1 (0.0–0.7)	—	—	—	—	—	—	—	—
Basophile granulocytes (%)	0.0 (0.0–1.4)	0–3	0.0–1.3	0.0–2.9	0.0–2.7	0–2	0–1	0.0–2.7	0.0–2.9
Basophile granulocytes ($\times 10^9$/L)	0.0 (0.0–0.2)	—	—	—	—	—	—	—	—
Platelets ($\times 10^9$/L)	807 (171.7–1280.6)	297–730	310–910	264–910	297–730	297–730	310–910	—	—
Reticulocytes (%)	—	—	—	2–14	1–12	1–12	2–14	—	—

Table 4
Summary of articles found through the literature review regarding normal biochemistry of ferrets

Article Type	Number of Articles
Repeated cross-sectional study	2[14,16]
Prospective descriptive observational study	2[17,18]
Narrative review	3
No access	1

no reference for normal thoracic radiograph in ferrets, with the exception of one conference proceeding that mentioned the existence of pleural lines in chest radiographs of healthy ferrets.[37]

One study found relevant anatomic variation of the vertebral column in ferrets.[38] In a group of 172 ferrets, about 2% of the ferrets had 15 thoracic vertebrae, 7% had 7 lumbar vertebrae, and 22% had 4 sacral vertebrae.

Ultrasound

Abdominal ultrasound

Ultrasonography has been used in ferrets for various diagnostic purposes, including adrenal gland visualization and measurement. Reference values for the size of specific anatomic structures are limited. Lymph nodes had a similar abdominal topography than the one expected in dogs and cats.[39] Healthy adrenal glands have been evaluated in 3 articles.[40–42] Only one of the articles assessed the health status of the adrenal glands with histopathology.[41] A sex-dependent size variation in adrenal glands has been reported, with adrenal glands being wider in males in 2 out of 3 studies **(Table 9)**.[40,41]

Echocardiography

Cardiac ultrasound has been extensively described in ferrets. Many variations among the studies were found either in the design (retrospective, prospective) or in the handling protocol (manual vs chemical restraint).[2–4,36] In only one study ferrets were evaluated without sedation.[2] Values in different studies were clinically comparable, although sedation was found to decrease fractional shortening in a similar way than in dogs **(Table 10)**.[43]

SPECIFIC DISEASES
Adrenal Gland Disease

Cause

Adrenal gland disease or adrenocortical disease (ACD) has been extensively studied in ferrets. The association between gonadectomy and adrenocortical neoplasm was first supported by a combined retrospective case series and owner survey published in the year 2000.[44] This finding was supported by further studies in ferrets demonstrating the key role of luteinizing hormone (LH) receptors in the pathogenesis of adrenal gland disease.[45] Most articles have focused on the role and effect of gonadectomy ever since.[46–50] The mechanism was investigated in 3 prospective descriptive cross-sectional studies.[44,45,49] Although classified with a very low level of evidence, this research is the only data found in the authors' search on the cause of ACD; responses to treatment (see later discussion) tend to confirm gonadectomy as a main cause.

The hypothalamus of the ferret secretes gonadotropin-releasing hormones (GnRHs), which stimulates the pituitary gland to secrete LH. Ferrets, as seen in

Table 5
Biochemical reference value

	Hein et al,[17] 2012	Lee et al,[16] 1982			Carpenter,[20] 2013	
Study design	Prospective descriptive observational study	Prospective descriptive observational study			Narrative review	
Blood sampling method	Vena saphena lateralis	Vena jugularis or cardiac puncture under ketamine anesthesia			—	—
Material	Serum	—				
Population	111 × Clinically healthy ferrets	5 × 4–8 mo Intact female	3 × 4–8 mo Intact male	5 × 4–8 mo Castrated males	Female	Male
Alanine aminotransferase (UI/L)	110.0 (49.0–242.8)	150.3 ± 49.3	157.6 ± 79.9	201.3 ± 142.0	54–280	54–289
Aspartate aspartate transaminase (UI/L)	74.0 (40.1–142.7)	—	—	—	40–120	28–248
Alkaline phosphatase (UI/L)	34.0 (13.3–141.6)	44.3 ± 11.3	52.4 ± 10.6	63.3 ± 29.2	3–62	11–120
Glutamate dehydrogenase (UI/L)	1.0 (0.0–2.5)	—	—	—	—	—
Gamma-glutamyl transpeptidase (UI/L)	4.0 (0.2–14.0)	—	—	—	0–5	0–5
Lactate dehydrogenase (UI/L)	325.0 (154.4–1780.6)	—	—	—	—	241–752
SDH (mU/mL)	—	2.6 ± 2.2	5.4 ± 4.5	3.3 ± 3.3	—	—
Creatinine kinase (UI/L)	203 (94.0–730.9)	—	—	—	—	—
Alpha-amylase (UI/L)	38.0 (19.4–61.9)	—	—	—	—	—
Lipase (UI/L)	204.0 (73.2–351.1)	—	—	—	—	0–200

(continued on next page)

Table 5
(continued)

	Hein et al[17] 2012		Lee et al[16] 1982		Carpenter[20] 2013	
Cholinesterase (UI/L)	526.0 (262.1–1017.5)	—	—	—	—	—
Glucose (mmol/L)	6.0 (3.0–8.5)	104.9 ± 16.4 mg/dL	104.0 ± 15.0 mg/dL	95.4 ± 17.0 mg/dL	85–207 mg/dL	62.5–198.0 mg/dL
Fructosamine (µmol/L)	163.0 (121.1–201.6)	—	—	—	—	—
Total protein (g/L)	67.8 (54.7–77.9)	60 ± 5	59 ± 3	58 ± 3	51–72	53–74
Globulin (g/L)	—	—	—	—	22–32	20–40
Albumin (g/L)	36.1 (28.0–43.9)	38 ± 2	37 ± 1	37 ± 2	32–41	28–42
Cholesterol (mmol/L)	4.9 (2.4–7.1)	—	—	—	122–296 mg/dL	64–221 mg/dL
Triglycerides (mmol/L)	1.0 (0.5–2.8)	—	—	—	—	—
Serum bile acids (µmol/L)	5.7 (0.0–28.9)	—	—	—	—	—
Bilirubin (µmol/L)	1.1 (0.0–3.3)	—	—	—	0–1 mg/dL	0.0–0.1 mg/dL
Urea (mmol/L)	9.8 (4.8–16.9)	BUN: 33.3 ± 7.6 mg/dL	BUN: 22.0 ± 6.3 mg/dL	BUN: 28.1 ± 7.6 mg/dL	BUN: 10–45 mg/dL	BUN: 11–42 mg/dL
Creatinine (µmol/L)	44.0 (23.0–76.7)	0.4 ± 0.1 mg/dL	0.4 ± 0.1 mg/dL	0.3 ± 0.0 mg/dL	0.2–1.0 mg/dL	0.2–1.0 mg/dL
Calcium (mmol/L)	2.3 (2.0–2.6)	9.0 ± 0.3 mg/dL	9.5 ± 0.6 mg/dL	9.3 ± 0.5 mg/dL	8.0–10.2 mg/dL	3.8–11.8 mg/dL
Phosphorus (mmol/L)	1.8 (1.0–3.1)	6.7 ± 0.6 mg/dL	6.7 ± 1.2 mg/dL	6.1 ± 0.6 mg/dL	4.2–10.1 mg/dL	4.0–8.7 mg/dL
Magnesium (mmol/L)	1.2 (0.9–1.6)	—	—	—	—	—
Sodium (mmol/L)	154.0 (140.1–169.7)	150.4 ± 1.5	154.4 ± 3.6	150.6 ± 3.3	142–156 mEq/L	137–162 mEq/L
Potassium (mmol/L)	5.0 (3.9–5.9)	4.9 ± 0.3	4.9 ± 0.2	4.9 ± 0.2	—	—
Chloride (mmol/L)	114.0 (108.9–119.9)	117.1 ± 1.9	112.5 ± 9.1	117.3 ± 2.2	112–124 mEq/L	102–126 mEq/L
Carbon dioxide	—	22.1 ± 3.1	23.4 ± 3.4	18.5 ± 3.2	16.5–27.8 mEq/L	12.2–28.0 mEq/L
Iron (µmol/L)	33.8 (11.7–56.3)	—	—	—	—	—
Thyroxine (nmol/L)	27.0 (15.9–42.0)	—	—	—	—	—
Cortisol (nmol/L)	6.6 (0.0–101.5)	—	—	—	—	—
Estradiol (pg/mL)	5.0 (0.0–12.2)	—	—	—	—	—
Progesterone (ng/mL)	0.0 (0.0–0.4)	—	—	—	—	—

Abbreviations: BUN, serum urea nitrogen; SDH, sorbitol dehydrogenase.

Table 6
Summary of urinalysis

	Male		Female	
Urine specific gravity	1.051 ± 0.009	1.034–1.070	1.042 ± 0.008	1.026 ± 1.060
pH	6.0 ± 0.3	5.0–6.5	6.1 ± 0.5	5.0–7.5
Protein	Frequency 22	Percent 92	Frequency 33	Percent 73
Blood	Frequency 11	Percent 46	Frequency 17	Percent 38
Bilirubin	Frequency 3	Percent 13	Frequency 8	Percent 18

Adapted from Eshar D, Wyre NR, Brown DC. Urine specific gravity values in clinically healthy young pet ferrets (Mustela furo). J Small Anim Pract 2012;53(2):117; with permission.

mice, express LH receptors in the zona reticularis of the adrenal cortex resulting in a secretion of sex hormones.[51] The most accepted mechanism is the lack of gonadal expression resulting in a lack of negative feedback causing a continuous release of GnRH and activation of adrenal LH receptors, which in turn induce tumorigenesis. This mechanism is reported independent from the age of neutering.[44]

The role of photoperiod and melatonin has been speculated as well as the genetic influence.[47] Neutered female ferrets exposed to prolonged photoperiod were not sensitive to estradiol implantation and produced an increase of LH, which may contribute to the disease.[52] Although expected, this effect was not investigated on the pathogenesis of adrenal neoplasia in ferrets. Genetic effect is well demonstrated in mice but has not been investigated in ferrets, and different oncogenic pathways are suspected.[50,53] This concept was originally strongly suspected because of the variation of incidence of adrenal neoplasia among the various ferret populations (European vs American ferret).[54]

Table 7
Summary of clinical pathology findings in the cerebrospinal fluid of healthy ferrets

Variables	All Samples
RBCs (cells per μL)	
Mean ± SD	1.041 ± 2.568
Range	0.0–11.560
95% CI	264.45–1.81785
WBCs (cells per μL)	
Mean ± SD	1.6 ± 1.8
Range	0–8
95% CI	1.05–2.14
Protein (mg/dL)	
Mean ± SD	31.4 ± 10.6
Range	20–68
95% CI	28.8–34.0

Abbreviations: CI, confidence interval; RBCs, red blood cells; WBCs, white blood cells.
Adapted from Platt SR, Dennis PM, McSherry LJ, et al. Composition of cerebrospinal fluid in clinically normal adult ferrets. Am J Vet Res 2004;65(6):759; with permission.

Table 8
Selected ferret ophthalmic data found through the literature review

IOP (rebound method)	14.07 ± 0.35 mm Hg
IOP (applanation method)	14.5 ± 3.27 mm Hg
Schirmer tear test (STT)	5.31 ± 1.32 mm/min
Central corneal thickness	0.337 ± 0.020 mm

Epidemiology

Many studies indicate that adrenal neoplasia is one of the most common tumors found in ferrets, with variable prevalence among countries. In the United States, one retrospective study over 30 years allowed a calculation of prevalence of about 2.2%.[55] In Japan, according to the data covered in one article over 5 years, the estimated prevalence was around 1.1%.[56] In the Netherlands, prevalence was reported to be 0.55% in the year 2000.[44] Some retrospective studies selected neoplasia as their inclusion criteria without mention of the global population studied, precluding population prevalence calculation. Most published articles were based on questionnaires, and results may have been biased by the collecting method. It should also be emphasized that adrenal gland disease is not reduced to neoplastic disease only.

Considering neoplastic disease in ferrets, adrenal gland neoplasia is definitely one of the most commonly mentioned in various studies varying from 16.7% to 36.6% of the neoplasia recorded in this species.[55–57] Schoemaker and colleagues[44] demonstrated that a linear correlation between age at neutering and age at time of diagnosis existed in a population of 50 ferrets. According to most studies, ferrets were affected between 3 and 6 years of age without sex predisposition, with the youngest specimen affected at 1 year of age.[44,55–57]

Proportions of adenoma and adenocarcinoma were variable among the studies found. Two main categories of articles were found: surgical case series and neoplastic disease survey. Surveys may have been biased by the lack of inclusion of hyperplasia, which is part of the ACD. In a recent Italian survey, 92% of the adrenal tumors were cortical carcinoma, which is higher than other sources reporting 18% to 30%.[55,57,58] From a clinical perspective, surgical case series give a better overview of the type of tumor found in practice. Carcinomas are found inconstantly from 10% to 40% of adrenal removed.[59,60] Leiomyomas and pheochromocytomas are found regularly but are rare compared with cortical tumors, except in one retrospective study

Table 9
Summary of ferret adrenal measurements found in the literature review

Article Named by First Author			Mean Measurement Left Adrenal (mm)	Mean Measurement Right Adrenal (mm)
Neuwirth et al,[41] 1997	Female	Length	7.5 + 1.2	7.4 + 1.0
		Width	3.7 + 0.6	3.7 + 0.4
	Male	Length	8.6 + 1.2	8.9 + 2.6
		Width	4.2 + 0.6	3.8 + 0.6
Kuijten et al,[42] 2007	Length		6.1 + 1.0	7.8 + 1.4
	Width		2.9 + 0.5	2.5 + 0.6
O'brien et al,[40] 1996	Length		7.2 ± 1.8	7.6 ± 1.8
	Width		2.8 ± 0.5	2.6 ± 0.4

Table 10
Selected ferret echocardiographic value found in the literature review

Article Named by First Author	Number of Ferrets	Sedation Protocol	LA (mm)	LVIDd (mm)	LVIDs (mm)	LVWd (mm)	Ao (mm)	FS (%)	IVSd (mm)
Dudas-Gyorki et al,[2] 2011	Male 19	None	10.0	13.0 + 1.2	8.9 + 1.2	3.3 + 0.3	5.5 + 0.6	32 + 7	3.1 + 0.3
	Female 27		8.9	10.4 + 1.6	7.1 + 1.5	2.8 + 0.4	4.6 + 0.4	34 + 6	2.6
Vastenburg et al,[3] 2004	Male 11	Isoflurane	6.0 + 1.3	9.7 + 1.6	7.0 + 1.4	2.6 + 0.5	4.5 + 0.7	27.6 + 7.9	3.3 + 0.4
	Female 18		5.7 + 0.7	9.9 + 1.3	6.9 + 1.2	2.8 + 0.5	4.3 + 0.5	30.6 + 7.9	3.4 + 0.5
Stepien et al,[4] 2000	30	Ketamine midazolam	7.1 + 1.8	8.8 + 1.5	5.9 + 1.5	4.2 + 1.1	5.3 + 1.0	33 + 14	3.6 + 0.7

Abbreviations: Ao, aortic diameter (short-axis view; end, systole); FS, fractional shortening; IVSd, interventricular septum in diastole; LA, left atrial diameter (left ventricular axis view); LVIDd, left ventricular diameter in diastole; LVIDs, left ventricular diameter in systole; LVWd, left ventricular wall thickness in diastole.

mentioning 44.7% of pheochromocytomas, which differs significantly from all other studies (**Table 11**).[61]

Diagnosis

Diagnosis of adrenal gland disease usually relies on a combination of diagnostic imaging, hormonal panel, and histology.

Ultrasonography

Ultrasonography has been extensively used because it is cost-effective and permits visualization of both adrenal glands. Adrenal ultrasonography has been described in 6 articles and correlation with ACD lesions in 4 articles.[41,42,63,64] One source suggests that shape alteration (deformation or rounder shape) is the most consistent sign to allow detection of abnormal adrenal gland.[42] Other signs may include heterogeneous structure and increased echogenicity.[42] However, the structure of normal and hyperplastic adrenal glands may not differ; adenomas cannot be differentiated from carcinomas based on ultrasonographic examination.[41,63] One surgical case series mentions that in 18 ferrets examined by ultrasound, 7 examinations were accurate, 6 abnormal adrenal glands were incorrectly diagnosed on the opposite side, and 5 adrenal glands were normal on ultrasound examination but were in fact abnormal surgically and histologically.[60]

Hormones

Use of a hormonal panel has been investigated in 3 articles.[65–67] In one article evaluating the level of various hormones, at least one among 17-hydroxy-progesterone, androstenedione, and estradiol was elevated in 96% of ferrets with ACD, suggesting that all 3 hormones should be tested for screening purposes. In other publications, 36% to 88% of the ferrets having ACD had elevated estradiol.[59,66] Proper diagnostic accuracy studies are lacking.

Use of the urinary corticoid/creatinine ratio (UCCR) was advocated because most ferrets with ACD in the cohort demonstrated a high UCCR.[68] However, the results of the study may have been biased because ferrets with ACD were compared with normal ferrets instead of with ferrets with other diseases. Dexamethasone injection was used to lower the UCCR, which seems insensitive in ferrets with ACD.

Cytologic examination of preputial epithelial cells can be used for detection of ACD because of the correlation of cornification and level of 17-hydroxy-progesterone.[69]

Treatment

Surgical treatment Historically, surgical excision of affected glands has been the standard treatment of ACD (**Table 12**). Surgical excision was also the only way to confirm the histologic nature of the adrenal lesion premortem. Seven case series were interested in the surgical removal of the affected glands.[60,62,70–73] Comparison between studies are extremely difficult because several factors varied between articles, including the surgical techniques (**Table 13**).

Regarding perioperative mortality, risk was reported from 2.0% to 5.5% depending on the series.

Long-term survival was good in all the studies, with 73.9% of ferrets surviving at least more than 6 months to 98% more than 1 year.[60,61,71] One study evaluated the effect of the technique (complete or partial removal) and the histologic nature on survival.[61] They found that the histologic nature of the lesion did not influence the survival rate, and that the use of cryosurgery was associated to poorer clinical outcomes.[60] However, this may be because more severe cases were treated with cryosurgery. Bilateral adrenalectomy was not associated with major complications (1%–5% of

Table 11
Summary and repartition of adrenocortical neoplasia found through the literature search

Article Named by First Author	Hyperplasia	Adenoma	Carcinoma	Pheochromocytoma	Nonspecified	Other
Weiss & Scott,[62] 1997	56% (61)	16% (18)	26% (29)	—	—	1 Normal
Rosenthal et al,[59] 1993	26% (13)	64% (32)	10% (5)	—	—	No metastasis
Miwa et al,[56] 2009	20% (41)	20% (41)	42% (87)	2	34	2 Leiomyoma
Jung et al,[61] 2014	12.8% (6)	14.9% (7)	2% (1)	21	—	5 Adrenalitis 1 Lymphoma 3 Adrenal hemorrhage 1 Adrenal infarction
Swiderski et al,[60] 2008	11% (15)	38% (50)	40% (53)	5	—	2 Cyst/1 vacuolation/1 teratoma 2 Leiomyoma 1 Fibro
Williams,[58] 2003	53% (439)	15% (129)	30% (251)	—	—	5 Leiomyoma
Avallone et al,[57] 2016	—	19% (61)	74% (228)	11	—	2 Neuroblastoma 3 Spindle cell 2 Leiomyosarcoma 1 Malignant not otherwise specified
Li et al,[55] 1998	—	30% (34)	18% (20)	4	53	1 Myelolipoma

Table 12
Summary of articles found through the literature review regarding surgical treatment of adrenocortical disease

Article Type	Number of Articles	Moderate	Low	Very Low
Retrospective cohort study	1[70,71]	2	8	5
Case series	3[60,61,72,73]			
Retrospective descriptive cross	1[62]			
Narrative review	8			
No access	1	—	—	—

the ferrets required mineralocorticoid or glucocorticoid supplementation).[72] The clinician should aim at removing all the affected adrenal gland whenever possible. When the size of the mass does not allow complete removal, debulking may be a palliative option. Ligation of the vena cava in order to excise the right adrenal gland may be

Table 13
Summary of findings and outcome of ferrets affected by adrenocortical disease classified by surgical treatment modalities through the literature search

Article Named by First Author	Number of Ferrets	Perioperative Mortality	Recurrence	Long-Term Survival
Miwa & Sasaki,[71] 2011	37 Cases 14 Cases surgery + medical 23 Cases surgery alone	1 (2%)	30.4% Recurrence Mean 7 mo (1–18 mo)	Surgical 73.9% >6 mo Surgical + medical 92.9% >6 mo
Weiss & Scott,[62] 1997	94 Cases 79 Unilateral 15 Bilateral	4 (4%)	— 2 of 79 Animals did not respond with unilateral adrenalectomy 17% Recurrence Mean 6 mo (3–14 mo) —	Not mentioned
Weiss et al,[72] 1999	56	1 (2%)	15% Recurrence	Not mentioned 3 of 56 Had hypocorticism
Swiderski et al,[60] 2008	130 78 Unilateral 10 Bilateral 17 Unilateral partial 16 Bilateral partial	Not mentioned	Not mentioned	4 of 28 Bilateral had hypoadrenocorticism 98% Survival at 1 y 88% Survival rate at 2 y 70% Survival rate at 5 y
Lennox & Wagner,[70] 2012	28	3 of 54 (5.5%)	Mean 13.6 (0–38 mo) 3 of 51 Animals did not respond to surgery	Not mentioned
Jung et al,[61] 2014	48	Not mentioned	Not mentioned	87.5% Survival at 1 y 74% Survival at 2 y

attempted. Collateral circulation seems to develop when the caudal vena cava is ligated.[74]

Resolution of signs was not systematically recorded, and effect of surgery was variable. In theory, surgery should achieve a definite cure of the disease. However, on the 4 articles that looked over recurrence, 17% to 30% of the ferrets recurred after surgical treatment (unilateral or bilateral adrenalectomy) and some ferrets did not respond to treatment.[71,72] Bilateral adrenalectomy also had a mild degree of recurrence (15%) comparable with other studies.[72] Median recurrence time was 6 to 7 month depending on the studies.[56,62]

In the study of Lennox and Wagner, all ferrets treated with surgery seemed to present recurrence.[70] The discrepancy between this study and others might be potentially explained by the very long follow-up of some cases: in some animals neoplasia relapsed 38 month after surgery. The lack of randomization strongly limits the interpretation of the findings.

Medical treatment Medical management was experimented with various drugs, especially GnRH agonist because they seemed to be the most effective in controlling the disease (**Table 14**). Four research articles have focused on medical management of ACD with 100 μg leuprolide acetate, 3 mg deslorelin acetate implant, and 4.7 mg deslorelin acetate implant.[75,77,78] The effect is systematic, but recurrence of clinical signs seems inevitable in all case series. Unfortunately, survival rates were not calculated in those articles. The survival time of ferrets treated with GnRH implants is expected to be at least 1 to 2 years because median time at recurrence extends from 13.7 to 17.5 months.[75,77]

Two research articles with a moderate level of evidence compared surgical and medical treatment.[70,72] Time to recurrence of clinical signs was longer with the use of a GnRH implant compared with the surgical group; 3 ferrets did not respond to surgery, whereas all ferrets responded to implants.[70] In the other study, the recurrence rate with leuprolide acetate treatment was similar to surgical treatment only (31.6% vs 30.4% respectively); but time to recurrence was shorter with the use of leuprolide than with surgery (median 3.8 vs 7.0 months respectively).

Another article mentioned a lower 6 months' survival rate for ferrets treated with surgery alone (73.9%) compared with ferrets treated with leuprolide acetate with (92.9%) and without surgery (100%) (**Table 15**).[71]

The melatonin implant effect was investigated in one trial supplementing ferrets with oral melatonin.[80] Clinical improvement was seen in most ferrets; but recurrence was seen in 6 out of 10 ferrets, and the treatment did not prevent adrenal glands from growing.[80] Melatonin implants were used in a case series involving 70 ferrets with clinical signs of ACD. All but one ferret had a clinical response.[79]

Table 14
Summary of articles found through the literature review regarding medical treatment of adrenocortical disease in ferrets

Article Type	Number of Articles	Moderate	Low	Very Low
Retrospective cohort study	1[70]	2	8	4
Before and after trial	2[75,76]			
Case series	3[77–79]			
Uncontrolled trial	1[80]			
Narrative review	8			
No access	2	—		

Table 15
Summary of findings and outcome of ferrets affected by adrenocortical disease classified by medical treatment modalities through the literature search

Treatment Type	Number of Individuals Tested	Median Time to Recurrence (mo)	Comments
Ferrets treated with leuprolide acetate injections[78]	20	3.7 ± 0.4 (1.5–8.0)	—
Ferrets treated with leuprolide acetate injections[71]	18	3.8 (1.5–20.0)	—
Ferrets treated with 3 mg deslorelin implant[77]	15	13.7 ± 3.5 (8.5–20.5)	—
Ferrets treated with 4.7 mg deslorelin implant[75]	30	17.5 ± 5.0 (8–30)	5 Ferrets died before recurrence
Ferrets treated with 4.7 mg deslorelin implant[70]	35	16.5 (3–30)	—

Use of a GnRH vaccine is mentioned in one article with a low level of evidence.[76] A trial for treatment against ACD showed a response in 5 of 9 ferrets and incomplete response in 4 of 9 ferrets. A trial for prevention showed a preventive effect of the vaccine, with 84% of untreated ferrets developing ACD versus 24% of vaccinated ferrets. It is noteworthy to stress that some ferrets still developed ACD.

Numerous treatments are reported in textbook and reviews, such as mitotane, trilostane, and ketoconazole; but none were evaluated in clinical or experimental research.

Based on this literature review, surgical management and medical management are difficult to compare because of the lack of comparative data on efficacy and long-term survival.

There are both clinical and research evidence that GnRH analogues have an effect on ACD, but there are limited data on median survival time with this treatment. Future research should test higher doses (eg, 9.4-mg implants). There is very strong evidence that GnRH analogues are suitable alternatives to surgical castration, but a preventive effect similar to the GnRH vaccine remains to be documented.[81,82] Medical treatment seems to provide a better clinical improvement and a longer time to recurrence than surgery.

Surgical management may eventually be curative for neoplastic cases. In a minority of ferrets, surgical treatment may lead to perioperative mortality, may result in no clinical improvement, or may result in ACD recurrence (even with bilateral adrenalectomy). Further studies should focus on the efficiency and evaluate whether the surgical technique used would have an influence on the alleviating the symptoms. Ultimately, a combined approach (surgery and implant) needs to be further studied.

Insulinoma

Cause
Insulinoma is a pancreatic islet β-cell tumor causing hypoglycemic syndrome in ferrets. Ferrets also exhibit other pancreatic neoplasia, such as pancreatic adenoma or adenocarcinoma. One theory on development of insulinoma is focused on the

type of diet offered, especially a kibble diet, which is higher in carbohydrates than natural prey.[83] One other support of this theory is the fact that black-footed ferrets (*Mustela nigripes*) do not present endocrine tumors such as seen in their domestic counterparts.[84] No peer-reviewed articles were found to corroborate this theory. Another theory includes a genetic component because of the prevalence difference between European and North American ferrets.[83] In an Italian survey, insulinoma accounted for 23.4% of the cases of neoplasia, which is comparable with the prevalence described in North American ferrets.[57]

Epidemiology

Insulinoma is recorded as the most common neoplasm in ferrets, ranging from 21.7% to 25.0% of all neoplasias found in this species.[55,56,58] It typically affects ferrets from 2 to 7 years old with a median age of 5 years.[85–87] It was reported to affect kittens as young as 2 weeks old.[55] Three distinct case series reported that males were more commonly affected than females.[85–87]

Lesions of the pancreatic islets are classified as hyperplasia, adenoma, and adenocarcinoma. One case series did not characterize the nature of the tumors. Another reported 59% of carcinoma, 38% had a combination of carcinoma and adenoma, and 1.7% adenomas.[86] The third report found 55% adenomas and 45% carcinomas.[87] A retrospective series focusing specifically on immunotyping pancreatic tumors showed most islet cell tumors expressing insulin and a vast minority expressing glucagon, somatostatin, and polypetide.[88]

Localization of the lesions varies depending on the study. The left lobe was the most commonly affected (34%–54% of the lesion), and the body of the pancreas was less commonly involved (3%–14%).[85,86] Disseminated lesions were common, with one study reporting 53% of ferrets presenting multiple lesions.[86]

Diagnosis

Diagnosis usually relies on hypoglycemic episode (<60 mg/dL) and ultrasonographic findings. The Whipple triad also provides clinical insights: low fasting glucose concentration, neurologic disturbance associated with hypoglycemia, and relief of neurologic disturbances with administration of glucose.

Three different case series of ferrets suffering from insulinoma were described. All cases of insulinoma had a fasting blood glucose concentration less than 70 mg/dL.[86,87] As previously noted, care must be taken before interpreting blood glucose obtained from a handheld point of care analyzer.

Insulinemia seems variable; hyperinsulinemia was documented in 83% of the ferrets affected with insulinoma in one series and in all ferrets in other case series.[86,89] Normal values of insulin have been published (4.6–43.3 µU/mL).[90]

Low insulin levels associated with hypoglycemia have been suggested as a method to exclude insulinoma, but no data were published to support that hypothesis. Serial blood glucose values have been recommended for diagnosis of insulinoma as well as fasting.[83,91] No documented research has demonstrated the added diagnostic value of this procedure over the Whipple triad.

The use of ultrasound for the diagnosis of pancreatic neoplasia in ferrets is underreported in the scientific literature.[83] One case series identified nodular lesion in 5 of 23 ferrets (21.7%). Exploratory laparotomy was the most common way described to confirm insulinoma through surgical biopsies or resection.

Treatment and prognosis

The authors found no research series focusing on medical management of insulinoma (apart from chemotherapy) (**Table 16**). All the published case series focused on

Table 16
Summary of articles found through the literature review regarding treatment of insulinoma in ferrets

Article Type	Number of Articles	Moderate	Low	Very Low
Retrospective cohort study	1[85]	1	7	8
Case series	4[86,87,89,92]			
Case report	4			
Narrative review	7			
No access	—		—	

surgical management, and the number of ferrets treated medically was low compared with the number of ferrets treated surgically. This bias is probably explained by the diagnostic method, which in essence relies on surgical removal and histologic examination (**Table 17**).

Several articles graded as very low evidence showed that surgical management achieved a reasonably good survival time (456–668 days) and a return to normal glycemia in the immediate postoperative period in most ferrets.[85] Hypoglycemic episodes

Table 17
Summary of findings and outcome of ferrets affected by insulinoma classified by treatment modalities through the literature search

Article Named by First Author	Treatment	Number of Ferrets	Mean Disease-Free Intervals	Survival Days (mo)	
Caplan et al,[86] 1996	Ferrets treated medically	3	Euthanasia 6.0–8.9 mo after surgery	—	
	Ferrets treated surgically	50	50% Remained hypoglycemic after surgery	532 (17.5)	517 (17)
			32% Recurrence (1.0–23.5 mo, median 10.6 mo)	487 (16)	
			16% Euglycemic 1 Persistent hyperglycemia	313 (10.3)	
	Ferrets nontreated	4	Euthanasia	—	
Weiss et al,[85] 1998	Ferrets treated medically	10	22 d (0–62)	186	
	Ferrets treated surgically with nodulectomy	27	234 d (0–546) 15% Remained hypoglycemic	456	
	Ferrets treated surgically with nodulectomy and pancreatectomy	29	365 d (0–690) 3.4% Remained hypoglycemic after surgery 3.4% Euglycemic	668	
Ehrart et al,[87] 1996	Ferrets treated medically	3	1 Necropsied 1 Euthanized after 9 d 1 Survived 504 d	—	
	Ferrets treated surgically	17	284 d (0–545)	563 (1–1100)	

reoccurred after surgery in 86% to 100% of the cases depending on the series.[85,86] More aggressive surgery tended to have a longer survival time as seen in the retrospective study by Weiss[85]; however, there was no evaluation of the association between the type of surgery and survival time in other studies. Apart from the minority of ferrets who remained euglycemic, all ferrets were also treated medically after surgery when clinical signs reoccurred. Therefore, the management is mainly based on a combination of medical and surgical treatment; survival times were calculated with this bias.

Textbooks and reviews have suggested medical management based on a small animal recommendation. This type of treatment alone in insulinoma remains to be evaluated in ferrets, especially considering treatment type (dietary management, type of steroid, diazoxide). One isolated case report refers to the use of glucagon continuous rate infusion for the management of hypoglycemic crisis.[93]

Chemotherapy is rarely reported, but a case series of 12 ferrets described the use of doxorubicin in cases of suspected insulinoma.[92] Eight ferrets improved with the doxorubicin injection and eventually became euglycemic at some point in the treatment. Three ferrets died during the study, one with dilated cardiomyopathy potentially related with chemotherapy, one from gastric ulceration, and one from lymphoma. No statistical analysis and no long-term follow-up were reported in this case series making conclusions uncertain. However, some clinical improvement was seen; therefore, this treatment deserves further scientific evaluation.

Lymphoma

Cause

Lymphoma is common in ferrets, being the third most common neoplasm in this species.[58] Characterization of lymphoma is constantly evolving in human and veterinary medicine. A proposal for standardized classification has been suggested by Mayer and Burgess.[94] The diversity of clinical presentation is reflected by the number of case reports found in the literature (19). Lymphomas affecting osseous, ocular, mediastinal, and visceral structures have been described.

Although spontaneous cases may occur, an infectious cause has been suggested and investigated in 3 articles. One article had a moderate level of evidence with a case-control study.[95] Cluster of lymphoma was demonstrated suggesting a viral origin, but feline leukemia virus and Aleutian disease virus were not isolated.[95] One other case series had similar findings.[96] Further research with a high level of evidence using a controlled trial demonstrated a horizontal transmission using fresh donor lymphoma cells and showed retroviral-like particles in affected ferrets.[97] Another infectious cause was mentioned in a case series of 4 ferrets suggesting a relationship between gastric mucosal associated lymphoid tissue lymphoma and helicobacter infection.[98] Those data were not further developed in more recent literature.

A genetic influence may play a role on oncogenesis in this species. In 2012, a novel endogenous lentivirus (ELVmpf) has been isolated.[99] Endogenous retrovirus is part of the ferret genome and may play a role in the pathogenesis of tumors, but there are no reports to date of the role of ELVmpf in the pathogenesis of lymphoma or other neoplasia in ferrets.[100]

Epidemiology

Lymphoma can occur at any age. Two retrospective case series mentioned 2 forms of the disease: one with a young lymphoblastic form (less than 1 year old) and one affecting older individuals (3 years old or older) with a slow progressing disease.[101,102] This age trend was not demonstrated by further case series.[57,103–105] In one series of cases, 2 ferrets less than 1 year of age were affected; both died within 1 day after diagnosis.[103] In a further series of cases, one ferret less than 1 year of age was affected, but the type of lymphoma and clinical outcome was not described.[104]

Immunohistochemistry (IHC) was used to classify the cell type involved in 4 different articles.[103,104,106,107] Monoclonal antihuman CD3 and CD79 alpha antibodies were used systematically. Other markers were searched occasionally.[104,107] Lymphoma of T-cell origin was most common in all reports, accounting for 80% to 90% of the cases.[103,104,106] The localization is differently recorded among the different surveys making comparison difficult. Cutaneous lymphoma was rarely reported (5%–7% of the case depending on the studies).[103,104] Gastrointestinal, multicentric, and to a lesser extent the mediastinal form seemed common.[57,58,103,106] One study using a different staging scheme suggested that more than half of the lymphomas were generalized to at least thoracic and abdominal cavities.[104]

Diagnosis
Currently, the reference standard for the diagnosis of lymphoma is achieved with a biopsy of the affected tissue. Fine-needle aspirate has been advocated for diagnostic purposes, but the accuracy of the technique has not been evaluated.[108] The diagnostic value of fine-needle aspirates has been reported in 4 cases with mesenteric node, liver, splenic, spinal, and/or cutaneous localization.[109–112] Concordance and comparative diagnostic value of cytology versus biopsy evidence is lacking.

Use of complete blood cell count is usually advocated either for diagnostic purposes or for staging. Leukemia was reported inconstantly and represented 2 of 27 (7.4%) cases in one of the series.[104] Reactive lymphocytosis is mentioned in one case series, up to 32% of ferrets affected with more young ferrets affected.[102]

Biochemistry is usually used for assessment and searching for paraneoplastic syndromes, such as hypercalcemia. This finding is reported in 2 of 28 (7.1%) and 3 of 41 (7.3%) cases in each study.[102,104]

Thoracic radiograph may help in identifying lesions, mainly mediastinal (20 of 60 cases) or thoracic (51% of the cases).[102,104] In one case series focusing on diagnostic imaging, pleural effusion was one of the reported findings (4 of 12).[105] Another interest of the radiograph would be to localize skeletal lesions. One case series reported bone lesions in 2 of 14 ferrets,[105] and 4 case reports showed bone involvement.[113–116]

Ultrasonography may help in identifying affected viscera. The enlargement of mesenteric lymph nodes was the most common ultrasonographic finding (40%–85%) as well as the enlargement of the spleen (57%–70%).[37,57,58,102]

Treatment and prognosis
Recommendations for the treatment of lymphoma in veterinary medicine follow the World Health Organization (WHO) Revised European American Lymphoma (REAL) classification scheme published in 2001, updated in 2008 and revised in 2016 (**Table 18**).[122] This system relies on several criteria. Since the emergence of IHC,

Table 18
Summary of articles found through the literature review regarding treatment of lymphoma in ferrets

Article Type	Number of Articles	Low	Very Low
Case series	3[101,102,104]	10	15
Descriptive observational	1[103]		
Case report	11[110–114,116–121]		
Narrative review	10		
No access	—	—	

Table 19
Summary of findings and outcome of ferrets affected by lymphoma classified by cell type through the literature search

Article Named by First Author	Type	Number of Ferrets	Median Survival Time (mo)
Ammersbach et al,[104] 2008	T small cell	12	5.6 (0.5–14.0)
	T large cell	2	1
	B cell	3	12.3 (7–19)
	Hodgkin	2	2.5 (2–3)
Onuma et al,[103] 2008	T small cell 1, 2, 5, 9, 10, 11, 16	7	1.56 (46.8 d [1–180])
	T large cell 7, 8, 12, 13	4	3.5 (105.25 d [10–210])
	B cell 4, 10	2	1.36 (41 d)
Erdman et al,[102] 1996	Immunoblastic large cell	19	6
	Diffuse small lymphocytic	8	8

characterization of the immunophenotype is the reference method to classify the disease. Other methods include tissue extension (single anatomic lesion, regional involvement, both sides of the diaphragm, and leukemic stage) and cytologic feature (nuclear size, nucleoli, shape, and mitotic activity).

Four case series reported the survival time associated with lymphoma classification. Two case reports were published before the WHO-REAL recommendations. The two remaining articles focused on histologic findings, survival time, and potential treatment.[103,104] One of the two articles used a different classification scheme based on the National Cancer Institute Working Formulation.[103] To allow indicative comparison because the Onuma and colleagues'[103] article presented raw data, the authors classified and integrated the ferrets of the cohort along with the WHO-REAL classification and extrapolated the median survival time. Ferrets classified with

Table 20
Summary of findings and outcome of ferrets affected by lymphoma classified by cell type through the literature search

Articles	Lymphoma Type and Treatment	Number of Ferrets		Median Survival Time (mo)
Ammersbach et al,[104] 2008	T cell + chemotherapy	9		4.3 (0.5–14.0)
	B cell + chemotherapy	4		8.8 (2–19)
	T cell nontreated	5		5.7
	B cell nontreated	1		7
Onuma et al,[103] 2008	T cell + chemotherapy	10		2.5 or 74.8 d (18–210)
	T cell nontreated	1		1 d
	B cell nontreated	1		37 d
	B cell treatment	1		45 d
Erdman et al,[102] 1996	21 Chemotherapy	3 Died of complication		10.6
		5 Lost		
		13 Ferrets		
	7 Surgery	Splenectomy		12
		Lymph node		
		Cutaneous		
	28 No treatment	16 Euthanized immediately		1.3–5.2 y
		8 Lost		
		4 Lived		

Table 21
Summary of case report involving ferrets affected by lymphoma and treatment modalities through the literature search (Case reports involving postmortem diagnosis or euthanasia immediately following diagnostic were excluded.)

Article	Lymphoma Type	Treatment	Outcome
"Focal Thoracolumbar Spinal Cord Lymphosarcoma in a Ferret (Mustela putorius furo)"[114]	Spinal null cell or natural killer cell lymphosarcoma (nonreactive to CD3, CD79alpha, and CD20)	Prednisone initially and no treatment after diagnosis	Euthanasia 6 mo after diagnosis
"A Case of Advanced Second-Degree Atrioventricular Block in a Ferret Secondary to Lymphoma"[110]	Cardiac lymphomatous infiltrate and liver infiltrate	Enalapril, furosemide, prednisone	Death 36 h after presentation
"Epitheliotropic Gastrointestinal T-cell Lymphoma with Concurrent Insulinoma and Adrenocortical Carcinoma in a Domestic Ferret (Mustela putorius furo)"[121]	Epitheliotropic gastrointestinal T-cell lymphoma	Prednisone	Death 15 mo after diagnosis
"Diagnosis and Treatment of Myelo-Osteolytic Plasmablastic Lymphoma of the Femur in a Domestic Ferret"[116]	Plasmablastic lymphoma of the femur	Hind limb amputation (Tufts protocol) L-asparaginase Cyclophosphamide Cytosine arabinoside	Survival 21 mo after the surgery
"Cutaneous Epitheliotropic Lymphoma in a Ferret"[120]	Cutaneous T-cell lymphoma	Isotretinoin Amoxicillin Clavulanate Shampoos Prednisone	Death of renal failure after 60 d

Study	Presentation	Treatment	Outcome
"Hypereosinophilic Syndrome with Hodgkin's-like Lymphoma in a Ferret"[118]	Hodgkin lymphoma in lung, mediastinum, liver, kidney, and lymph node	Prednisone, Furosemide, Aminophylline	Euthanasia 3 wk after initial presentation
"Splenic Lymphosarcoma in a Ferret"[124]	Splenic	Splenectomy	Euthanasia after 2 wk postoperatively
"Chemotherapeutical Remission of Multicentric Lymphosarcoma in a Ferret"[125]	Mediastine, liver, and spleen biopsy	L-asparaginase, Cyclophosphamide, Prednisone	Survival 11 mo after diagnosis
"Use of a Vascular Access System for Administration of Chemotherapeutic Agents to a Ferret with Lymphoma"[126]	Multicentric lymphoma	L-asparaginase, Vincristine, Doxorubicin, Cyclophosphamide, Methotrexate, Chlorambucil, Prednisone	Survival 10 mo after diagnosis
"T Cell Lymphoma in the Lumbar Spine of a Domestic Ferret (Mustela putorius furo)"[113]	Spinal T-cell lymphoma	Prednisone	Death 2 wk after diagnosis
"Combination Doxorubicin and Orthovoltage Radiation Therapy, Single-Agent Doxorubicin, and High-Dose Vincristine for Salvage Therapy of Ferret Lymphosarcoma"[119]	Multicentric lymphoma	Doxorubicin, Radiation therapy, Vincristine	Survival 23 mo

intermediate grade with small-medium cell and low mitotic index were classified as small cell lymphoma. Ferrets with intermediate grade with medium-large cell and intermediate-high mitotic index were classified as large cell lymphoma. Two cases of the series could not be classified, and 4 cases were excluded because the survival was not mentioned.

Influence of immunohistochemistry type and mitotic index The first study by Ammersbach and colleagues[104] presents a trend with B-cell lymphomas having a better survival time than T-cell lymphomas. This case series excluded euthanized animals from survival analysis, which may artificially increase the survival time for the T-cell lymphomas group (**Table 19**). In the other series from Onuma and colleagues,[103] low survival time for B-cell lymphomas (<50 days) was observed. B-cell lymphomas are rare in ferrets, so it may be difficult to define a prognosis based on those two series (total number n = 4). Two distinct case reports involving B-cell lymphomas were found in the literature review.[111,116] One had a survival of more than 21 month but the other ferret was euthanized shortly after presentation. Based on cytologic examination, 2 studies found that small lymphocytic type had longer survival time than large cell lymphoma.[102,104]

Influence of extension One study allowed differentiation of systemic dissemination of lymphoma versus localized neoplastic transformation (spleen, superficial lymph node, intestinal). Calculated median survival time was 109.75 days (21–210) in localized lymphoma versus disseminated lymphoma 35.5 days (1–180).[103] This same cohort included 4 cases with total or partial remission of lymphoma restricted to one organ (spleen, mediastinum, skin, cervical lymph node); but the exact survival times were not mentioned, so inclusion in calculation could not be achieved.[103] Focal lymphomas were mentioned several times in the literature and survival times were variable (15 days to 21 months). One case of plasmablastic lymphoma of the femur achieved remission, and one patient with epitheliotropic gastrointestinal T-cell lymphoma died 15 months after diagnosis.[116,121]

Influence of treatment The use of chemotherapy was very variable among the case series and the case report, and combined protocol was very diverse. The first case series of 29 ferrets reported the use of chemotherapy (without protocol description) and higher median survival time for nontreated ferrets.[104] The authors extracted the case from the second cohort by Onuma and colleagues.[103] This second case series included most ferrets with chemotherapy (mainly prednisone), and comparison with nontreated ferrets cannot be made. No recommendation toward chemotherapy or absence of treatment can be made (**Table 20**).

There are multiple case reports with detailed description of the treatment. Medical treatment alone is usually based on prednisone and achieve very variable results. One report of alternative medicine is mentioned in a textbook (**Table 21**).[123]

In a review article, the survival of ferrets with a combined chemotherapy protocol was 437 days (36–1178) compared with all lymphoma cases, which was 242 days (0–1199); but no mention of classification was made.[127] Two case reports used combined chemotherapy protocols, one using a venous access port (VAP), and achieved survival at least 10 months after diagnosis.[125,126] The combined protocol used a combination of prednisone, L-asparaginase, and cyclophosphamide.[125,126] With the use of the VAP, vincristine and doxorubicin were added in the protocol; but the ferret probably died of secondary immunosuppression.[126]

A report combining chemotherapy and radiation therapy allowed survival of 23 months in a 2-year-old ferret.[119]

The combination of surgical treatment and chemotherapy was used in 5 cases and yielded apparent remission.[103,116] Four cases were described in the series by Onuma and colleagues,[103] combining surgical treatment and either melphalan or lomustine.[103] One patient with plasmablastic lymphoma has undergone a hind-limb amputation and a combined chemotherapy protocol.[116]

Currently based on this literature review, no recommendation on therapy can be made for lymphoma treatment, although some isolated cases of complete remission and feasibility of various treatment modalities were demonstrated. Determination of an efficient and safe dose of chemotherapeutic drugs in ferrets is needed. Specific ferret calculation of body surface area has been investigated to enhance the chemotherapy dosing regimen.[128]

SUMMARY

This review article aims to give some insight into the current literature and the level of evidence associated with diagnosis and treatment of common disease in ferrets. Unfortunately, most data have a low level of evidence, mainly because of the scarcity of information, even for very common diseases. Low-level evidence does not mean that the scientific information is not accurate but that further studies are likely to change in the understanding of the disease. Randomized trials are still uncommon in ferret literature because of economic and ethical reasons. Clinical research could be stimulated through individual methodology and statistics but also the creation of an international working group in order to progress in more efficient medicine for our ferret patients.

REFERENCES

1. Kociba GJ, Caputo CA. Aplastic anemia associated with estrus in pet ferrets. J Am Vet Med Assoc 1981;178(12):1293–4.
2. Dudas-Gyorki Z, Szabo Z, Manczur F, et al. Echocardiographic and electrocardiographic examination of clinically healthy, conscious ferrets. J Small Anim Pract 2011;52(1):18–25.
3. Vastenburg MH, Boroffka SA, Schoemaker NJ. Echocardiographic measurements in clinically healthy ferrets anesthetized with isoflurane. Vet Radiol Ultrasound 2004;45(3):228–32.
4. Stepien RL, Benson KG, Wenholz LJ. M-mode and Doppler echocardiographic findings in normal ferrets sedated with ketamine hydrochloride and midazolam. Vet Radiol Ultrasound 2000;41(5):452–6.
5. Bublot I, Wayne Randolph R, Chalvet-Monfray K, et al. The surface electrocardiogram in domestic ferrets. J Vet Cardiol 2006;8(2):87–93.
6. Quesenberry KE, Carpenter JW. Ferrets, rabbits and rodents: clinical medicine and surgery. 3rd edition. St Louis (MO): Elsevier; 2012.
7. Lewington JH. Ferret husbandry medicine and surgery. 2nd edition. Philadelphia: Saunders Elsevier; 2007.
8. Bone L, Battles AH, Goldfarb RD, et al. Electrocardiographic values from clinically normal, anesthetized ferrets (Mustela putorius furo). Am J Vet Res 1988; 49(11):1884–7.
9. Johnson-Delaney CA, Orosz SE. Ferret respiratory system: clinical anatomy, physiology, and disease. Vet Clin North Am Exot Anim Pract 2011;14(2): 357–67, vii.
10. Maxwell BM, Brunell MK, Olsen CH, et al. Comparison of digital rectal and microchip transponder thermometry in ferrets (Mustela putorius furo). J Am Assoc Lab Anim Sci 2016;55(3):331–5.

11. Kastner D, Apfelbach R. Effects of cyproterone acetate on mating behavior, testicular morphology, testosterone level, and body temperature in male ferrets in comparison with normal and castrated males. Horm Res 1987;25(3):178–84.
12. Friedrichs KR, Harr KE, Freeman KP, et al. ASVCP reference interval guidelines: determination of de novo reference intervals in veterinary species and other related topics. Vet Clin Pathol 2012;41(4):441–53.
13. Marini RP, Jackson LR, Esteves MI, et al. Effect of isoflurane on hematologic variables in ferrets. Am J Vet Res 1994;55(10):1479–83.
14. Hoover JP, Baldwin CA. Changes in physiologic and clinicopathologic values in domestic ferrets from 12 to 47 weeks of age. Companion Anim Pract 1988;2(1): 40–4.
15. Böttle M, Ewringmann A, Göbel T. Haematological examinations of the ferret (Mustela putorius furo). Kleintierpraxis 1999;44(9):673–82.
16. Lee EJ, Moore WE, Fryer HC, et al. Haematological and serum chemistry profiles of ferrets (Mustela putorius furo). Lab Anim 1982;16(2):133–7.
17. Hein J, Spreyer F, Sauter-Louis C, et al. Reference ranges for laboratory parameters in ferrets. Vet Rec 2012;171(9):218.
18. Ohwada K, Katahira K. Reference values for organ weight, hematology and serum chemistry in the female ferret (Mustela putrius furo). Jikken Dobutsu 1993;42(2):135–42.
19. Smith SA, Zimmerman K, Moore DM. Hematology of the domestic ferret (Mustela putorius furo). Vet Clin North Am Exot Anim Pract 2015;18(1):1–8.
20. Carpenter JW. Exotic animal formulary. 4th edition. Saint Louis (MO): Elsevier Saunders; 2013.
21. Siperstein LJ. Ferret hematology and related disorders. Vet Clin North Am Exot Anim Pract 2008;11(3):535–50, vii.
22. Gerber KL, Freeman KP. ASVCP guidelines: quality assurance for portable blood glucose meter (glucometer) use in veterinary medicine. Vet Clin Pathol 2016;45(1):10–27.
23. Hagvik J. Glucose measurement: time for a gold standard. J Diabetes Sci Technol 2007;1(2):169–72.
24. Petritz OA, Antinoff N, Chen S, et al. Evaluation of portable blood glucose meters for measurement of blood glucose concentration in ferrets (Mustela putorius furo). J Am Vet Med Assoc 2013;242(3):350–4.
25. Summa NM, Eshar D, Lee-Chow B, et al. Comparison of a human portable glucometer and an automated chemistry analyzer for measurement of blood glucose concentration in pet ferrets (Mustela putorius furo). Can Vet J 2014;55(9):865–9.
26. Benson KG, Paul-Murphy J, Hart AP, et al. Coagulation values in normal ferrets (Mustela putorius furo) using selected methods and reagents. Vet Clin Pathol 2008;37(3):286–8.
27. Takahashi S, Hirai N, Shirai M, et al. Comparison of the blood coagulation profiles of ferrets and rats. J Vet Med Sci 2011;73(7):953–6.
28. Hirai N, Takahashi S, Kaji N, et al. Comparison of the blood coagulation profiles of female ferrets with those of rats and dogs. J Vet Med Jpn 2012;65(7):563–6.
29. Eshar D, Wyre NR, Brown DC. Urine specific gravity values in clinically healthy young pet ferrets (Mustela furo). J Small Anim Pract 2012;53(2):115–9.
30. Platt SR, Dennis PM, McSherry LJ, et al. Composition of cerebrospinal fluid in clinically normal adult ferrets. Am J Vet Res 2004;65(6):758–60.
31. Di Girolamo N, Andreani V, Guandalini A, et al. Evaluation of intraocular pressure in conscious ferrets (Mustela putorius furo) by means of rebound tonometry and comparison with applanation tonometry. Vet Rec 2013;172(15):396.

32. Montiani-Ferreira F, Mattos BC, Russ HH. Reference values for selected ophthalmic diagnostic tests of the ferret (Mustela putorius furo). Vet Ophthalmol 2006;9(4):209–13.

33. Onuma M, Kondo H, Ono S, et al. Radiographic measurement of cardiac size in 64 ferrets. J Vet Med Sci 2009;71(3):355–8.

34. Stepien RL, Benson KG, Forrest LJ. Radiographic measurement of cardiac size in normal ferrets. Vet Radiol Ultrasound 1999;40(6):606–10.

35. Ono S, Onuma M, Ueki M, et al. Radiographic measurement of cardiac size in ferrets with heart disease. Adv Anim Cardiol 2008;41(2):37–43.

36. Malakoff RL, Laste NJ, Orcutt CJ. Echocardiographic and electrocardiographic findings in client-owned ferrets: 95 cases (1994-2009). J Am Vet Med Assoc 2012;241(11):1484–9.

37. Suran JN, La Toya L, Wyre NR. Radiographic and ultrasonographic measurements in healthy domestic companion ferrets. Paper presented at: Association of Exotic Mammal Veterinarians Conference. Orlando, October 19–23, 2014.

38. Proks P, Stehlik L, Paninarova M, et al. Congenital abnormalities of the vertebral column in ferrets. Vet Radiol Ultrasound 2015;56(2):117–23.

39. Garcia DAA, Silva LCS, Lange RR, et al. Anatomia ultrassonográfica dos linfonodos abdominais de furões europeus hígidos. Pesquisa Veterinária Brasileira 2011;31:1129–32.

40. O'Brien RT, Paul-Murphy J, Dubielzig RR. Ultrasonography of adrenal glands in normal ferrets. Vet Radiol Ultrasound 1996;37(6):445–8.

41. Neuwirth L, Collins B, Calderwood-Mays M, et al. Adrenal ultrasonography correlated with histopathology in ferrets. Vet Radiol Ultrasound 1997;38(1):69–74.

42. Kuijten AM, Schoemaker NJ, Voorhout G. Ultrasonographic visualization of the adrenal glands of healthy ferrets and ferrets with hyperadrenocorticism. J Am Anim Hosp Assoc 2007;43(2):78–84.

43. Sousa MG, Carareto R, De-Nardi AB, et al. Effects of isoflurane on echocardiographic parameters in healthy dogs. Vet Anaesth Analg 2008;35(3):185–90.

44. Schoemaker NJ, Schuurmans M, Moorman H, et al. Correlation between age at neutering and age at onset of hyperadrenocorticism in ferrets. J Am Vet Med Assoc 2000;216(2):195–7.

45. Schoemaker NJ, Teerds KJ, Mol JA, et al. The role of luteinizing hormone in the pathogenesis of hyperadrenocorticism in neutered ferrets. Mol Cell Endocrinol 2002;197(1–2):117–25.

46. Wagner S, Kiupel M, Peterson RA 2nd, et al. Cytochrome b5 expression in gonadectomy-induced adrenocortical neoplasms of the domestic ferret (Mustela putorius furo). Vet Pathol 2008;45(4):439–42.

47. Bielinska M, Kiiveri S, Parviainen H, et al. Gonadectomy-induced adrenocortical neoplasia in the domestic ferret (Mustela putorius furo) and laboratory mouse. Vet Pathol 2006;43(2):97–117.

48. Schillebeeckx M, Pihlajoki M, Gretzinger E, et al. Novel markers of gonadectomy-induced adrenocortical neoplasia in the mouse and ferret. Mol Cell Endocrinol 2015;399:122–30.

49. de Jong MK, ten Asbroek EE, Sleiderink AJ, et al. Gonadectomy-related adrenocortical tumors in ferrets demonstrate increased expression of androgen and estrogen synthesizing enzymes together with high inhibin expression. Domest Anim Endocrinol 2014;48:42–7.

50. de Jong MK, Schoemaker NJ, Mol JA. Expression of sfrp1 and activation of the Wnt pathway in the adrenal glands of healthy ferrets and neutered ferrets with hyperadrenocorticism. Vet J 2013;196(2):176–80.

51. Bielinska M, Parviainen H, Kiiveri S, et al. Review paper: origin and molecular pathology of adrenocortical neoplasms. Vet Pathol 2009;46(2):194–210.

52. Ryan KD. Hormonal correlates of photoperiod-induced puberty in a reflex ovulator, the female ferret (Mustela furo). Biol Reprod 1984;31(5):925–35.

53. Beuschlein F, Galac S, Wilson DB. Animal models of adrenocortical tumorigenesis. Mol Cell Endocrinol 2012;351(1):78–86.

54. Simone-Freilicher E. Adrenal gland disease in ferrets. Vet Clin North Am Exot Anim Pract 2008;11(1):125–37, vii.

55. Li X, Fox JG, Padrid PA. Neoplastic diseases in ferrets: 574 cases (1968-1997). J Am Vet Med Assoc 1998;212(9):1402–6.

56. Miwa Y, Kurosawa A, Ogawa H, et al. Neoplastic diseases in ferrets in Japan: a questionnaire study for 2000 to 2005. J Vet Med Sci 2009;71(4):397–402.

57. Avallone G, Forlani A, Tecilla M, et al. Neoplastic diseases in the domestic ferret (Mustela putorius furo) in Italy: classification and tissue distribution of 856 cases (2000-2010). BMC Vet Res 2016;12(1):275.

58. Williams B. Neoplasia. In: Quesenberry KE, Carpenter JW, editors. Ferrets, rabbits and rodents: clinical medicine and surgery. 2nd edition. St Louis (MO): Elsevier Saunders; 2003. p. 91–107.

59. Rosenthal KL, Peterson ME, Quesenberry KE, et al. Hyperadrenocorticism associated with adrenocortical tumor or nodular hyperplasia of the adrenal gland in ferrets: 50 cases (1987-1991). J Am Vet Med Assoc 1993;203(2):271–5.

60. Swiderski JK, Seim HB 3rd, MacPhail CM, et al. Long-term outcome of domestic ferrets treated surgically for hyperadrenocorticism: 130 cases (1995-2004). J Am Vet Med Assoc 2008;232(9):1338–43.

61. Jung JW, Choi YM, Yoon HY, et al. Clinical outcomes of 48 pet ferrets with adrenal disease. J Vet Clin 2014;31(5):389–93.

62. Weiss CA, Scott MV. Clinical aspects and surgical treatment of hyperadrenocorticism in the domestic ferret: 94 cases (1994-1996). J Am Anim Hosp Assoc 1997;33(6):487–93.

63. Besso JG, Tidwell AS, Gliatto JM. Retrospective review of the ultrasonographic features of adrenal lesions in 21 ferrets. Vet Radiol Ultrasound 2000;41(4):345–52.

64. Ackermann J, Carpenter JW, Godshalk CP, et al. Ultrasonographic detection of adrenal gland tumors in two ferrets. J Am Vet Med Assoc 1994;205(7):1001–3.

65. Rosenthal KL, Peterson ME. Evaluation of plasma androgen and estrogen concentrations in ferrets with hyperadrenocorticism. J Am Vet Med Assoc 1996;209(6):1097–102.

66. Wagner RA, Dorn DP. Evaluation of serum estradiol concentrations in alopecic ferrets with adrenal gland tumors. J Am Vet Med Assoc 1994;205(5):703–7.

67. Schoemaker NJ, Mol JA, Lumeij JT, et al. I plasma concentrations of adrenocorticotrophic hormone and alpha-melanocyte-stimulating hormone in ferrets (Mustela putorius furo) with hyperadrenocorticism. Am J Vet Res 2002;63(10):1395–9.

68. Schoemaker NJ, Wolfswinkel J, Mol JA, et al. Urinary glucocorticoid excretion in the diagnosis of hyperadrenocorticism in ferrets. Domest Anim Endocrinol 2004;27(1):13–24.

69. Protain HJ, Kutzler MA, Valentine BA. Assessment of cytologic evaluation of pre-putial epithelial cells as a diagnostic test for detection of adrenocortical disease in castrated ferrets. Am J Vet Res 2009;70(5):619–23.
70. Lennox AM, Wagner R. Comparison of 4.7-mg deslorelin implants and surgery for the treatment of adrenocortical disease in ferrets. J Exot Pet Med 2012;21(4): 332–5.
71. Miwa Y, Sasaki N. Prognosis after surgery and/or leuprolide acetate administration in Ferrets with adrenal diseases. J Jpn Vet Med Assoc 2011;64:554–8.
72. Weiss CA, Williams BH, Scott JB, et al. Surgical treatment and long-term outcome of ferrets with bilateral adrenal tumors or adrenal hyperplasia: 56 cases (1994-1997). J Am Vet Med Assoc 1999;215(6):820–3.
73. Lawrence HJ, Gould WJ, Flanders JA, et al. Unilateral adrenalectomy as a treat-ment for adrenocortical tumors in ferrets: five cases (1990-1992). J Am Vet Med Assoc 1993;203(2):267–70.
74. Calicchio KW, Bennett RA, Laraio LC, et al. Collateral circulation in ferrets (Mus-tela putorius) during temporary occlusion of the caudal vena cava. Am J Vet Res 2016;77(5):540–7.
75. Wagner RA, Finkler MR, Fecteau KA, et al. The treatment of adrenal cortical dis-ease in ferrets with 4.7-mg deslorelin acetate implants. J Exot Pet Med 2009; 18(2):146–52.
76. Miller LA, Fagerstone KA, Wagner RA, et al. Use of a GnRH vaccine, GonaCon, for prevention and treatment of adrenocortical disease (ACD) in domestic fer-rets. Vaccine 2013;31(41):4619–23.
77. Wagner RA, Piche CA, Jochle W, et al. Clinical and endocrine responses to treatment with deslorelin acetate implants in ferrets with adrenocortical disease. Am J Vet Res 2005;66(5):910–4.
78. Wagner RA, Bailey EM, Schneider JF, et al. Leuprolide acetate treatment of adrenocortical disease in ferrets. J Am Vet Med Assoc 2001;218(8):1272–4.
79. Murray J. Melatonin implants: an option for use in the treatment of adrenal dis-ease in ferrets. J Exot Mammal Med Surg 2005;3(1):1–6.
80. Ramer JC, Benson KG, Morrisey JK, et al. Effects of melatonin administration on the clinical course of adrenocortical disease in domestic ferrets. J Am Vet Med Assoc 2006;229(11):1743–8.
81. van Zeeland YR, Pabon M, Roest J, et al. Use of a GnRH agonist implant as alternative for surgical neutering in pet ferrets. Vet Rec 2014;175(3):66.
82. Schoemaker NJ, van Deijk R, Muijlaert B, et al. Use of a gonadotropin releasing hormone agonist implant as an alternative for surgical castration in male ferrets (Mustela putorius furo). Theriogenology 2008;70(2):161–7.
83. Chen S. Pancreatic endocrinopathies in ferrets. Vet Clin North Am Exot Anim Pract 2008;11(1):107–23, vii.
84. Lair S, Barker IK, Mehren KG, et al. Epidemiology of neoplasia in captive black-footed ferrets (Mustela nigripes), 1986-1996. J Zoo Wildl Med 2002;33(3): 204–13.
85. Weiss CA, Williams BH, Scott MV. Insulinoma in the ferret: clinical findings and treatment comparison of 66 cases. J Am Anim Hosp Assoc 1998;34(6):471–5.
86. Caplan ER, Peterson ME, Mullen HS, et al. Diagnosis and treatment of insulin-secreting pancreatic islet cell tumors in ferrets: 57 cases (1986-1994). J Am Vet Med Assoc 1996;209(10):1741–5.
87. Ehrhart N, Withrow SJ, Ehrhart EJ, et al. Pancreatic beta cell tumor in ferrets: 20 cases (1986-1994). J Am Vet Med Assoc 1996;209(10):1737–40.

88. Andrews GA, Myers NC 3rd, Chard-Bergstrom C. Immunohistochemistry of pancreatic islet cell tumors in the ferret (Mustela putorius furo). Vet Pathol 1997;34(5):387–93.

89. Marini RP, Ryden EB, Rosenblad WD, et al. Functional islet cell tumor in six ferrets. J Am Vet Med Assoc 1993;202(3):430–3.

90. Mann F, Stockham S, Freeman M, et al. Reference intervals for insulin concentrations and insulin: glucose ratios in the serum of ferrets. J Small Exot Anim Med 1993;57:543–7.

91. Quesenberry KE, Rosenthal KL. Endocrine diseases. In: Quesenberry KE, Carpenter JW, editors. Ferrets, rabbits and rodent: clinical medicine and surgery. St Louis (MO): Elsevier Saunders; 2003. p. 79–90.

92. Dutton MA. Case studies on doxorubicin for the treatment of ferret insulinoma (12 cases). J Exot Mammal Med Surg 2004;2(1):5–7.

93. Bennett KR, Gaunt MC, Parker DL. Constant rate infusion of glucagon as an emergency treatment for hypoglycemia in a domestic ferret (Mustela putorius furo). J Am Vet Med Assoc 2015;246(4):451–4.

94. Mayer J, Burgess K. An update on ferret lymphoma: a proposal for a standardized classification of ferret lymphoma. J Exot Pet Med 2012;21(4):343–6.

95. Erdman SE, Kanki PJ, Moore FM, et al. Clusters of lymphoma in ferrets. Cancer Invest 1996;14(3):225–30.

96. Batchelder MA, Erdman SE, Li X, et al. A cluster of cases of juvenile mediastinal lymphoma in a ferret colony. Lab Anim Sci 1996;46(3):271–4.

97. Erdman SE, Reimann KA, Moore FM, et al. Transmission of a chronic lymphoproliferative syndrome in ferrets. Lab Invest 1995;72(5):539–46.

98. Erdman SE, Correa P, Coleman LA, et al. Helicobacter mustelae-associated gastric MALT lymphoma in ferrets. Am J Pathol 1997;151(1):273–80.

99. Cui J, Holmes EC. Endogenous lentiviruses in the ferret genome. J Virol 2012; 86(6):3383–5.

100. Kassiotis G. Endogenous retroviruses and the development of cancer. J Immunol 2014;192(4):1343–9.

101. Erdman SE, Moore FM, Rose R, et al. Malignant lymphoma in ferrets: clinical and pathological findings in 19 cases. J Comp Pathol 1992;106(1):37–47.

102. Erdman SE, Brown SA, Kawasaki TA, et al. Clinical and pathologic findings in ferrets with lymphoma: 60 cases (1982-1994). J Am Vet Med Assoc 1996; 208(8):1285–9.

103. Onuma M, Kondo H, Ono S, et al. Cytomorphological and immunohistochemical features of lymphoma in ferrets. J Vet Med Sci 2008;70(9):893–8.

104. Ammersbach M, Delay J, Caswell JL, et al. Laboratory findings, histopathology, and immunophenotype of lymphoma in domestic ferrets. Vet Pathol 2008;45(5): 663–73.

105. Suran JN, Wyre NR. Imaging findings in 14 domestic ferrets (Mustela putorius furo) with lymphoma. Vet Radiol Ultrasound 2013;54(5):522–31.

106. Coleman LA, Erdman SE, Schrenzel MD, et al. Immunophenotypic characterization of lymphomas from the mediastinum of young ferrets. Am J Vet Res 1998; 59(10):1281–6.

107. Hammer AS, Williams B, Dietz HH, et al. High-throughput immunophenotyping of 43 ferret lymphomas using tissue microarray technology. Vet Pathol 2007; 44(2):196–203.

108. Rakich PM, Latimer KS. Cytologic diagnosis of diseases of ferrets. Vet Clin North Am Exot Anim Pract 2007;10(1):61–78, vi.

109. Beaufrere H, Neta M, Smith DA, et al. Demodectic mange associated with lymphoma in a ferret. J Exot Pet Med 2009;18(1):57–61.
110. Menicagli F, Lanza A, Sbrocca F, et al. A case of advanced second-degree atrioventricular block in a ferret secondary to lymphoma. Open Vet J 2016;6(1):68–70.
111. Gupta A, Gumber S, Schnellbacher R, et al. Malignant B-cell lymphoma with Mott cell differentiation in a ferret (Mustela putorius furo). J Vet Diagn Invest 2010;22(3):469–73.
112. Li X, Fox G, Erdman SE, et al. Cutaneous lymphoma in a ferret (Mustela putorius furo). Vet Pathol 1995;32(1):55–6.
113. Hanley CS, Wilson GH, Frank P, et al. T cell lymphoma in the lumbar spine of a domestic ferret (Mustela putorius furo). Vet Rec 2004;155(11):329–32.
114. Ingrao JC, Eshar D, Vince A, et al. Focal thoracolumbar spinal cord lymphosarcoma in a ferret (Mustela putorius furo). Can Vet J 2014;55(7):667–71.
115. Long H, di Girolamo N, Selleri P, et al. Polyostotic lymphoma in a ferret (Mustela putorius furo). J Comp Pathol 2016;154(4):341–4.
116. Eshar D, Wyre NR, Griessmayr P, et al. Diagnosis and treatment of myeloosteolytic plasmablastic lymphoma of the femur in a domestic ferret. J Am Vet Med Assoc 2010;237(4):407–14.
117. Saunders GK, Thomsen BV. Lymphoma and Mycobacterium avium infection in a ferret (Mustela putorius furo). J Vet Diagn Invest 2006;18(5):513–5.
118. Blomme EA, Foy SH, Chappell KH, et al. Hypereosinophilic syndrome with Hodgkin's-like lymphoma in a ferret. J Comp Pathol 1999;120(2):211–7.
119. Hutson CA, Kopit MJ, Walder EJ. Combination doxorubicin and orthovoltage radiation therapy, single agent doxorubicin and high dose vincristine for salvage therapy of ferret lymphosarcoma. J Am Anim Hosp Assoc 1992;28:365–8.
120. Rosenbaum MR, Affolter VK, Usborne AL, et al. Cutaneous epitheliotropic lymphoma in a ferret. J Am Vet Med Assoc 1996;209(8):1441–4.
121. Sinclair KM, Eckstrand C, Moore PF, et al. Epitheliotropic gastrointestinal T-cell lymphoma with concurrent insulinoma and adrenocortical carcinoma in a domestic ferret (Mustela putorius furo). J Exot Pet Med 2016;25(1):34–43.
122. Arber DA, Orazi A, Hasserjian R, et al. The 2016 revision to the World Health Organization classification of myeloid neoplasms and acute leukemia. Blood 2016;127(20):2391–405.
123. Lewington JH. General neoplasia. In: Lewington JH, editor. Ferret husbandry, medicine and surgery. Philadelphia: Saunders Elsevier; 2007. p. 318–46.
124. Flock M. Splenic lymphosarcoma in a ferret. Can Vet J 1989;30(7):597.
125. Dugan SJ, Center SA, Randolph JF, et al. Chemotherapeutical remission of multicentric lymphosarcoma in a ferret (Mustela putorius furo). J Am Anim Hosp Assoc 1989;25:69–74.
126. Rassnick KM, Gould WJ 3rd, Flanders JA. Use of a vascular access system for administration of chemotherapeutic agents to a ferret with lymphoma. J Am Vet Med Assoc 1995;206(4):500–4.
127. Antinoff N, Hahn K. Ferret oncology: diseases, diagnostics, and therapeutics. Vet Clin North Am Exot Anim Pract 2004;7(3):579–625, vi.
128. Jones KL, Granger LA, Kearney MT, et al. Evaluation of a ferret-specific formula for determining body surface area to improve chemotherapeutic dosing. Am J Vet Res 2015;76(2):142–8.

Evidence-Based Advances in Rodent Medicine

Vladimir Jekl, DVM, PhD, DECZM (Small Mammal)*, Karel Hauptman, DVM, PhD,
Zdenek Knotek, DVM, PhD, DECZM (Herpetogy)

KEYWORDS

- Guinea pig • Rat • Dental disease • Mammary gland tumor • Deslorelin

KEY POINTS

- In case of hyperadrenocorticism diagnostics in guinea pigs, an adrenocorticotropic hormone stimulation test and analyses of saliva cortisol concentrations are recommended.
- Uroliths in guinea pigs are mostly of calcium carbonate origin, so other factors than dietary need to be considered in case of urolithiasis.
- In guinea pigs, itopride can be used as a potent gastrointestinal motility stimulant.
- In case of dental diseases in rodents, more attention should be focused on phosphorus dietary content, altered tooth structure, and jaw calcification.
- Prevention of mammary gland tumors is based on ovariectomy before 7 months of age and on weight management.

INTRODUCTION

The number of exotic companion pet rodents seen in veterinary practices is growing very rapidly. According to the American Veterinary Medical Association's surveys, more than 2,093,000 pet rodents were kept in US households in 2007 and in 2012 it was more than 2,349,000 animals.[1] The most commonly kept species are guinea pigs (*Cavia porcellus*), hamsters (*Mesocricetus auratus, Phodopus sp, Cricetulus sp*), gerbils (*Meriones unguiculatus*), rats (*Rattus norvegicus*), and chinchillas (*Chinchilla lanigera*). All of these species have been used in experimental research as models for human diseases for decades. The number of publications in scientific journals dealing with the aforementioned species is tremendous. When searching Web of Knowledge[2] for the last 10 years (2006–2016), it was found that a rat in the title or topic was used in 558,792 publications. In the case of a guinea pig, hamster, gerbil, and

Disclosure statement: The authors have nothing to disclose.
This article is supported by the institutional research of the Faculty of Veterinary Medicine (2017) University of Veterinary and Pharmaceutical Sciences Brno.
Avian and Exotic Animal Clinic, Faculty of Veterinary Medicine, University of Veterinary and Pharmaceutical Sciences Brno, Palackého tr. 1946/1, Brno 61242, Czech Republic
* Corresponding author.
E-mail address: VladimirJekl@gmail.com

chinchilla, it was 21,633, 18,415, 3412, and 921, respectively. Because of the spread of exotic companion mammal societies, conferences, and specialty colleges, the number of publications in veterinary medicine also increased, especially in the last 10 years.

However, only a small part of the literature is composed of properly designed research. This article summarizes the most important evidence-based knowledge in exotic pet rodents. The information presented is graded based on the Grades of Recommendation, Assessment, Development, Evaluation guidelines.[3]

EVIDENCE-BASED ADVANCES IN DIAGNOSIS
Diagnosis of Hyperadrenocorticism in Guinea Pigs

Hyperadrenocorticism (Cushing syndrome) was recently described as the third most common endocrinopathy in guinea pigs. Both adrenal-dependent hyperadrenocorticism and pituitary-dependent hyperadrenocorticism can be present.[4,5] The clinical signs include nonpruritic, bilateral symmetric alopecia (**Fig. 1**), thinner skin, polyuria, polydipsia, muscle weakness, and weight loss.[6] Diagnosis was previously based on clinical and ultrasonic findings, on high plasma cortisol levels, and by using adrenocorticotropic hormone (ACTH) response test. However, as guinea pigs have relatively large adrenal glands and their size estimation abased on body weight or other physiologic/anatomic parameters is not published and high levels of circulating cortisol,[7] which fluctuate diurnally and can be influenced by many other factors, the diagnostic accuracy of these techniques is likely limited.[8]

Similarly to the study by Fenske,[9,10] Nemeth and colleagues[11] revealed a high biological relevance of noninvasive cortisol measurements in saliva and fecal samples (fecal glucocorticoid metabolites [FGM]) of domestic guinea pigs. Saliva cortisol and FGM levels measured in samples adjusted to the appropriate gut passage time were both significantly increased in response to the social confrontations and were highly correlated to the actual circulating cortisol levels in plasma. Saliva cortisol concentrations were exclusively affected by the experimental conditions, with no day-related effects. Only saliva cortisol concentrations proved successful in predicting plasma cortisol levels, which was not the case for FGM levels. As saliva can be easily sampled with much less disturbance than blood sampling procedures, repeated saliva cortisol measurements can also be used for long-term cortisol level monitoring.[12] In case of an ACTH response test in healthy animals, after the intramuscular administration of the ACTH (20 IU), salivary cortisol concentration increased from 2.2 ng/mL to

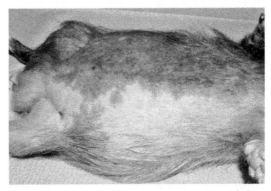

Fig. 1. Alopecia of the ventral abdomen in a male guinea pig with hyperadrenocorticism.

47 ng/mL (1 hour), 72 ng/mL (2 hours), 137 ng/mL (3 hours), and 170 ng/mL (4 hours), respectively.[10]

Therefore, for the final diagnosis of hyperadrenocorticism in guinea pigs, ACTH response test and salivary cortisol levels determination is recommended. The American College of Veterinary Internal Medicine's guidelines for hyperadrenocorticism[13] should be followed. However, sensitivity, specificity, and positive and negative predictive values of these test are not yet established. Other causes of alopecia in guinea pigs, such is dermatophytosis, ectoparasitoses, hypovitaminosis C, and barbering, need to be excluded.

Dental imaging

In the scientific literature, dental disease in chinchillas, guinea pigs, and degus has been primarily referred to as elongation and malocclusion of the cheek teeth. Periodontal disease, caries, and tooth resorptive lesions are also very common, especially in guinea pigs and chinchillas. For this reason, the physical examination must be followed by radiologic diagnosis with standard radiography and/or computed tomography (CT) and thorough oral cavity inspection, ideally with an endoscopy-guided intraoral examination.[14,15] CT has been found to have more diagnostic value; it bypasses the intrinsic limit of standard radiography whereby anatomic structures are superimposed on a single 2-dimensional plane.[16–19] A recent study showed that the diagnostic accuracy of CT was superior in 24 patients (80.0%) in diagnosis and prognosis and in 17 patients (56.6%) for guiding extraoral dental and surgical treatment and that extraoral radiography provided superior accuracy in 5 patients (16.6%) for guiding intraoral dental treatment.[16] Micro-CT is used rarely in clinical veterinary practice; however, it provides superior resolution over conventional CT and will show dental pathologies in detail.[20–23] In an experimental method comparison study, the in vivo and ex vivo micro-CT examination of rat femurs in sham and ovariectomized animals were compared.[24] At a voxel size of 18 μm, scanning in vivo or ex vivo had no effect on any of the outcomes measured. When compared with a 9-μm voxel size scan, imaging at 18 μm resulted in significant underestimation of the connectivity density of the trabecular bone and a significant overestimation of the trabecular indices (trabecular thickness, degree of anisotropy) and of the cortical indices (cortical bone area, cortical area fraction, cortical thickness). These results suggest the benefit to scanning the proximal tibia of rats at a voxel size as low as 9 μm. Further studies with hard outcomes (eg, overall survival time) are required in order to account for the increased acquisition time, anesthesia, and radiation exposure associated with lower voxel size in vivo.[24] Guidelines for the assessment of bone microstructure in rodents should be followed when micro-CT images of rodent bones are evaluated.[25]

Pituitary tumor imaging

Pituitary tumors are very common in aging rats, especially pituitary adenomas (**Fig. 2**).[26] The incidence of pituitary tumors differ between sex, rat strains, and body condition. The incidence of the tumor in untreated male Fischer rats (F344) was reported to be 30.4%, and in untreated female F344 it was 54.2%. Dinse and colleagues[27] described 45%, and 39% incidence of pituitary tumors in Fischer rats (F344/N) and Sprague Dawley (SD) rats, respectively. In a study by Haseman and colleagues,[28] the pituitary tumors had significantly higher incidence in rats with increased body weight. However, in pet rats these tumors are commonly diagnosed post mortem, as the described incidence of these tumors in clinical practice seems to be underestimated (8 rats from 375 animals).[29] Diagnosis is based on the use of

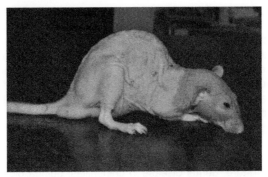

Fig. 2. Hunched posture, cachexia, and discoordination in a rat with adenohypophyseal adenoma.

advanced imaging modalities, especially CT[30] and MRI.[31,32] Although a high-resolution CT scanner might also be effective in detecting large pituitary lesions, its relatively poor contrast resolution may hamper detection of small pituitary adenomas in rats. There is a comparative study of pituitary volume variations and clinical signs in humans but not in rats.[33] Recent studies showed that manganese MRI of calcium influx in spontaneous rat pituitary adenomas[34] and PET, a nuclear medicine, functional imaging technique can be used for the imaging of the pituitary tumors in rats, which can be more effective in the pituitary tumor detection.

Mineral Composition of Urinary Stones

Urolithiasis is a relatively common health disorder in pet guinea pigs; however, only one study is published as cross-sectional[35] and one retrospective[36]; other articles are presented in the form of case reports.[37–40] An outbreak of *Streptococcus pyogenes* infection and associated urolith formation was also described in a colony of 800 experimentally bred Dunkin-Hartley guinea pigs resulting in 364 deaths. The mineral analyses of the urinary calculi showed the presence of calcium oxalate.[41]

Mineral analyses of the uroliths from 2 studies in pet guinea pigs showed that the most common urinary calculi are calcium carbonate (calcite), which is in contrast with previous studies (**Fig. 3**).

A study by Hawkins and colleagues[35] suggested that differences in calculus composition are likely attributable to the methods used to identify the various

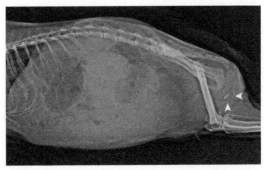

Fig. 3. Lateral abdominal radiograph of a female guinea pig with ureterolith (*arrowheads*).

crystalline components. However, most of the published data are in the form of case reports or as a disorder of the guinea pig colony, which was fed by the same diet.

As the main crystals in the urine of the guinea pigs are of calcium carbonate origin as in rabbits,[42] additional studies are needed to evaluate risk factors for urolithiasis, such as diet and environment, so the pathophysiology of urolithiasis in pet guinea pigs can be better understood.

EVIDENCE-BASED ADVANCES IN THERAPEUTICS
Peristalsis

There are several *drugs used for stimulation of peristalsis* used in herbivorous rodents with gastrointestinal stasis/postoperative ileus. In guinea pigs and rats, recent experimental evidence-based data exist for itopride, cisapride, mosapride,[43] and prucalopride[44] as drugs used for small intestine and colonic stimulation. Itopride accelerated colonic transit dose dependently in both guinea pigs and rats, and significant acceleration was observed at 10 mg/kg by mouth in both animals. However, cisapride did not affect colonic transit significantly up to 10 mg/kg in guinea pigs and rats nor did mosapride in guinea pigs. Mosapride slightly delayed colonic transit in rats, the delay being statistically significant at a dose of 1 mg/kg and greater. In rats, itopride, cisapride, and mosapride all enhanced gastric emptying dose dependently, with statistically significant effects being observed at doses of 10, 1, and 1 mg/kg, respectively. Therefore, itopride exerted stimulatory effects on gastric emptying and colonic transit at the same dose, whereas cisapride and mosapride were found not to accelerate colonic transit at 10 mg/kg by mouth, a dose that was 10 times higher than that required to accelerate gastric emptying.[43] In guinea pigs, prucalopride administered orally at a dose of 10 mg/kg restores both upper and lower gastrointestinal transit after experimental laparotomy.[44]

Providing appropriate analgesia is essential in minimizing pain and maintaining optimal animal care and welfare in all animal species. Nonsteroidal antiinflammatory drugs (eg, meloxicam) and opioids (eg, butorphanol, buprenorphine) are the most commonly used analgesics in veterinary practices. Recently, a *sustained-release formulation of buprenorphine* (Bup-SR) showed an analgesic effect for 48 hours (Bup-SR 0.6, 1.2, or 2.2 mg/kg) in mice[45,46] and 48 to 72 hours (Bup-SR 1.2 mg/kg) in rats[47,48] and guinea pigs.[49] Gross pathologic examination revealed no signs of toxicity.[48] The current studies demonstrated that the clinical efficacy of Bup-SR is superior to that of immediate-release buprenorphine (buprenorphine hydrochloride) according to results from the ethogram of assessing postoperative pain in mice.[50]

Use of Surgical Laser Devices

The use of laser devices during surgery
The use of laser devices during surgery is becoming popular in laboratory and clinical rodent medicine. In mice in which tumors were excised by means of laser, scalpel blade, and diathermy, the group exposed to laser surgery experienced significantly lower tumor recurrence and significantly lower perioperative mortality rates.[51] Furthermore, in laboratory rodents, carbon dioxide laser provided rapid postoperative healing of skin incisions.[52] One of the life-threatening complications, apart from mucosal edema and accidental burns, is the ignition. As most pet rodents are not intubated during surgeries, in case of ignition, the severe burns on the head and proximal parts of the body can be expected.[53] A recent study showed that in 400 surgeries performed on 100 rat carcasses, 11 fire events occurred.[54] Ignition was associated with procedures on the head and when using open mask systems. In case of using laser, but also

electrocautery, the use of open masks by the addition of a latex diaphragm, which significantly reduced the occurrence of fire ignition during laser surgery, is recommended. As the inhalation anesthetic and oxygen are 2 of the main factors of potential ignition, surgical lasers should be avoided for facial surgery of nonintubated anesthetized rodents.

Contraceptive Medications

Deslorelin acetate

Deslorelin acetate (4.7-mg implant), a gonadotropin-releasing hormone agonist, is commonly used to prevent folliculogenesis in several species. In the case of pet rodents, some information is available for rats and guinea pigs. In the case of female rats, it was shown that after 6 months, the implant interfered with the normal estrous cycle of female rats and affected the preantral follicle population.[55] The study by Grosset and colleagues[56] indicated that the deslorelin contraceptive effect can be at least 10 months. The contraceptive effect was also proved for males for 6 months after treatment.[57] However, the exact duration of action has not yet been determined in both males and females. In a study by Kohutova and colleagues,[58] 15 female guinea pigs were followed for 2 estrous cycles before and 12 months after deslorelin implantation. Four female guinea pigs were included in a study by Forman and colleagues,[59] whereby the effect of deslorelin was followed for 196 days. In both of these studies, deslorelin had a contraceptive effect. However, in a study by Kohutova and colleagues,[58] all of the deslorelin-treated animals developed ovarian and uterine pathologies. In the case of male guinea pigs, treatment had no effect on testicular volume, male behavior, and testosterone concentrations; all females that mated with deslorelin-treated males got pregnant. Therefore, deslorelin had no contraceptive effect in male guinea pigs. Further studies are needed before recommending the use of deslorelin as contraception in female guinea pigs.

EVIDENCE-BASED ADVANCES IN COMMON DISORDERS
Dental Disease in Guinea Pigs and Degus

Dental disease is one of the most common diseases in guinea pigs and degus.[15,60–62] These strictly herbivorous rodents have complete hypsodont aradicular/elodont dentition. Most animals with dental disease are presented for weight loss, reduced food intake or anorexia, and drooling. Degus are also commonly presented for dyspnea associated with elodontoma formation or due to cheek teeth elongation in the nasal cavity.[20,60]

Pathophysiology of the dental disease is associated with less abrasive properties of the diet, alteration of the chewing pattern, reduction of the chewing duration, and mineral dietary imbalances. It was found that guinea pig teeth can adapt to the diet with different abrasiveness and that the rate of eruption and attrition changes.[63] In a study by Müller and colleagues,[63] cheek tooth angle did not become shallower with decreasing diet abrasiveness, suggesting that a lack of dietary abrasiveness does not cause the typical bridge formation of anterior cheek teeth frequently observed in guinea pigs. These findings suggested that other factors than diet abrasiveness, such as mineral imbalances and hereditary malocclusion, are more likely causes for dental problems observed in this species. The study by Müller and colleagues[63] was short-term (14 days), and long-term studies are not available for this species.

In a study by Jekl and colleagues,[64] it was shown that degus fed a high-phosphorus diet for 14 months developed severe dental disease. Based on macroscopic observation, histopathologic examination, transmission, and scanning electron microscopy, animals fed with a calcium/phosphorus ratio of 1:1 had enamel depigmentation, enamel hypoplasia, enamel pitting, and altered dentin morphology (**Fig. 4**).[65] Such a diet was responsible for the rapid development of dental disease (apical and coronal crown elongation of all cheek teeth) with subsequent severe health impairment. All the ill degus had decalcified jaws.

These results suggest that, in the case of dental diseases in rodents, more attention should be focused on phosphorus dietary content, altered tooth structure, and jaw calcification.

Mammary Gland Tumors in Rats

Mammary gland tumors (**Fig. 5**) are the most common tumors in pet rats.[29] In the case of laboratory rats, analyses of 18 National Toxicology Program chronic rodent carcinogenicity bioassays: 9 Harlan SD rat bioassays and 9 F344/N rat bioassays showed that female SD rats had higher incidence rates for spontaneous mammary gland fibroadenoma (67.4% vs 48.4%) and mammary gland carcinoma (10.2% vs 2.4%) relative to female F344/N rats. The age of presentation of privately kept rodents ranged from 5 to 48 months (25.3±8.7 months)[29] in one study and in another ranged from 8 to 54 months (mean 24 months).[66]

Mammary gland tumors are more common in sexually intact animals.[27,66,67] Previous studies have shown that there is also a positive correlation between the presence of a pituitary tumor and body weight and the incidence and time of onset of mammary gland tumors.[26,67,68] Development of these tumors is mediated through increased levels of estrogens, and adipose tissue is considered to be one of the major sources of extraglandular estrogen.[69] In a study by Dinse and colleagues,[27] the body condition was more related to the mammary gland tumor development.

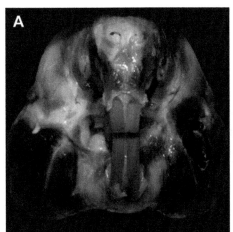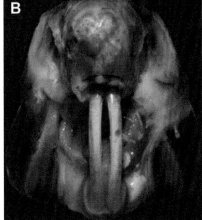

Fig. 4. Incisors of degus (A) fed with 13.2 g/kg calcium and with 6.3 g/kg phosphorus of dry matter basis and (B) fed with 9.1 g/kg calcium and with 9.5 g/kg phosphorus of dry matter basis for 14 months. (B) In degus fed with high phosphorus content, the incisor enamel was depigmented and had rough surface: enamel hypoplasia. All tooth structures were affected. Maxillary incisors are fractured. (*From* Jekl V, Krejcirova L, Buchtova M, et al. Effect of high phosphorus diet on tooth microstructure of rodent incisors. Bone 2011;49(3):480, with permission.)

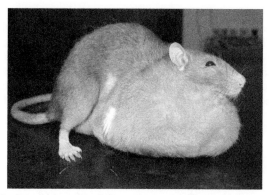

Fig. 5. Large inguinal mammary gland fibroadenoma in the intact female rat.

One of the preventative measures for mammary gland tumor development in female rats is neutering, as it was described in SD rats that ovariectomy before 7 months of age inhibited development of spontaneous mammary tumors by 95% in comparison with intact females.[70] Another important part of prevention of these spontaneous tumors is weight management, as weight reduction decreases the estrogen levels via a decrease in body fat.[69]

CURRENT CONTROVERSIES AND CLINICAL TOPICS REQUIRING ADDITIONAL EVIDENCE

Deslorelin acetate can be used as a prevention of mammary gland neoplasia in rats. The use of deslorelin acetate (deslorelin implant 4.7 mg) in rats showed that this therapy interferes with the normal cyclicity of female rats and affects the preantral follicle population for at least 1 year.[55] No mammary gland tumor development was described, but experimental design in that study was focused on uterine and ovarian changes only. Deslorelin implants also have no effect on mammary gland tumors.[56] Further studies are needed to prove the positive effect of deslorelin on mammary gland tumor development in rats.

REFERENCES

1. AVMA. US pet ownership & demographics sourcebook: 2012 edition. Schaumburg (IL): AVMA; 2012.
2. Web of Knowledge. Availbale at: https://apps.webofknowledge.com. Accessed February 1, 2017.
3. Grades of Recommendation, Assessment, Development, Evaluation (GRADE) Working Group. Grading quality of evidence and strength of recommendations. BMJ 2004;328:1490–4.
4. Nowotny I. Hyperadrenokortizismus beim Meerschweinchen. (Hyperadrenocorticism in the Guinea pig). Thesis. Vienna (Austria): Diploma of Veterinary Medicine, University of Veterinary Medicine; 2010.
5. Zeugswetter F, Fenske M, Hassan J, et al. Cushing's syndrome in a guinea pig. Vet Rec 2007;160:878–80.
6. Künzel F, Mayer J. Endocrine tumours in the guinea pig. Vet J 2015;206(3): 268–74.
7. Keightley MC, Fuller PJ. Cortisol resistance and the guinea pig glucocorticoid receptor. Steroids 1995;60(1):87–92.

8. Liu L, Matthews SG. Adrenocortical response profiles to corticotrophin releasing hormone and adrenocorticotrophin challenge in the chronically catheterized adult guinea-pig. Exp Physiol 1999;84:971–7.

9. Fenske M. Saliva cortisol and testosterone in the guinea pig: measures for the endocrine function of adrenals and testes? Steroids 1996;61:647–50.

10. Fenske M. The use of salivary cortisol measurements for the non-invasive assessment of adrenal cortical function in guinea pigs. Exp Clin Endocrinol Diabetes 1997;105:163–8.

11. Nemeth M, Pschernig E, Wallner B, et al. Non-invasive cortisol measurements as indicators of physiological stress responses in guinea pigs. PeerJ 2016;4:e1590.

12. Nemeth M, Millesi E, Wagner KH, et al. Effects of diets high in unsaturated fatty acids on socially induced stress responses in guinea pigs. PLoS One 2014;9: e116292.

13. Behrend EN, Kooistra HS, Nelson R, et al. Diagnosis of spontaneous canine hyperadrenocorticism: ACVIM consensus statement (small animal). J Vet Intern Med 2012;27:1292–304.

14. Legendre L. Anatomy and disorders of the oral cavity of guinea pigs. Vet Clin North Am Exot Anim Pract 2016;19(3):825–42.

15. Mans C, Jekl V. Anatomy and disorders of the oral cavity of chinchillas and degus. Vet Clin North Am Exot Anim Pract 2016;19(3):843–69.

16. Capello V, Cauduro A. Comparison of diagnostic consistency and diagnostic accuracy between survey radiography and computed tomography of the skull in 30 rabbits with dental disease. J Exot Pet Med 2016;25(2):115–27.

17. Capello V, Lennox A. Advanced diagnostic imaging and surgical treatment of an odontogenic retromasseteric abscess in a guinea pig. J Small Anim Pract 2015; 56(2):134–7.

18. Capello V, Lennox A, Ghisleni G. Elodontoma in two guinea pigs. J Vet Dent 2015; 32(2):111–9.

19. Schweda MC, Hassan J, Böhler A, et al. The role of computed tomography in the assessment of dental disease in 66 guinea pigs. Vet Rec 2014;175(21):538.

20. Jekl V, Zikmun T, Hauptman K. Dyspnea in a degu (*Octodon degu*) associated with maxillary cheek teeth elongation. J Exot Pet Med 2016;25(2):128–32.

21. Morkmued S, Hemmerle J, Mathieu E, et al. Enamel and dental anomalies in latent-transforming growth factor beta-binding protein 3 mutant mice. Eur J Oral Sci 2017;125(1):8–17.

22. Souza MJ, Greenacre CB, Avenell JS, et al. Diagnosing a tooth root abscess in a guinea Pig (Cavia porcellus) using micro computed tomography Imaging. J Exot Pet Med 2006;15(4):274–7.

23. Minarikova A, Fictum P, Zikmund T, et al. Dental disease and periodontitis in a guinea pig (Cavia porcellus). J Exot Pet Med 2016;25:150–6.

24. Longo AB, Salmon PL, Ward WE. Comparison of ex vivo and in vivo microcomputed tomography of rat tibia at different scanning settings. J Orthop Res 2016. http://dx.doi.org/10.1002/jor.23435.

25. Bouxsein ML, Boyd SK, Christiansen BA, et al. Guidelines for assessment of bone microstructure in rodents using micro-computed tomography. J Bone Miner Res 2010;25(7):1468–86.

26. McComb DJ, Kovacs K, Beri J, et al. Pituitary adenomas in old Sprague-Dawley rats: a histologic, ultrastructural, and immunocytochemical study. J Natl Cancer Inst 1984;73:1143–66.

27. Dinse GE, Peddada SD, Harris SF, et al. Comparison of historical control tumor incidence rates in female Harlan Sprague-Dawley and Fischer 344/N rats from

two-year bioassays performed by the National Toxicology Program. Toxicol Pathol 2010;38(5):765–75.

28. Haseman JK, Hailey JR, Morris RW. Spontaneous neoplasm incidences in Fischer 344 rats and B6C3F, mice in two-year carcinogenicity studies: a National Toxicology Program update. Toxicol Pathol 1998;26(3):428–41.

29. Rey F, Bulliot C, Bertin N, et al. Morbidity and disease management in pet rats: study of 375 cases. Vet Rec 2015;176(15):385.

30. Casanueva FF, Gordon WL, Friesen HG. Computerized cranial tomography in the evaluation of pituitary tumours in rats. Acta Endocrinol (Copenh) 1983;103(4): 487–91.

31. van Nesselrooij JH, Bruijntjes JP, van Garderen-Hoetmer A, et al. Magnetic resonance imaging compared with hormonal effects and histopathology of estrogen-induced pituitary lesions in the rat. Carcinogenesis 1991;12:289–97.

32. Mayer J, Sato A, Kiupel M, et al. Extralabel use of cabergoline in the treatment of a pituitary adenoma in a rat. J Am Vet Med Assoc 2011;239(5):656–60.

33. Soni BK, Joish UK, Sahni H, et al. A comparative study of pituitary volume variations in MRI in acute onset of psychiatric conditions. J Clin Diagn Res 2017;11(2): TC01–4.

34. Cross DJ, Flexman JA, Anzai Y, et al. In vivo manganese MR imaging of calcium influx in spontaneous rat pituitary adenoma. AJNR Am J Neuroradiol 2007;28(10): 1865–71.

35. Hawkins MG, Ruby AL, Drazenovich TL, et al. Composition and characteristics of urinary calculi from guinea pigs. J Am Vet Med Assoc 2009;234(2):214–20.

36. Rogers KD, Jones B, Roberts L, et al. Composition of uroliths in small domestic animals in the United Kingdom. Vet J 2011;188(2):228–30.

37. Eshar D, Lee-Chow B, Chalmers HJ. Ultrasound-guided percutaneous antegrade hydropropulsion to relieve ureteral obstruction in a pet guinea pig (Cavia porcellus). Can Vet J 2013;54(12):1142–5.

38. Pizzi R. Cystoscopic removal of a urolith from a pet guinea pig. Vet Rec 2009; 165(5):148–9.

39. Ramakrishnan NK, Rybczynska AA, Visser AK, et al. Small-animal PET with a σ-ligand, 11C-SA4503, detects spontaneous pituitary tumors in aged rats. J Nucl Med 2013;54(8):1377–83.

40. Stieger SM, Wenker C, Ziegler-Gohm D, et al. Ureterolithiasis and papilloma formation in the ureter of a guinea pig. Vet Radiol Ultrasound 2003;44(3):326–9.

41. Okewole PA, Odeyemi PS, Oladunmade MA, et al. An outbreak of Streptococcus pyogenes infection associated with calcium oxalate urolithiasis in guinea pigs (Cavia porcellus). Lab Anim 1991;25:184–6.

42. Buss S, Bourdeau JE. Calcium balance in laboratory rabbits. Miner Electrolyte Metab 1984;10:127–32.

43. Tsubouchi T, Saito T, Mizutani F, et al. Stimulatory action of itopride hydrochloride on colonic motor activity in vitro and in vivo. J Pharmacol Exp Ther 2003;306(2): 787–93.

44. Park SJ, Choi EJ, Yoon YH, et al. The effects of prucalopride on postoperative ileus in guinea pigs. Yonsei Med J 2013;54(4):845–53.

45. Clark TS, Clark DD, Hoyt RF Jr. Pharmacokinetic comparison of sustained-release and standard buprenorphine in mice. J Am Assoc Lab Anim Sci 2014;53(4): 387–91.

46. Jirkof P, Tourvieille A, Cinelli P, et al. Buprenorphine for pain relief in mice: repeated injections vs sustained-release depot formulation. Lab Anim 2015; 49(3):177–87.

47. Foley PL, Liang H, Crichlow AR. Evaluation of a sustained-release formulation of buprenorphine for analgesia in rats. J Am Assoc Lab Anim Sci 2011;50(2): 198–204.
48. Seymour TL, Adams SC, Felt SA, et al. Postoperative analgesia due to sustained-release buprenorphine, sustained-release meloxicam, and carprofen gel in a model of incisional pain in rats (Rattus norvegicus). J Am Assoc Lab Anim Sci 2016;55(3):300–5.
49. Smith BJ, Wegenast DJ, Hansen RJ, et al. Pharmacokinetics and paw withdrawal pressure in female guinea pigs (*Cavia porcellus*) treated with sustained-release buprenorphine and buprenorphine hydrochloride. J Am Assoc Lab Anim Sci 2016;55(6):789–93.
50. Kendall LV, Wegenast DJ, Smith BJ, et al. Efficacy of sustained-release buprenorphine in an experimental laparotomy model in female mice. J Am Assoc Lab Anim Sci 2016;55(1):66–73.
51. Peled I, Shohat B, Gassner S, et al. Excision of epithelial tumors: CO_2 laser versus conventional methods. Cancer Lett 1976;2:41–5.
52. Wang Z, Devaiah AK, Feng L, et al. Fiber-guided CO_2 laser surgery in an animal model. Photomed Laser Surg 2006;24:646–50.
53. Collarile T, Di Girolamo N, Nardini G, et al. Fire ignition during laser surgery in pet rodents. BMC Vet Res 2012;8:177.
54. Selleri P, Di Girolamo N. A randomized controlled trial of factors influencing fire occurrence during laser surgery of cadaveric rodents under simulated mask anesthesia. J Am Vet Med Assoc 2015;246(6):639–44.
55. Cetin Y, Alkis I, Sendag S, et al. Long-term effect of deslorelin implant on ovarian pre-antral follicles and uterine histology in female rats. Reprod Domest Anim 2013;48(2):195–9.
56. Grosset C, Peters S, Peron F, et al. Contraceptive effect and potential side-effects of deslorelin acetate implants in rats (*Rattus norvegicus*): preliminary observations. Can J Vet Res 2012;76(3):209–14.
57. Edwards B, Smith A, Skinner DC. Dose and durational effects of the gonadotropin-releasing hormone agonist, deslorelin: the male rat (*Rattus norvegicus*) as a model. J Zoo Wildl Med 2013;44(4 Suppl):S97–101.
58. Kohutova S, Jekl V, Knotek Z, et al. The effect of deslorelin acetate on the oestrous cycle of female guinea pigs. Vet Med 2015;60(3):155–60.
59. Forman C, Wehrend A, Goericke-Pesch S. A Deslorelin implants are suitable for contraception in female, but not male guinea pigs. In: Proceedings of the VIII International Symposium on Canine and Feline Reproduction. Paris (France), June 22–25, 2016. p. 135.
60. Jekl V, Gumpenberger M, Jeklova E, et al. Impact of pelleted diets with different mineral compositions on the crown size of mandibular cheek teeth and mandibular relative density in degus (Octodon degus). Vet Rec 2011;168(24):641.
61. Long CV. Common dental disorders of the degu (*Octodon degus*). J Vet Dent 2012;29(3):158–65.
62. Minarikova A, Hauptman K, Jeklova E, et al. Diseases in pet guinea pigs: a retrospective study in 1000 animals. Vet Rec 2015;177:200.
63. Müller J, Clauss M, Codron D, et al. Tooth length and incisal wear and growth in guinea pigs (Cavia porcellus) fed diets of different abrasiveness. J Anim Physiol Anim Nutr (Berl) 2015;99(3):591–604.
64. Jekl V, Hauptman K, Knotek Z. Diseases in pet degus: a retrospective study in 300 animals. J Small Anim Pract 2011;52(2):107–12.

65. Jekl V, Krejcirova L, Buchtova M, et al. Effect of high phosphorus diet on tooth microstructure of rodent incisors. Bone 2011;49(3):479–84.
66. Vergneau-Grosset C, Keel MK, Goldsmith D, et al. Description of the prevalence, histologic characteristics, concomitant abnormalities, and outcomes of mammary gland tumors in companion rats (Rattus norvegicus): 100 cases (1990-2015). J Am Vet Med Assoc 2016;249(10):1170–9.
67. Hotchkiss CE. Effect of the surgical removal of subcutaneous tumors on survival of rats. J Am Vet Med Assoc 1995;206:1575–9.
68. Thurman JD, Bucci TJ, Hart RW, et al. Survival, body weight, and spontaneous neoplasms in ad libitum-fed and food restricted Fischer-344 rats. Toxicol Pathol 1994;22:1–9.
69. Rao GN. Influence of diet on tumors of hormonal tissues. Prog Clin Biol Res 1996; 394:41–56.
70. Planas-Silva MD, Rutherford TM, Stone MC. Prevention of age-related spontaneous mammary tumors in outbred rats by late ovariectomy. Cancer Detect Prev 2008;32:65–71.

Evidence-Based Advances in Avian Medicine

Noémie M. Summa, Dr Med Vet, IPSAV[a],
David Sanchez-Migallon Guzman, LV, MS, DECZM (Avian, Small Mammal), DACZM[b],*

KEYWORDS

- Avian • Diagnosis • Cardiology • Prognosis • Atherosclerosis • Avian bornavirus
- Reproductive disorders • Pharmacokinetics studies

KEY POINTS

- Fecal Gram stains should be use as a parallel testing strategy with fecal culture, because many of the bacteria identified in cytology might ultimately not be isolated in culture.
- For the assessment of the fractures of the pectoral girdle, addition of a caudoventral-craniodorsal oblique radiographic view made at 45° to the frontal plane improves sensitivity and specificity of ventrodorsal radiographs.
- Rocuronium bromide topically results in safe and reliable mydriasis in the multiple species of birds evaluated, which might be advantageous for evaluation of the posterior chamber during ophthalmic examination.
- Avian bornavirus can be transmitted vertically, whereas horizontal transmission by direct contact appears to be an inefficient route of infection in immunocompetent fully fledged domestic canaries and cockatiels in experimental conditions.
- Deslorelin acetate implants successfully prevent egg laying in cockatiels, pigeons, and Japanese quails with variable efficacy and duration between species and without apparent adverse effects.

INTRODUCTION

This article presents relevant advances in avian medicine and surgery over the past 5 years. New information has been published to improve clinical diagnosis in avian diseases, especially in diagnostic imaging, cardiovascular medicine, and ophthalmology. This article also describes new pharmacokinetic studies on antimicrobial, antifungal,

Disclosure Statement: The authors have nothing to disclose.
[a] Department of Clinical Sciences, School of Veterinary Medicine, University of Montreal, 3200, rue Sicotte, Saint-Hyacinthe, QC J2S 7M2, Canada; [b] Department of Medicine and Epidemiology, School of Veterinary Medicine, University of California, Davis, 1 Garrod Drive, Davis, CA 95616, USA
* Corresponding author.
E-mail address: guzman@ucdavis.edu

cardiac, anticonvulsant, and psychotropic drugs, with a direct application on therapeutic management of a large number of disorders and diseases. Advances in the understanding and treatment of common avian disorders, including proventricular dilation disease, atherosclerosis, and reproductive disorders, are presented in this article as well. This article does not cover advances in avian pain management and anesthesia, despite being one of the most remarkable areas in which avian medicine has progressed, because they are covered elsewhere in this issue. Although important progress has been made over the past years, there is still much research that needs to be done regarding the etiology, pathophysiology, diagnosis, and treatment of avian diseases to support an evidence-based approach (**Table 1**).

EVIDENCE-BASED ADVANCES IN DIAGNOSIS
Laboratory Testing

The normal gastrointestinal flora of healthy psittacine birds is composed predominately of gram-positive bacteria. Pathogenic bacteria are usually gram-negative, and normal percentage of gram-negative is usually controversial among clinicians. In a recent study in healthy Hispaniolan Amazon parrots fed 100% pelleted diet, fecal Gram stains from cloacal swabs showed 97% of gram-positive bacteria with 86.2% of gram-positive rods, and 14.7% of gram-positive cocci.[1] Although 70% of the birds had 100% of gram-positive bacteria, 30% of the parrots had from 3% to 15% of gram-negative bacteria on Gram stains. *Escherichia coli* was the only gram-negative bacteria identified on cloacal swab culture. Overall, agreement between Gram stain and culture was fair, with a tendency for culture to underestimate the true diversity of bacterial flora. This study highlights that gram-negative bacteria are not uncommon in healthy Hispaniolan Amazon parrots and that Gram stains may be of higher value than culture as screening tests for health assessment. Culture should be performed with abnormal Gram stains and/or digestive clinical signs.

Liver enzymes and bile acids are commonly used to evaluate the liver in birds. To determine the threshold for detecting acute liver injury by plasma biochemical testing, liver enzymes were measured in fasted Indian ring-necked parakeets (*Psittacula krameri manillensis*) after experimental induction of liver injury through hepatic biopsy or crush injury.[2] Plasma sorbitol dehydrogenase (SDH) activity was the most specific indicator of liver injury in this species, increased above 12 U/L at 12 hours, and returned to normal values after. Bile acid concentrations and c-glutamyl transferase activity were not affected. Increases in serum aminotransferase, lactate dehydrogenase, and alkaline phosphatase in the first 24 hours were assumed to be related to muscle injury as the creatinine kinase was elevated. Further studies are needed to evaluate the use of SDH in liver injury diagnosis in other avian species.

Acute phase proteins (APP), such as serum amyloid A (SAA), are used to assess acute and chronic inflammation.[3–6] APPs are classified as negative and positive, and major, moderate, and minor.[3–6] Positive APPs increase and decrease shortly after an inflammatory event but continued inflammatory stimulus results in persistent and progressive increases.[3–6] A significant increase in SAA was observed in falcons with inflammatory diseases compared with healthy birds or birds with noninflammatory disease.[3] Surprisingly, SAA activity was not associated with amyloidosis in these falcons, possibly because liver failure had already compromised the production of SAA. SAA levels remained significantly increased in falcons with chronic pododermatitis or fungal pneumonia/airsacculitis. In another study, falcons with confirmed aspergillosis showed significantly lower prealbumin values.[4] These APPs could be used as a prognostic factor to assess treatment response in this species. However, interspecies

Table 1
Grading system presenting the overall quality evidence of the main articles presented in this article

Reference	Type of Evidence	Grade	Intervention	Outcome
1				
2	Prospective blind study: Experimental animal	2	Liver enzymes measurement after acute live injury in Indian ring-necked parakeets.	Sorbitol dehydrogenase activity was the most specific indicator of liver injury in this species.
3–6	Prospective study: Experimental animal	3	Effects of rocuronium in European kestrels, common buzzards, little owls, tawny owls, and Hispaniolan Amazon parrots.	Rocuronium was safe and effective in these species.
7,8	Prospective study: Experimental animal	2	Thromboelastography values in different avian species.	Thromboelastography could be useful in avian species if provided appropriate species-specific reference ranges.
9	Observational study: Case series	1	Evaluation of the pectoral girdle via radiographs in birds of prey.	H view is recommended to assess the pectoral girdle.
10	Observational study: Case series	2	Normal computed tomography (CT) structures of the bird of several avian species.	CT could represent the imaging technique of choice to assess head lesions in birds.
11	Prospective blind study: Experimental animal	2	Echocardiographic measurements via 3 different techniques in red-tailed hawks.	Poor agreement between techniques and between observers.
12	Prospective blind study: Experimental animal	3	Measurement of large vessels via CT angiography in Hispaniolan Amazon.	Development of reference ranges, good agreement between observers.
13	Prospective study: Experimental animal	3	Effects of hooding on physiologic parameters in red-tailed hawks.	Hooded hawks had a lower heart rate and respiratory rate. No effects on stress-induced hyperthermia.
14–18	Prospective study: Experimental animal	2	Mydriatic effects of topical rocuronium in different species.	Topical rocuronium induced mydriasis with species-variation regarding effects on diameter and duration.
19–21	Prospective study: Experimental animal	3	Pharmacokinetics of a single intramuscular injection of ceftiofur-crystalline-free acid in different avian species.	Establishment of pharmacokinetics parameters of ceftiofur-crystalline-free acid in different avian species.

(continued on next page)

Table 1
(continued)

Reference	Type of Evidence	Grade	Intervention	Outcome
22–25	Prospective study: Experimental animal	3	Pharmacokinetics of enrofloxacin, danofloxacin, and marbofloxacin in Japanese quail and common pheasants.	Marbofloxacin and danofloxacin should be used over enrofloxacin for treatment of susceptible bacterial infection in Japanese quail and common pheasants.
26	Randomized trial: Experimental animal	3	Pharmacokinetics of fluconazole in drinking water in cockatiels.	Establishment of pharmacokinetics parameters of fluconazole in cockatiels.
27–30	Prospective study: Experimental animal	3	Pharmacokinetics of terbinafine in Hispaniolan Amazon parrots and red-tailed hawk.	Establishment of pharmacokinetics parameters of terbinafine in Hispaniolan Amazon parrots and red-tailed hawk.
31,32	Prospective study: Experimental animal	3	Effect of itraconazole nanosuspension in Japanese quail inoculated with aspergillosis.	Once daily 30-min inhalation of a 10% itraconazole nanosuspension is recommended for treatment of pulmonary aspergillosis in birds.
33–38	Prospective study: Experimental animal	3	Pharmacokinetics of voriconazole in avian species.	Establishment of pharmacokinetics parameters of voriconazole in different avian species.
39,40	Prospective study: Experimental animal	2	Treatment protocols of voriconazole in pigeons and falcons.	Voriconazole was effective to reduce the lesions of aspergillosis in these 2 species.
41	Case series	1	Toxicity of voriconazole in penguins.	Importance of species-specific dosing of voriconazole in penguins and plasma therapeutic drug monitoring.
42	Prospective study: Experimental animal	3	Pharmacokinetics of pimobendan in Hispaniolan Amazon parrot.	Establishment of pharmacokinetics parameters of pimobendan in Hispaniolan Amazon parrots.

(continued on next page)

Table 1
(continued)

Reference	Type of Evidence	Grade	Intervention	Outcome
43	Prospective study: Experimental animal	3	Pharmacokinetics of orally administered phenobarbital in African gray parrots.	Establishment of pharmacokinetics parameters of phenobarbital in African gray parrots.
44	Randomized trial: Experimental animal	3	Pharmacokinetics of levetiracetam in Hispaniolan Amazon parrots.	Establishment of pharmacokinetics parameters of levetiracetam in Hispaniolan Amazon parrots.
45	Prospective study: Experimental animal	3	Pharmacokinetics of paroxetine in African gray parrots.	Establishment of pharmacokinetics parameters of paroxetine in Gray parrots.
46	Prospective study: Experimental animal	3	Pharmacokinetics of amitriptyline HCl and its metabolites in African gray parrots and cockatoos.	High variation of pharmacokinetic parameters between avian species and among individuals.
47–50	Prospective study: Experimental animal	3	Assessment of transmission modalities in bornavirus.	Vertical transmission is possible in avian species affected with bornavirus.
51	Prospective study: Experimental animal	3	Effects of meloxicam on bornavirus-infected cockatiels.	Meloxicam at 0.5 mg/kg every 12 h is not recommended for the management of bornavirus-affected cockatiels.
52–54	Retrospective studies	2	Prevalence and risk factors of atherosclerosis in avian species.	Atherosclerosis was significantly associated with several factors including species, sex, age, and plasma cholesterol.
55	Randomized trial: Experimental animal	2	Experimental induction of atherosclerosis in Quaker parrots with diet changes.	Diet high in cholesterol induced advanced atherosclerotic lesions by 4 mo.
56–58	Prospective study: Experimental animal	3	Evaluation of plasma lipids in avian species.	Establishment of reference ranges.
59	Prospective study: Experimental animal	2	Effects of diet changes on plasma lipids in avian species.	Variable effects on plasma concentration of HDL-C and LDL-C.

(continued on next page)

Table 1
(continued)

Reference	Type of Evidence	Grade	Intervention	Outcome
60	Prospective study: Experimental animal	2	Effects of exercise on the plasma lipid profile in Hispaniolan Amazon parrots.	HDL-C concentrations were significantly higher in exercised parrots at 61 d and returned to near baseline by 105 d.
61–64	Randomized trial: Experimental animal	3	Evaluation of the effects deslorelin acetate implants on egg production in Japanese quail, pigeons, and cockatiels.	Deslorelin acetate implant decreased or stopped egg production these species.
65–68	Prospective study: Experimental animal	2	Evaluation of blood glucometers in avian species.	The used of blood glucometers was not recommended in avian species except in pigeons.
69	Retrospective study	3	Survey and critical appraisal of the use of statistics in avian medicine.	Overall 35.3% (128/363) of articles were considered statistically unacceptable.
70	Case report	1	Advancement flap as a novel treatment for a pododermatitis lesion in a red-tailed hawk.	Successful outcome.
71	Case report	1	Use of a vascular access port for antibiotic administration in the treatment of pododermatitis in a chicken.	Successful outcome.

variations are highly likely to affect the interpretation of APP levels. Sick or injured red-tailed hawks showed higher plasma haptoglobin and ceruloplasmin activities, 2 positive APPs, and lower plasma iron concentrations compared with healthy free-living or healthy captive birds.[6] In American flamingos, albumin was a marker for pododermatitis as a negative APP, whereas mild and chronic pododermatitis was not reflected in positive APPs.[5]

In avian species, available methods to assess coagulation for the avian practitioner include thrombocyte number estimation and measures of bleeding time and whole-blood clotting time, and both methods yield important limitations. Other diagnostic tests for dogs and cats are not available in birds, as they typically require avian-specific reagents that are not commercially available. Thromboelastography (TEG) provides a global assessment of coagulation, including the rate of clot initiation, clot kinetics, achievement of maximum clot strength, and fibrinolysis,[7] and has known a recent interest in avian species through recent publication and conference presentations. In 2 recent studies, kaolin-activated TEG was used to assess the applicability of TEG in Hispaniolan Amazon parrots,[7] as well as in scarlet ibis (*Eudocimus ruber*), American flamingos, helmeted Guinea fowl, Humboldt penguins (*Spheniscus humboldti*), and domestic chickens.[8] The studies concluded TEG with specific reference intervals could prove useful in evaluating avian hemostatic disorders and further studies are needed to develop reference ranges in avian species.

Imaging

Fractures of the pectoral girdle are frequently reported in wild birds in association with high-velocity frontal impact, such as collision with a window or vehicle. Although commonly used to diagnose fracture of the pectoral girdle, ventrodorsal (VD) and lateral views allow a limited assessment of the coracoid, scapula, and clavicle integrity due to superimposition. A new caudoventral-craniodorsal oblique radiographic view made at 45° to the frontal plane, called H view, was recently described to provide a more accurate evaluation of the thoracic girdle.[9] The combination of the H view with the standard VD view allowed detection of fractures in the pectoral girdle in 9 of 9 raptors with a sensitivity of 100% (95% confidence interval 66–100) and a specificity of 93% (68–100), whereas only 7 of 9 were detected with the standard VD alone with a sensitivity of 89% (52–100) and a specificity of 80% (52–96). The H view alone had the higher specificity of 100% (66–100) but the lowest sensitivity of 78% (40–97).[9]

Plain radiographs can be limited in the diagnosis of lesions of heads in birds. In a recent study, an atlas of normal computed tomography (CT) anatomy of the head was established in blue-and-gold macaws (*Ara ararauna*), African gray parrots (*Psittacus erithacus*), and monk parakeets (*Myiopsitta monachus*).[10] Optimal visibility of the bony structures of the head was achieved via CT with a standard soft tissue filter and pulmonary window.[10] Reconstitution of CT images in a dorsal plane provided a better visualization of some complex head structures.[10] Soft tissue structures could be assessed adequately with the use of contrast medium (Optiray [350 mg/mL], 660 mg/kg; Covidien Spa, Segrate, Italy) injected in the jugular vein.[10] The investigators suggested that CT would be the imaging technique of choice in the evaluation of lesions of the heads of birds.

Cardiology and Vascular Medicine

In a study comparing the transcoelomic, contrast transcoelomic, and transesophageal echocardiographic evaluations in red-tailed hawks (*Buteo jamaicensis*), echocardiographic measurements were deemed unreliable due to low agreement between observers and between techniques, except with the left ventricle measured by the same observer.[11] Better agreement was observed with the transesophageal approach. Measurements of the aortic diameter could not be obtained in any hawks. As a result, the same echographer should perform follow-up echocardiographic measurements, and only 20% difference from initial measurements should be considered significant.

Reference limits for the apparent diameter of the ascending aorta, abdominal aorta, pulmonary arteries, and brachiocephalic trunk in Hispaniolan Amazon parrots (*Amazona ventralis*) via CT angiography are now available.[12] Arterial diameter measurements at the described locations were reliable, and agreement between the 2 observers was good, except for the brachiocephalic trunk, and could have a diagnostic value for vascular diseases (eg, atherosclerosis). Motion artifact was a limiting factor for the accuracy of measurement. The investigators recommended performing angiography immediately after intravenous injection of 3 mL/kg iohexol (Omnipaque 240 mg/mL; GE Healthcare Inc, Princeton, NJ).

In a recent study, the effects of hooding on physiologic parameters was evaluated in red-tailed hawks (*Buteo jamaicensis*) manually restrained for 15 minutes.[13] Hooded birds had a significantly lower respiratory and heart rate compared with birds restrained without a hood.[13] There was no effect of hooding on stress-induced hyperthermia.[13]

Ophthalmology

Achievement of mydriasis for complete ophthalmic examination is challenging in birds, because of the presence of striated muscle in the iris. The effects on pupil dilation and adverse effects of the neuromuscular blocking agent rocuronium bromide were assessed in European kestrels (Falco tinnunculus),[14] common buzzards (Buteo buteo),[15] little owls (Athene noctua),[15] tawny owls (Strix aluco),[16] and in Hispaniolan Amazon parrots,[17,18] with a single topical instillation in each eye of 0.12 mg, 0.40 mg, 0.35 mg, 0.20 mg, and 0.15 to 0.20 mg of rocuronium bromide, respectively. Maximal pupillary diameter (MPD) was observed at 40 minutes in little owls,[16] 50 minutes in parrots,[17] 90 minutes in kestrels,[14] and 110 minutes in buzzards.[15] In tawny owls, 2 instillations of rocuronium did not significantly change the MPD compared with a single instillation, but shortened the onset of MPD from 80 minutes to 60 minutes and increased the duration of mydriasis.[16] Pupillary reflexes (PLR) were absent at 10 minutes in all parrots,[17] and at 20 minutes in all kestrels.[14] The pupillary light reflex never completely disappeared during the time evaluated in the study in some tawny owls, possibly related to the heavy iris pigmentation.[16] Pigment-binding effect of heavily pigmented iris could cause an initial accumulation of the drug with a delay of mydriasis onset followed by a slow release within the eye with a prolonged duration of action.[15] PLR was normal in parrots after 420 minutes or 24 hours,[17,18] whereas PLR was normal at 270 minutes in kestrels,[14] and at 240 minutes in tawny owls after a single instillation.[16] Ocular irritation, local and systemic muscle paralysis, and respiratory distress were not observed. Superficial corneal ulceration was observed at 24 hours in 2 of 10 parrots[17] and 3 of 8 parrots had transient inferior eyelid paresis after receiving rocuronium that resolved within 24 hours in the other study.[18] Theses variable results could be related to interspecies variations or to study design differences. The third eyelid was retracted for 1 minute following rocuronium instillation in all studies, except in 1 study in parrots.[17] In this study, the Amazon parrots received a topical administration of proparacaine to avoid third eyelid movement during rocuronium application.[17] In the other study in parrots, the birds were manually restrained in lateral recumbency with the apex of the cornea positioned upward for 2 minutes following administration in each eye.[18]

EVIDENCE-BASED ADVANCES IN THERAPEUTICS
Antimicrobial Drugs

Ceftiofur is a third-generation cephalosporin with bactericidal activity against gram-positive and gram-negative, aerobic and anaerobic bacteria, by inhibiting bacterial cell wall synthesis. It is available as ceftiofur crystalline-free acid (CCFA), a sustained-release formulation with an oil base. In red-tailed hawks, when targeting a plasma ceftiofur concentration of 4 μg/mL, CCFA administration should be repeated every 36 or 45 hours for the 10 mg/kg dose and every 96 or 120 hours for the 20 mg/kg dose intramuscularly (IM) for gram-negative and gram-positive infections, respectively.[19] In American flamingos (Phoenicopterus ruber) receiving 10 mg/kg of CCFA IM, plasma ceftiofur concentrations remained above the target minimum inhibitory concentration (MIC) (1 μg/mL) for 72 hours in all birds and 96 hours in 82% of birds.[20] Little to no inflammation at the sites of injection was observed 10 days after a single CCFA administration in hawks using a 25-gauge needle,[19] and no palpable abnormalities were noted at the site of injection in flamingos.[20] Pharmacokinetics studies of CCFA have been performed in other avian species (**Table 2**).[21,22]

Table 2
Pharmacokinetic parameters of ceftiofur-crystalline-free acid after a single intramuscular injection in red-tailed hawks (n = 10), American flamingos (n = 11), helmeted Guinea fowl (n = 14), and American black ducks (n = 20) analyzed by compartmental methods

Species	Tested Recommended Dosage	Mean Cmax, μg/mL	Mean Tmax, h	$T_{1/2}$, h	Target Plasma Concentration, μg/mL	Reference
Red-tailed hawk (*Buteo jamaicensis*)	10, 20 mg/kg IM Gram–: q36 h at 10 mg/kg q96 h at 20 mg/kg Gram+: q45 h at 10 mg/kg q120 h at 20 mg/kg	10 mg/kg: 6.8 20 mg/kg: 15.1	10 mg/kg: 6.4 20 mg/kg: 6.7	10 mg/kg: 29 20 mg/kg: 50	>4.0	[19]
American flamingos (*Phoenicopterus ruber*)	10 mg/kg IM, q72–96 h	7.49	27	39.9	>1	[20]
Helmeted Guinea fowl (*Numida meleagris*)	10 mg/kg IM, q72 h	5.6	19.3	29	≤1	[21]
American black ducks (*Anas rubripes*)	10 mg/kg IM, q72 h	13.1	24	32	>4.0	[22]

Abbreviations: Cmax, maximal concentration; IM, intramuscular; q, every; Tmax, time of maximal concentration; T1/2, terminal half-life.

Fluoroquinolones are bactericidal concentration-dependent antimicrobials with activity against gram-negative organisms, less activity against gram-positive organisms, minimal activity against anaerobic bacteria, and occasional activity against *Chlamydia* spp, *Mycoplasma* spp, and *Mycobacterium* spp. In Japanese quail (*Coturnix japonica*) receiving a separate intravenous and oral dose of enrofloxacin at 10 mg/kg, danofloxacin at 10 mg/kg, and marbofloxacin at 5 mg/kg, the highest bioavailability was observed for danofloxacin followed by marbofloxacin, with low intersubject variability.[23] In contrast, bioavailability for enrofloxacin was low, with high intersubject variability, possibly related to significant metabolism of enrofloxacin to ciprofloxacin with a first-pass effect. Similar findings were found in other pharmacokinetics of enrofloxacin and marbofloxacin in Japanese quail and common pheasants (*Phasianus colchicus*),[24] whereas danofloxacin had a good oral bioavailability in pheasants.[25] Based on these results, danofloxacin or marbofloxacin would be preferred over enrofloxacin for treatment of infections with susceptible bacteria in Japanese quail and pheasants in those countries in which they can be legally administered in food-producing animals.

Antifungal Drugs

Fungal infections, such as candidiasis or aspergillosis are commonly reported in avian species. Fluconazole inhibits ergosterol synthesis in the fungal cell membranes and possesses activity against *Candida* spp, *Cryptococcus* spp, *Blastomyces* spp, *Coccidiodes* spp, and *Histoplasma* spp. In cockatiels (*Nymphicus hollandicus*), treatment with fluconazole administered orally at a dosage of 5 mg/kg once daily or 10 mg/kg every 48 hours or administered in the drinking water at a concentration of 100 mg/L resulted in plasma concentrations in most cockatiels that exceeded the human MIC of most strains of *Candida albicans*.[26] This study provides a valuable alternative option to the frequent oral treatment administration required with other antifungal drugs.

Terbinafine, an allylamine thought to be fungicidal that inhibits the synthesis of ergosterol by blocking the enzyme squalene monooxygenase, has an activity against *Microsporum* spp, *Trichophyton* spp, *Candida* spp, *Aspergillus* spp, *Blastomyces* spp, and *Histoplasma* spp. In Hispaniolan Amazon parrots, plasma terbinafine concentrations were maintained above in vitro MIC for approximately 1 hour and 4 hours in birds nebulized with a crushed tablet solution and a raw powder solution, respectively, using a nebulizer with 0.5 to 10 μm particles, over 15 minutes.[27] Higher concentrations of solution, longer nebulization, or more frequent administration are likely required to reach therapeutic plasma concentrations. Although neither formulation provided systemic plasma concentrations for a clinically relevant period, tissue concentrations could have heavier clinical implications. In the same species, a single dose of oral terbinafine hydrochloride at 60 mg/kg showed a peak concentration within the range for the in vitro MIC for *Aspergillus flavus* (0.01–0.5 μg/mL) and *Aspergillus fumigatus* (0.02–5.0 μg/mL) with no adverse effect.[28] The pharmacokinetics of terbinafine have also been evaluated in red-tailed hawks following administration of 15, 30, and 60 mg/kg orally, and have shown that the volume of distribution of oral terbinafine decreased with increasing doses, suggesting an accumulation in deep tissues.[29] As the drug eliminates slowly in this species, long-term administration of terbinafine should be done with caution (**Table 3**).[30]

Itraconazole is a triazole antifungal agent, commonly used in birds for treatment of aspergillosis. Japanese quails were inoculated in the trachea with a low-spore and high-spore dose of *A fumigatus* in a study evaluating the efficacy of itraconazole nanosuspensions.[31] Starting 2 hours after inoculation, the birds were nebulized with 2 nanosuspensions (mean particle size of 180–230 nm) of 10% or 4% of itraconazole,

Table 3
Pharmacokinetic parameters of terbinafine after a single oral administration in red-tailed hawks (n = 10), African penguins (n = 10), and Hispaniolan Amazon parrots (n = 6) analyzed by compartmental methods

Species	Recommended Dose	Tested Doses, mg/kg	Cmax, µg/mL	Tmax, h	$T_{1/2}$, h	Target Plasma Concentration, µg/mL	Reference
Red-tailed hawk (Buteo jamaicensis)	22 mg/kg IM, q24 h	15 30 60	0.3 1.2 2	5.4 3.4 5.1	14.7 17.5 13.3	>1	29
African penguin (Spheniscus demersus)	15 mg/kg IM, q24 h	3 7 15	0.1 0.2 0.2	2.7 1.6 2.4	10 13 17	0.8–1.6 (Aspergillus fumigatus)	30
Hispaniolan Amazon parrots (Amazona ventralis)	≥60 mg/kg, PO, q8h	60	353	6.4	8.7	Failed to reach 1–4 µg/mL	28

Abbreviations: Cmax, maximal concentration; IM, intramuscular; q, every; Tmax, time of maximal concentration; T1/2, terminal half-life.

once daily for 30 minutes and for 6 days.[31] Inhalation of 10% itraconazole suspension completely blocked the development of aspergillosis in the quails exposed to the low-spore dose, and retarded the disease course without preventing lethality in birds inoculated with a high-spore dose. Inhalation of 4% itraconazole suspension was less effective than the 10% suspension.[31] The same investigators showed in a previous study that the administration of 10% itraconazole nanosuspension for 5 days resulted in tissue concentration of the primary active metabolite hydroxyl-itraconazole within the range of 1 μg/g lung tissue for 72 hours following the last dose, reaching the MIC of *A fumigatus* of 0.5 μg/mL.[32] However, at this concentration, systemic absorption of itraconazole and its primary metabolite were observed; therefore, this route may not prevent systemic adverse effects related to the azoles in birds.[32] The study concluded that once-daily 30-minute inhalation of a 10% itraconazole nanosuspension is required to obtain active tissue concentrations of itraconazole and its metabolite and for the treatment of pulmonary aspergillosis in birds.

Voriconazole inhibits ergosterol synthesis in fungal cell membranes by inhibiting the fungal cytochrome P450 enzyme. In a study in red-tailed hawks receiving single and multiple dosing of 10 mg/kg, voriconazole concentrations exceeded at least 4 times the MIC to inhibit 90% (MIC90) of *Aspergillus* spp (1 μg/mL) and remained above the MIC90 for 8.8 ± 1.1 hours after single dosing and 6.5 ± 1.5 hours after multiple dosing, suggesting a dosing every 8 hours for prolonged therapy.[33] Pharmacokinetic studies of voriconazole have also been performed in other avian species **(Table 4)**.[33–37,39,40] Toxicity of voriconazole resulting in neurologic clinical signs has been reported in penguins.[41] Caution should be applied when extrapolating a dose from a different avian species, because voriconazole shows saturable and nonlinear pharmacokinetics in most species; therefore, the drug's pharmacokinetics are dependent on the administered dose. Dose extrapolation is further complicated because voriconazole induces its own metabolism enzymes after repeated administration in some species but not in others.[34]

Cardiovascular Drugs

Pimobendan is a novel cardiotonic vasodilator with a positive inotropic effect via mobilization of intracellular calcium, calcium-sensitizing effect on cardiac myofibril, and pulmonary arterial and venous dilation. Its bioavailability is much lower in parrots than other species and a dose of 10 mg/kg is recommended in Hispaniolan Amazon parrots to reach target pimobendan plasma concentrations based on human studies.[42] In this study, oral absorption was better when using a crushed tablet over raw powder mixture, with a terminal half-life of 2.1 hours and a mean plasma concentration peak of 8.26 ng/mL at 3 hours.

Anticonvulsant Drugs

Phenobarbital is an anticonvulsant barbiturate that inhibits seizures at doses lower than those that produce anesthesia.[43] It is effective as an anticonvulsant in part because of its potentiating action on the inhibitory neurotransmitter gamma aminobutyric acid, which increases the seizure threshold and lowers the electrical activity of the seizure focus.[43] In a pharmacokinetic study in African gray parrots,[72] at a dosage of 20 mg/kg orally, Cmax values were much lower than the targeted plasma concentrations of 30 μg/mL, and the study concluded that treatment of seizure disorders in African gray parrots with phenobarbital at the doses described in the study may not produce therapeutic control.

Levetiracetam is a newer antiepileptic drug that acts by inhibiting the excitatory neurotransmitter release via binding to the synaptic vesicle protein, by modulating

Table 4
Pharmacokinetic parameters of voriconazole after a single or multiple oral administration in red-tailed hawks (n = 8–12), African gray parrots (n = 12), Hispaniolan Amazon parrots (n = 12–15), Mallard ducks (n = 6), pigeons (n = 6), Falcons (n-6), chickens (n = 12), and Japanese quail

Species	Recommended Dose	Dosage	Mean Cmax, µg/mL	Mean Tmax, h	$T_{1/2}$, h	Target Plasma Concentration, µg/mL	Reference
Red-tailed hawk (Buteo jamaicensis)	10 mg/kg PO q8 h	10 mg/kg PO	4.7	2.0	2.8	>>1	33
		10 mg/kg PO q12 for 14 d	4.5	2.4	2.1		
African gray parrots (Psittacus erithacus timneh)	12–18 mg/kg PO q12 h	6 mg/kg PO diluted in water	0.54	2	1.11	>0.4	34
		12 mg/kg PO diluted in water	1.89	4	1.59		
		12 mg/kg PO diluted in suspending agent	3.02	2	1.07		
		18 mg/kg PO diluted in water	5.67	2	1.59		
Hispaniolan Amazon parrots (Amazona ventralis)	18 mg/kg PO q8 h	12 mg/kg PO	2.49	1.00	0.90	>0.4	35
		24 mg/kg PO	5.08	2.00	1.25		
Mallard ducks (Anas platyrhynchos)	20 mg/kg PO q8-12 h with or without food	10 mg/kg PO	3.94	0.77	1.11	>0.5	36
		20 mg/kg PO without liquid diet	11.06	1.33	1.01		
		20 mg/kg PO with liquid diet	10.91	2	1.79		
Racing pigeons (Columba livia domestica)	10 mg/kg PO q12 h	10 mg/kg PO q12 h for 14 d	N/A	N/A	N/A	> 0.25	39
		20 mg/kg PO q24 h for 14 d	N/A	N/A	N/A	Improvement of in situ lesions of aspergillosis	
Falcons	12.5 mg/kg PO q12 h in meat	12.5 mg/kg PO q12 h for 14 d without meat	1.9–7.5	N/A	N/A	>1	40
		12.5 mg/kg PO q12 h for 14 d with meat	0.2–1.7	N/A	N/A		
Chickens	10 mg/kg PO q12 h	10 mg/kg PO	0.88	0.75	1.45	>0.25	37
Japanese quail (Coturnix japonica)	40 mg/kg PO < q24 h	20 mg/kg PO	5.8	2	N/A	>0.5	38
		40 mg/kg PO	6.9	2	N/A		

Abbreviations: Cmax, maximal concentration; N/A, non applicable; PO, by mouth; q, every; Tmax, time of maximal concentration; T1/2, terminal half-life.

calcium-dependent exocytosis of neurotransmitters, and by suppressing the inhibitory effect of Zn^{2+} on GABA and glycine-gated currents. In Hispaniolan Amazon parrots, oral administration of levetiracetam at 50 mg/kg every 8 hours or 100 mg/kg every 12 hours is recommended as a starting dosage based on levetiracetam plasma concentrations.[44]

Psychotropic Drugs

Paroxetine is a psychoactive drug that is functionally classified as a selective serotonin reuptake inhibitor (SSRI). SSRIs exhibit their action by blocking the presynaptic receptors responsible for the reuptake of serotonin (5-hydroxytryptamine [5-HT]), thereby increasing serotonergic activity at the postsynaptic membrane. Paroxetine is one of the most potent, with a twofold to threefold greater affinity for the serotonin receptor than serotonin itself, as well as being very selective. In a pharmacokinetic study in African gray parrots,[45] it was found that paroxetine had a rapid distribution and elimination after intravenous administration. Oral administration of paroxetine HCl dissolved in water resulted in a relatively slow absorption with a Tmax of 5.9 ± 2.6 hours and low oral bioavailability of 31% ± 15%. Repeated administration resulted in higher rate of absorption, most likely due to a saturation the cytochrome P450-mediated first-pass metabolism. This study concluded that oral administration of paroxetine HCl at 4 mg/kg every 12 hours in parrots results in plasma concentrations within the therapeutic range recommended for the treatment of depression in humans. Further studies are needed to demonstrate the clinical efficacy of this dosage regimen in parrots with behavioral disorders.

Amitriptyline is a tricyclic antidepressant, used to manage feather-destructive behavior in psittacine birds. The oral administration of a single dose of 1.5 mg/kg, 4.5 mg/kg, and 9 mg/kg of amitriptyline in African gray parrots and cockatoos (Cacatua spp) resulted in highly variable disposition among and within species.[46] The current recommended dosage of 1 to 5 mg/kg every 12 hours in psittacine birds appears insufficient to achieve serum concentrations within the human therapeutic range (60 ng/mL) and did not yield predictable concentrations.[46] Doses of up to 9 mg/kg may be necessary to achieve human therapeutic range; however, it was associated with clinical signs of toxicity in one bird.[46] In addition, elimination half-life varied from 1.6 to 91.2 hours, preventing determination of safe dosing intervals.[46] Therefore, therapeutic drug monitoring combined with response to therapy is indicated to determine individual therapeutic ranges.

EVIDENCE-BASED ADVANCES IN COMMON DISORDERS
Advances in Avian Bornavirus

Avian bornaviruses (ABVs) are causative agents of proventricular dilatation disease (PDD), a widely distributed disease in avian species associated with central nervous system clinical signs and impaired gastrointestinal motility and function.[47] The transmission is thought to be through ingestion of contaminated drop. Recent efforts have been made to understand the transmission of these viruses among birds.[48] In a study with experimental infection of cockatiels with ABV-4 and canaries (Serinus canaria forma domestica) with ABV-C1, horizontal transmission of ABV by direct contact between adult infected and healthy cockatiels or canaries was inefficient, suggesting that horizontal transmission of ABV by direct contact is inefficient in immunocompetent fully fledged domestic canaries and cockatiels.[48] Using fertilized eggs obtained from 4 pairs of sun conures (Aratinga solstitialis) infected with ABV-2, ABV RNA could be detected in early embryos of all pairs, in brain, liver, and eyes of late-stage embryos of one of the pairs and in blood of a 2-week-old hatchling of this pair, demonstrating that vertical transmission could occur in this species.[47] In another study with eggs obtained from wild Canada geese (*Branta canadensis*) in an endemic area, ABV RNA was found in the yolk of one egg.[49] However, ABV RNA was not detected in any embryos or newly hatched goslings, and none of the newly hatched goslings showed ABV antibodies.

As PDD is a significant cause of morbidity and mortality in captive birds, better understanding of pathogenicity is primordial. In one study, psittacine birds with a high ABV RNA load in crop and cloaca combined with high anti-ABV antibodies were at higher risk to develop clinical signs of PDD, suggesting that humoral antibodies do not protect against the disease.[50] The meaning of the detection of ABV RNA and antibodies at a low and inconsistent level for a single bird is still unclear.

Treatment options are still limited for this disease. In experimental inoculation of cockatiels with ABV-4, all meloxicam-treated ABV-challenged birds receiving 0.5 mg/kg of meloxicam orally every 12 hours for 130 days, died or were euthanized because of severe weight loss and depression between 60 to 118 days after challenge, whereas all untreated ABV-challenged birds survived to 150 days after challenge, despite reverse-transcriptase polymerase chain reaction positive for ABV-4.[51] Meloxicam-treated birds without ABV inoculation survived to the end of study, in apparent good health. Other treatment options are under investigation, including immunomodulating therapy or other anti-inflammatory drugs, such as robenacoxib.

Advances in Atherosclerosis

Atherosclerosis is a chronic inflammatory fibroproliferative vascular disease characterized by vascular inflammation and buildup of cholesterol, fibrin, calcium, and cellular waste products within the intima of the vessel wall.[52–54] Atherosclerosis is considered the most common vascular disease in captive psittacine birds. Clinical signs are associated with flow-limiting stenosis. A large retrospective case-control study in North America showed that the overall prevalence of type IV to VI atherosclerotic lesions was 6.8% in psittacine birds.[52] Older age and female sex were important risk factors, and the risk increased dramatically in birds of 20 to 30 years of age.[52] Reproductive diseases were the only identified modifiable risk factor.[52] Association between *Chlamydia* spp and atherosclerosis is controversial based on published data.[52,53] African gray parrots (*P erithacus*), Amazon parrots (*Amazona* spp), and cockatiels (*N hollandicus*) were more likely to develop atherosclerotic lesions, whereas cockatoos (*Cacatua* spp) and macaws (*Ara* spp) were less likely.[52]

The differences observed in prevalence among psittacine genera was found to be possibly explained in part by differences in plasma total cholesterol concentrations.[54] In an experimental study in Quaker parrots (*Myiopsitta monachus*), atherosclerotic lesion severity and arterial cholesterol content increased linearly with time, and both were significantly correlated with plasma cholesterol concentration.[55] Similar findings were reported in another study, in which psittacine birds with atherosclerosis had significantly higher cholesterol level than control birds.[54] However, according to certain investigators, cholesterol can be problematic as a bio-indicator of cardiovascular disease in parrots, due to its variation related to the female reproductive cycle.[54] Association between atherosclerotic lesions and low-density lipoprotein (LDL-C) or high-density lipoprotein (HDL-C) cholesterol levels is controversial. In Quaker parrots, atherosclerosis was associated with increased LDL-C levels and dyslipidemia, with a shift from HDL-C to LDL-C as the main plasma lipoproteins,[55] whereas a high correlation with atherosclerosis prevalence was found with increasing HDL-C but not LDL-C in a large retrospective study with multiple psittacine birds.[54] Interpretation of lipid panel profile can be challenging, especially as reference intervals in psittacine birds have been established in Amazon parrots, African gray parrots (*P erithacus*) and pionus.[57,58]

Effects of diet and exercise on plasma lipid level have also been investigated. In Quaker parrots, diet increased in cholesterol (1%) induced advanced atherosclerotic lesions by 4 months and increased plasma cholesterol concentrations.[55] However, no apparent effect of pelleted versus seed-based diets was observed on plasma cholesterol or triglyceride concentrations in Quaker parrots in another study.[56] African gray parrots fed a high-fat diet rich in saturated fatty acids had significantly higher plasma cholesterol levels than parrots on a low-fat diet or high-fat diet enriched in omega-6 unsaturated fatty acids,[59] whereas there was no significant difference in cholesterol and lipoprotein plasma concentrations between African gray parrots fed a pelletized versus seed-based diet in another study.[57] Although evaluating the effects of exercise on plasma lipid profiles in Hispaniolan Amazon parrots with naturally occurring hypercholesterolemia, HDL-C concentrations were significantly higher in exercised parrots at 61 days, which is associated with reduced risk of cardiovascular disease in humans.[60] However, HDL-C concentrations returned to near baseline by 105 days, possibly related to declining participation in aviary flight sessions in the latter part of the study.[60] No significant effect of exercise on LDL-C or total cholesterol concentration was observed and the parrots remained hypercholesterolemic during the study.[60]

Advances in Reproductive Inhibition

Reproductive disorders, such as chronic egg laying or dystocia, are one of the most common diseases in companion birds. Surgical management can be challenging, especially in smaller species, and medical therapy is often preferred. Several studies have been recently performed to assess the effect of deslorelin acetate implant, a gonadotropin-releasing hormone agonist. In Japanese quail, 6 of 10 quails ceased laying eggs for approximately 70 days after receiving a 4.7-mg deslorelin acetate implant, whereas 7 of 10 quails ceased laying eggs for 100 days and for at least 182 days after receiving two 4.7-mg and one 9.4-mg implant of deslorelin acetate, respectively.[61,62] Administration of a 4.7-mg deslorelin implant in pigeons (n = 10) completely ceased egg production in all birds in the treatment groups from 49 to 63 days.[63] In cockatiel receiving 4.7-mg deslorelin acetate implants, none of the deslorelin-implanted birds laid eggs within the first 180 days of the study, whereas 11 of 13 placebo-implanted birds laid eggs between 12 and 42 days following implantation.[64] After 180 days, only 5 of 13 deslorelin-implanted birds laid their first egg between 192 and 230 days following implant placement. The effect of deslorelin acetate implants on sex hormones has also been evaluated. In Japanese quail, plasma androstenedione, 17β-estradiol, and testosterone concentrations did not correlate with the efficacy of deslorelin acetate.[61,62] In female pigeons, deslorelin administration significantly reduced serum luteinizing hormone concentrations compared with pretreatment levels at 7, 28, 56, and 84 days.[63] Overall, deslorelin acetate implants appear safe in avian species. No adverse effects were observed in Japanese quail on histopathology following administration of a 4.7-mg, 2 × 4.7-mg, or 9.4-mg deslorelin implants.[61,62] No effect on weight was observed in female pigeons and Japanese quail following the administration of deslorelin implant.[61-63] Mild transient erythema and soft tissue swelling were observed following implant placement in both control and treatment groups in cockatiels, and resolved within 72 hours.

CURRENT CONTROVERSIES AND CLINICAL TOPICS REQUIRING ADDITIONAL EVIDENCE
Blood Glucometer Use

In a study in domestic pigeons (*Columba livia domestica*), a commercial, handled, human glucometer (Accu-check; Roche Diagnostics, Mannheim, Germany) underestimated systematically blood glucose (BG) concentrations in normoglycemic, hypoglycemic, and hyperglycemic birds compared with a standard autoanalyzer, following experimental induction of hypoglycemia and hyperglycemia.[65] As there was a significant correlation between results measured by the glucometer and the autoanalyzer, the investigators concluded that the real BG concentrations in pigeons could be predicted based on results obtained by this glucometer. In Hispaniolan Amazon parrots,[66,67] the bias between the readings of veterinary-handled and human-handled glucometers and auto-analyzers for BG concentrations was shown to be inconsistent. Therefore, the use of glucometer was not recommended in this species, similarly to rhinoceros auklets in an older study.[68] Further studies are needed to evaluate the efficacy of blood glucometers in birds.

Statistical Analysis

A recent study performed by Dr Beaufrère and colleagues[69] reviewed all avian research articles that were published in 8 veterinary journals from 2007 to 2011 for the quality of their statistical use, following standardized statistical guidelines. This study showed that an overall 35.3% (128/363) of articles were considered statistically unacceptable. A mild positive effect of the presence of a PhD degree holder or a specialty board diplomate and the journal impact factor were observed on the quality of statistics. This article highlights the tremendous need to improve statistical quality of published avian research articles.

NEW IDEAS

The use of a single advancement flap was described in a case report for the treatment of a chronic, nonresponsive grade V/VII pododermatitis of the right metatarsal pad in a red-tailed hawk.[70] The interdigital skin between digits 3 and 4 was used to perform the flap. Two months after surgery, the pododermatitis was healed and the hawk was released into the wild. This technique can present an interesting alternative to current techniques for management of these lesions in avian species.

Another case report presents the use of a vascular access port for antibiotic administration in the treatment of pododermatitis in a chicken with a class IV/V pododermatitis associated with a multidrug-resistant *E coli* bacterium.[71] Due to concern with injection volume and duration of treatment, placement of a vascular access port in the right jugular vein was elected. The port was kept for 5 months without complication and the infection resolved.

REFERENCES

1. Evans EE, Mitchell MA, Whittington JK, et al. Measuring the level of agreement between cloacal Gram's stains and bacterial cultures in Hispaniolan Amazon parrots (*Amazona ventralis*). J Avian Med Surg 2014;28:290–6.
2. Williams SM, Holthaus L, Barron HW, et al. Improved clinicopathologic assessments of acute liver damage due to trauma in Indian ring-necked parakeets (*Psittacula krameri manillensis*). J Avian Med Surg 2012;26:67–75.
3. Caliendo V, McKinney P, Bailey T, et al. Serum amyloid A as an indicator of health status in falcons. J Avian Med Surg 2013;27:83–9.

4. Kummrow M, Silvanose C, Di Somma A, et al. Serum protein electrophoresis by using high-resolution agarose gel in clinically healthy and *Aspergillus* species-infected falcons. J Avian Med Surg 2012;26:213–20.

5. Delk KW, Wack RF, Burgdorf-Moisuk A, et al. Acute phase protein and electrophoresis protein fraction values for captive American flamingos (*Phoenicopterus ruber*). J Zoo Wildl Med 2015;46:929–33.

6. Lee KA, Goetting VS, Tell LA. Inflammatory markers associated with trauma and infection in red-tailed hawks (*Buteo jamaicensis*) in the USA. J Wildl Dis 2015;51: 860–7.

7. Keller KA, Sanchez-Migallon Guzman D, Acierno MJ, et al. Thromboelastography values in Hispaniolan Amazon parrots (*Amazona ventralis*): a pilot study. J Avian Med Surg 2015;29:174–80.

8. Strindberg S, Nielsen TW, Ribeiro ÂM, et al. Thromboelastography in selected avian species. J Avian Med Surg 2015;29:282–9.

9. Visser M, Hespel AM, de Swarte M, et al. Use of a caudoventral-craniodorsal oblique radiographic view made at 45° to the frontal plane to evaluate the pectoral girdle in raptors. J Am Vet Med Assoc 2015;247:1037–41.

10. Veladiano IA, Banzato T, Bellini L, et al. Computed tomographic anatomy of the heads of blue-and-gold macaws (*Ara ararauna*), African grey parrots (*Psittacus erithacus*), and monk parakeets (*Myiopsitta monachus*). Am J Vet Res 2016;77: 1346–56.

11. Beaufrere H, Pariaut R, Rodriguez D, et al. Comparison of transcoelomic, contrast transcoelomic, and transesophageal echocardiography in anesthetized red-tailed hawks (*Buteo jamaicensis*). Am J Vet Res 2012;73:1560–8.

12. Beaufrere H, Rodriguez D, Pariaut R, et al. Estimation of intrathoracic arterial diameter by means of computed tomographic angiography in Hispaniolan Amazon parrots. Am J Vet Res 2011;72:210–8.

13. Doss GA, Mans C. Changes in physiologic parameters and effects of hooding in red-tailed hawks (*Buteo jamaicensis*) during manual restraint. J Avian Med Surg 2016;30(2):127–32.

14. Barsotti G, Briganti A, Spratte JR, et al. Safety and efficacy of bilateral topical application of rocuronium bromide for mydriasis in European Kestrels (*Falco tinnunculus*). J Avian Med Surg 2012;26:1–5.

15. Barsotti G, Briganti A, Spratte JR, et al. Bilateral mydriasis in common buzzards (*Buteo buteo*) and little owls (*Athene noctua*) induced by concurrent topical administration of rocuronium bromide. Vet Ophthalmol 2010;13:35–40.

16. Barsotti G, Briganti A, Spratte JR, et al. Mydriatic effect of topically applied rocuronium bromide in tawny owls (*Strix aluco*): comparison between two protocols. Vet Ophthalmol 2010;13:9–13.

17. Baine K, Hendrix DV, Kuhn SE, et al. The efficacy and safety of topical rocuronium bromide to induce bilateral mydriasis in Hispaniolan Amazon parrots (*Amazona ventralis*). J Avian Med Surg 2016;30:8–13.

18. Petritz OA, Guzman DSM, Gustavsen K, et al. Evaluation of the mydriatic effects of topical administration of rocuronium bromide in Hispaniolan Amazon parrots (*Amazona ventralis*). J Am Vet Med Assoc 2016;248:67–71.

19. Sadar MJ, Hawkins MG, Byrne BA, et al. Pharmacokinetics of a single intramuscular injection of ceftiofur crystalline-free acid in red-tailed hawks (*Buteo jamaicensis*). Am J Vet Res 2015;76:1077–84.

20. Kilburn JJ, Cox SK, Backues KA. Pharmacokinetics of ceftiofur crystalline free acid, a long-acting cephalosporin, in American flamingos (*Phoenicopterus ruber*). J Zoo Wildl Med 2016;47:457–62.

21. Wojick KB, Langan JN, Adkesson MJ, et al. Pharmacokinetics of long-acting cef-
    tiofur crystalline-free acid in helmeted guineafowl (*Numida meleagris*) after a sin-
    gle intramuscular injection. Am J Vet Res 2011;72:1514–8.
22. Hope K, Tell L, Byrne B, et al. Pharmacokinetics of a single intramuscular injection
    of ceftiofur crystalline-free acid in American black ducks (*Anas rubripes*). Am J
    Vet Res 2012;73:620–7.
23. Haritova A, Dimitrova D, Dinev T, et al. Comparative pharmacokinetics of enro-
    floxacin, danofloxacin, and marbofloxacin after intravenous and oral administra-
    tion in Japanese quail (*Coturnix coturnix japonica*). J Avian Med Surg 2013;27:
    23–31.
24. Lashev L, Dimitrova D, Milanova A, et al. Pharmacokinetics of enrofloxacin and
    marbofloxacin in Japanese quails and common pheasants. Br Poult Sci 2015;
    56:255–61.
25. Dimitrova D, Haritova A, Dinev T, et al. Comparative pharmacokinetics of dano-
    floxacin in common pheasants, guinea fowls and Japanese quails after intrave-
    nous and oral administration. Br Poult Sci 2014;55:120–5.
26. Ratzlaff K, Papich MG, Flammer K. Plasma concentrations of fluconazole after a
    single oral dose and administration in drinking water in cockatiels (*Nymphicus
    hollandicus*). J Avian Med Surg 2011;25:23–31.
27. Emery LC, Cox SK, Souza MJ. Pharmacokinetics of nebulized terbinafine in His-
    paniolan Amazon parrots (*Amazona ventralis*). J Avian Med Surg 2012;26:161–6.
28. Evans EE, Emery LC, Cox SK, et al. Pharmacokinetics of terbinafine after oral
    administration of a single dose to Hispaniolan Amazon parrots (*Amazona ventra-
    lis*). Am J Vet Res 2013;74:835–8.
29. Bechert U, Christensen JM, Poppenga R, et al. Pharmacokinetics of terbinafine
    after single oral dose administration in red-tailed hawks (*Buteo jamaicensis*).
    J Avian Med Surg 2010;24:122–30.
30. Bechert U, Christensen JM, Poppenga R, et al. Pharmacokinetics of orally admin-
    istered terbinafine in African penguins (*Spheniscus demersus*) for potential treat-
    ment of aspergillosis. J Zoo Wildl Med 2010;41:263–74.
31. Wlaź P, Knaga S, Kasperek K, et al. Activity and safety of inhaled itraconazole
    nanosuspension in a model pulmonary aspergillus fumigatus infection in inocu-
    lated young quails. Mycopathologia 2015;180:35–42.
32. Rundfeldt C, Wyska E, Steckel H, et al. A model for treating avian aspergillosis:
    serum and lung tissue kinetics for Japanese quail (*Coturnix japonica*) following
    single and multiple aerosol exposures of a nanoparticulate itraconazole suspen-
    sion. Med Mycol 2013;51:800–10.
33. Gentry J, Montgerard C, Crandall E, et al. Voriconazole disposition after single
    and multiple, oral doses in healthy, adult red-tailed hawks (*Buteo jamaicensis*).
    J Avian Med Surg 2014;28:201–8.
34. Flammer K, Osborne JAN, Webb DJ, et al. Pharmacokinetics of voriconazole after
    oral administration of single and multiple doses in African grey parrots (*Psittacus
    erithacus timneh*). Am J Vet Res 2008;69:114–21.
35. Guzman DSM, Flammer K, Papich MG, et al. Pharmacokinetics of voriconazole
    after oral administration of single and multiple doses in Hispaniolan Amazon par-
    rots (*Amazona ventralis*). Am J Vet Res 2010;71:460–7.
36. Kline Y, Clemons KV, Woods L, et al. Pharmacokinetics of voriconazole in adult
    mallard ducks (*Anas platyrhynchos*). Med Mycol 2011;49:500–12.
37. Burhenne J, Haefeli WE, Hess M, et al. Pharmacokinetics, tissue concentrations,
    and safety of the antifungal agent voriconazole in chickens. J Avian Med Surg
    2008;22:199–207.

38. Tell LA, Clemons KV, Kline Y, et al. Efficacy of voriconazole in Japanese quail (*Coturnix japonica*) experimentally infected with *Aspergillus fumigatus*. Med Mycol 2010;48:234–44.

39. Beernaert LA, Pasmans F, Baert K, et al. Designing a treatment protocol with voriconazole to eliminate *Aspergillus fumigatus* from experimentally inoculated pigeons. Vet Microbiol 2009;139:393–7.

40. Schmidt V, Demiraj F, Di Somma A, et al. Plasma concentrations of voriconazole in falcons. Vet Rec 2007;161:265–8.

41. Hyatt MW, Georoff TA, Nollens HH, et al. Voriconazole toxicity in multiple penguin species. J Zoo Wildl Med 2015;46:880–8.

42. Guzman DSM, Beaufrère H, KuKanich B, et al. Pharmacokinetics of single oral dose of Pimobendan in Hispaniolan Amazon parrots (*Amazona ventralis*). J Avian Med Surg 2014;28:95–101.

43. Powers L, Papich M. Pharmacokinetics of orally administered phenobarbital in African grey parrots (*Psittacus erithacus erithacus*). J Vet Pharmacol Ther 2011;34: 615–7.

44. Schnellbacher R, Beaufrere H, Vet DM, et al. Pharmacokinetics of levetiracetam in healthy Hispaniolan Amazon parrots (*Amazona ventralis*) after oral administration of a single dose. J Avian Med Surg 2014;28:193–200.

45. van Zeeland YR, Schoemaker NJ, Haritova A, et al. Pharmacokinetics of paroxetine, a selective serotonin reuptake inhibitor, in Grey parrots (*Psittacus erithacus erithacus*): influence of pharmaceutical formulation and length of dosing. J Vet Pharmacol Ther 2013;36:51–8.

46. Visser M, Ragsdale MM, Boothe DM. Pharmacokinetics of amitriptyline HCl and its metabolites in healthy African grey parrots (*Psittacus erithacus*) and cockatoos (*Cacatua* species). J Avian Med Surg 2015;29:275–81.

47. Kerski A, De Kloet AH, De Kloet SR. Vertical transmission of avian bornavirus in Psittaciformes: avian bornavirus RNA and anti-avian bornavirus antibodies in eggs, embryos, and hatchlings obtained from infected sun conures (*Aratinga solstitialis*). Avian Dis 2012;56:471–8.

48. Rubbenstroth D, Brosinski K, Rinder M, et al. No contact transmission of avian bornavirus in experimentally infected cockatiels (*Nymphicus hollandicus*) and domestic canaries (*Serinus canaria forma domestica*). Vet Microbiol 2014;172:146–56.

49. Delnatte P, Nagy É, Ojkic D, et al. Investigation into the possibility of vertical transmission of avian bornavirus in free-ranging Canada geese (*Branta canadensis*). Avian Pathol 2014;43:301–4.

50. Heffels-Redmann U, Enderlein D, Herzog S, et al. Follow-up investigations on different courses of natural avian bornavirus infections in psittacines. Avian Dis 2012;56:153–9.

51. Hoppes S, Heatley JJ, Guo J, et al. Meloxicam treatment in cockatiels (*Nymphicus hollandicus*) infected with avian bornavirus. J Exot Pet Med 2013;22:275–9.

52. Beaufrère H, Ammersbach M, Reavill DR, et al. Prevalence of and risk factors associated with atherosclerosis in psittacine birds. J Am Vet Med Assoc 2013; 242:1696–704.

53. Pilny AA, Quesenberry KE, Bartick-Sedrish TE, et al. Evaluation of *Chlamydophila psittaci* infection and other risk factors for atherosclerosis in pet psittacine birds. J Am Vet Med Assoc 2012;240:1474–80.

54. Beaufrère H, Cray C, Ammersbach M, et al. Association of plasma lipid levels with atherosclerosis prevalence in psittaciformes. J Avian Med Surg 2014;28:225–31.

55. Beaufrère H, Nevarez J, Wakamatsu N, et al. Experimental diet-induced atherosclerosis in Quaker parrots (*Myiopsitta monachus*). Vet Pathol 2013;50:1116–26.

56. Belcher C, Heatley JJ, Petzinger C, et al. Evaluation of plasma cholesterol, triglyceride, and lipid density profiles in captive monk parakeets (*Myiopsitta monachus*). J Exot Pet Med 2014;23:71–8.
57. Stanford M. Significance of cholesterol assays in the investigation of hepatic lipidosis and atherosclerosis in psittacine birds. Exot DVM 2005;7:28.
58. Ravich M, Cray C, Hess L, et al. Lipid panel reference intervals for Amazon parrots (*Amazona* species). J Avian Med Surg 2014;28:209–15.
59. Bavelaar F, Beynen A. Plasma cholesterol concentrations in African grey parrots fed diets containing psyllium. J Appl Res Vet Med 2003;1:97–104.
60. Gustavsen KA, Stanhope KL, Lin AS, et al. Effects of exercise on the plasma lipid profile in Hispaniolan amazon parrots (*Amazona ventralis*) with naturally occurring hypercholesterolemia. J Zoo Wildl Med 2016;47:760–9.
61. Petritz OA, Sanchez-Migallon Guzman D, Hawkins MG, et al. Comparison of two 4.7-milligram to one 9.4-milligram deslorelin acetate implants on egg production and plasma progesterone concentrations in Japanese quail (*Coturnix coturnix japonica*). J Zoo Wild Med 2015;46(4):789–97.
62. Petritz OA, Sanchez-Migallon Guzman D, Paul-Murphy J, et al. Evaluation of the efficacy and safety of single administration of 4.7-mg deslorelin acetate implants on egg production and plasma sex hormones in Japanese quail (*Coturnix coturnix japonica*). Am J Vet Res 2013;74:316–23.
63. Cowan ML, Martin GB, Monks DJ, et al. Inhibition of the reproductive system by deslorelin in male and female pigeons (*Columba livia*). J Avian Med Surg 2014;28:102–8.
64. Summa N, Guzman DS, Larrat S, et al. Evaluation of high dosages of oral meloxicam in American kestrels (*Falco sparverius*). J Avian Med Surg, in press.
65. Mohsenzadeh MS, Zaeemi M, Razmyar J, et al. Comparison of a point-of-care glucometer and a laboratory autoanalyzer for measurement of blood glucose concentrations in domestic pigeons (*Columba livia domestica*). J Avian Med Surg 2015;29:181–6.
66. Acierno MJ, Mitchell MA, Schuster PJ, et al. Evaluation of the agreement among three handheld blood glucose meters and a laboratory blood analyzer for measurement of blood glucose cocentration Hispaniolan Amazon parrots (*Amazona ventralis*). Am J Vet Res 2009;70:172–5.
67. Acierno MJ, Schnellbacher R, Tully TN. Measuring the level of agreement between a veterinary and a human point-of-care glucometer and a laboratory blood analyzer in Hispaniolan Amazon parrots (*Amazona ventralis*). J Avian Med Surg 2012;26:221–4.
68. Lieske CL, Ziccardi MH, Mazet JAK, et al. Evaluation of 4 handheld blood glucose monitors for use in seabird rehabilitation. J Avian Med Surg 2002;16:277–85.
69. Beaufrère H, Kearney MT, Tully TN. Can we trust the avian medical literature: survey and critical appraisal of the use of statistics in avian medicine from 2007 to 2011. J Exot Pet Med 2015;24:415–26.
70. Sander S, Whittington JK, Bennett A, et al. Advancement flap as a novel treatment for a pododermatitis lesion in a red-tailed hawk (*Buteo jamaicensis*). J Avian Med Surg 2013;27:294–300.
71. Doneley RJT, Smith BA, Gibson JS. Use of a vascular access port for antibiotic administration in the treatment of pododermatitis in a chicken. J Avian Med Surg 2015;29:130–5.
72. Plumb D. Phenobarbital. In: Plumb D, editor. Veterinary drug handbook. Stockholm (WI): PharmaVetInc; 2011. p. 805–9.

Evidence-Based Advances in Aquatic Animal Medicine

Claire Vergneau-Grosset, med vet, IPSAV, CES, DACZM[a],
Sylvain Larrat, med vet, MSc, DES, DACZM[b],*

KEYWORDS

- Aquatic • Evidence-based medicine • Fish • Scientific evidence

KEY POINTS

- Evidence-based medicine is in its infancy in aquatic animal medicine regarding diagnostic techniques, especially because environmental parameters may be confounding factors influencing reference intervals in clinical pathology.
- Antiinfectious therapeutic agents have been studied extensively owing to commercial and ecological implications in aquaculture.
- Emerging diseases are commonly described in aquatic animal medicine; new diseases favored by environmental changes should be differentiated from newly discovered diseases.

INTRODUCTION

Piscine species are the most numerous and diverse group among vertebrates with more than 27,000 species.[1,2] Information derived from other vertebrates is usually not appropriate for the medical care of aquatic species. Although extrapolation may be possible among fish species, the reader should be aware that differences between 2 piscine species may be as great as between a cat and a rabbit. Hence, there is the need of species-specific evidence. Invertebrate aquatic species, included shrimps, snails, urchins, crabs, and corals, may be found in hobbyist aquaria and deserve the same level of medicine, whenever possible, as other animals.

Evidence-Based Advances in Diagnosis

Diagnostics tests available in aquatic animal medicine include blood tests, imaging, microbiology, and histopathology results. A recent article evaluated whether studies published between 2006 and 2012 about teleost diagnostic tests accuracy followed

The authors have nothing to disclose.
[a] Zoological Medicine Service, Aquarium du Québec, Faculté de médecine vétérinaire, Université de Montréal, 3200 Sicotte, Saint-Hyacinthe, Quebec J2S 2M2, Canada; [b] Clinique Vétérinaire Benjamin Franklin, 38 Rue Du Danemark Za Porte Océane 2, Brech/Auray 56400, France
* Corresponding author.
E-mail address: sylvainlarrat@yahoo.fr

http://dx.doi.org/10.1016/j.cvex.2017.04.003
1094-9194/17/© 2017 Elsevier Inc. All rights reserved.
vetexotic.theclinics.com

Standards for Reporting of Diagnostic Accuracy. Out of 66 peer-reviewed studies, only 11 complied with these guidelines, emphasizing the need for more rigorous validation of diagnostic tests in teleost fish.[3]

HEMATOLOGY AND THE INFLUENCE OF ENVIRONMENTAL PARAMETERS

Hematology reference intervals have been published for certain fish species.[4] However, environmental parameters and nutritional status have been shown to significantly affect these values, as exemplified in wild-caught and aquarium-housed lake sturgeon (*Acipenser fulvescens*), where specimens displayed different reference intervals in an observational study.[4] In contrast, parasitic infestation in wild-caught pike have been shown to influence hematology results only marginally, with a significant increase of mean corpuscular volume among all hematologic parameters investigated in a case-control study.[5] These findings highlight that blood tests may not be sensitive or specific in fish and should be further investigated to confirm their clinical relevance. Other conditions may cause more hematologic abnormalities, with significant hematologic changes associated with cyprinid herpesivrus 2 infection in 10 moribund Prussian carp (*Carassius gibelio*),[6] or with trematode experimental infection in Bluegill (*Lepomis macrochirus*).[7] Clinicians should be aware of the lack of evidence supporting direct extrapolation from domestic mammal clinical pathology results in fish.

MICROBIOLOGY

Microbiological tests, including bacterial and fungal cultures, are used extensively in aquatic animals. In invertebrates displaying an open vascular system in constant and direct contact with the environment, such as echinoderms, the interpretation of these tests is particularly challenging. Of note, some healthy fish normally display positive blood cultures.[8] The environmental conditions used for in vitro cultures are also critical to evaluate. The temperature of incubation should be close to the fish temperature to avoid in vitro selection of different germs. In addition, different incubation media may result in different results; for instance, marine agar, which contains salt and minerals close to marine water content, should be favored when dealing with samples collected from marine fish species. In addition, a precise identification of cultured colonies may be challenging and development of molecular diagnostic techniques, including matrix-assisted desorption ionization time-of-flight mass spectrometry is a recent advance in fish medicine.[9,10] This technology is based on ionization of biomolecules, identified by mass spectrometry:protein profile is then compared with a database created for the species of interest.[11] An increasing number of fish pathogens are being added to the available database for aquatic animal species.[12]

HISTOPATHOLOGY

Histopathology is a commonly used diagnostic test in fish. However, clinicians should be aware the limitations of immunohistochemistry using mammalian antibodies. The challenges of immunohistochemistry use in fish have been suggested in case reports[13–15] and experimental studies are needed to validate the use of immunohistochemistry in piscine species.

Evidence-Based Advances in Therapeutics

Pharmacokinetic and pharmacodynamic studies are available for certain fish species using various routes, including enteral, parenteral, and immersion treatments (**Tables 1** and **2**). The best route of parenteral administration is debated and likely depends on

Table 1
Some recent pharmacokinetic studies available for invertebrate species

Drug	Species	n	Temperature	Route	Recommended Dosage	Reference
Florfenicol	Pacific white shrimp (*Litopenaeus vannamei*)	72	25°C	PO	10 mg/kg	Fang et al,[16] 2003
Enrofloxacin	Green sea urchin (*Strongylocentrotus droebachiensis*)	12 12	10.4–11.5°C	Bath IC	10 mg/L for 6 h 10 mg/kg q4–5 d	Phillips et al,[17] 2016
Enrofloxacin	Ridgetail white prawn (*Exopalaemon carinicauda*)	81 81	18°C 18°C	PO Bath	10 mg/kg q 24 h 10 mg/mL q24 h for 5 d	Liang et al,[18] 2014
Enrofloxacin	Manila clam (*Ruditapes philippinarum*)	88	16–22°C	Bath	5 μg/mL for 24 h	Chang et al,[19] 2012

Abbreviations: IC, intracoelomic; PO, per os.

Table 2
Selected studies documenting the effect of probiotics and prebiotics in aquatic animals

Type of Evidence	Product	Species	Duration	Outcome	Reference
Nonrandomized, controlled trial	Beta-glucan 6 mg/kg body weight	Koi	25 d	Significant increase of basal C-reactive protein and alternative complement activity and after lipopolysaccharide administration.	Pionnier et al,[20] 2014
Randomized, controlled trial	Beta-glucan 0.2%–0.3% in feed	Persian sturgeon (Acipenser persicus)	6 wk	Significant increase of lysozyme activity and alternative complement activity. No effect on seric immunoglobulin concentration.	Aramli et al,[21] 2015
Randomized, controlled trial	Mannan oligosaccharide 2–8 g/kg	Pacific white shrimp	8 wk	Increased survival to ammonia stress, increased superoxide dismutase activity >4 g/kg.	Zhang et al,[22] 2012
Randomized trial	Garlic 50 g/kg feed	Koi	6 wk	Decreased protein and lipid tissue oxidation, decreased seric ASAT and ALP activity.	Shahsavani et al,[23] 2011
Nonrandomized, controlled trial	Garlic 1% in feed	Indian prawn (Fenneropenaeus indicus)	1 h–5 d	Decreased mortality rate to 30% vs 100% in the control group after inoculation with multiresistant Vibrio harveyi.	Vaseeharan et al,[24] 2011
Randomized trial	Bee propolis and Aloe barbadensis: 0%–2% in feed	Nile tilapia (Oreochromis niloticus)	2 wk	Increased thrombocyte count, no effect on phagocytic activity nor lysozyme activity.	Dotta et al,[25] 2014
Randomized, controlled trial			2 wk	Significant decrease of monogenean gill parasites in treated group.	Dotta et al,[26] 2015
Randomized trial			2 wk	Increased acute inflammation associated with macrophages after induction of swim bladder inflammation.	Dotta et al,[27] 2015
Randomized, controlled trial	Bee propolis 0.5%–1% in feed	Japanese eel (Anguilla japonica)	12 wk	Increased serum lysosome activity. Decreased activity with higher supplementation rates.	Bae et al,[28] 2012

Randomized, controlled trial	Ethanolic extract of bee propolis 0–4 g/kg in feed	Rainbow trout (Oncorhynchus mykiss)	10 wk	Significant increase of antioxidant enzymes, decrease of triglycerides, decrease of plasmatic ASAT and ALAT, increase of growth rate.	Deng et al,[29] 2011
Randomized, controlled trial	Bee propolis 0–9 g/kg in feed		8 wk	No significant effect on biochemistry parameters or growth rate.	Beyraghdar Kashkooli et al,[30] 2011
Nonrandomized, controlled trial	Bee propolis 10 mg/kg body weight	Koi	2 wk	Alleviates hematologic toxic effects of trichlorfon.	Yonar et al,[31] 2015
Randomized, controlled trial	Bee pollen 2.5% in feed	Nile tilapia	20–30 d	Significant increase of phagocytic activity, serum bactericidal activity against Aeromonas hydrophila, hematocrit, leukocyte count, neutrophil and monocytes percentages, 7% mortality after intracoelomic inoculation of A hydrophila vs 100% in control group.	El-Asely et al,[32] 2014
Randomized, controlled trial	Peppermint 3%	Rainbow trout	8 wk	Dose-dependent increase of hematocrit and white blood cell count, 46% mortality after inoculation with Yersinia vs 75% in control group.	Adel et al,[33] 2016
Randomized, controlled trial	Peppermint 3%	Caspian brown trout (Salmo trutta caspius)	8 wk	Significant increase of skin mucus lysozyme activity, increased intestinal lactic acid bacteria.	Adel et al,[34] 2015

Abbreviations: ALAT, alanine aminotransferase; ALP, alkaline phosphatase; ASAT, aspartate aminotransferase.

the drug used. Intracoelomic injections may be accidentally performed into a coelomic organ, including the gonads in reproductive fish, resulting in modified pharmacokinetic parameters.[35] Conversely, intramuscular (IM) injections may result in leakage of suspensions from the injection site and partial delivery.[36,37] Other studies have found similar pharmacokinetic results via IM or intracoelomic administrations.[38]

Interspecific variability may be high; for example, the elimination half-life of florfenicol is 12 hours in koi (Cyprinus carpio) versus 4 hours in threespot gourami (Trichopodus trichopterus).[39] In some instances, randomized, controlled trials enrolling numerous fish individuals are available in aquaculture species, and results may be extrapolated to ornamental species.[40] For instance, results obtained from Channel catfish (Ictalurus punctatus) may be extrapolated to common plecos (Hypostomus plecostomus) among Siluriformes.[41] Ornamental fish are considered minor food-producing animal species in the United States and in Europe, and appropriate laws should apply regarding treatment choice. Clinicians should also keep in mind that water quality parameters, such as salinity, pH, and temperature, will impact pharmacokinetic results in aquatic animals.[19,42]

Aquatic animal treatment methods may harbor risks for the environment and public heath, because as excess of drugs can enter waterways, resulting in the potential development of resistant bacteria.[43,44] Pharmacokinetic and residue studies about sustained-release antibiotics are useful to refine antibiotic dosages and minimize antibiotic resistance. Recommended dosages may be much higher than described in other ectotherm species. For example, after an IM injection of 60 mg/kg of ceftiofur crystallin-free acid (Excede For Swine, Pfizer Animal Health, New York, NY), active metabolites remained above the target concentration from 0.4 to 2.5 weeks in three-quarters of fish.[35] This dosage is twice as high as the dosage described in reptiles with the same formulation.[45] When using IM injections, it may be important to administer the drug in the cranial part of the body because many piscine species display a renal and hepatic portal system,[46,47] but this remains to be evaluated systematically. Fish also display 2 types of muscles—white and dark muscle—and different pharmacokinetic profiles have been reported depending on the type of muscles at the site of injection.[48] Again, variations among fish species may be important. In common stingrays (Dasyatis pastinaca), cefovecin (Convenia, Zoetis, Florham Park, NJ) administered at 8 mg/kg IM did not remain above therapeutic concentration for more than 24 hours,[49] whereas in white bamboo sharks (Chiloscyllium plagiosum), cefovecin administered at the same dosage subcutaneously was detected for 4 days after administration.[50] This difference may be owing to species-specific protein-binding abilities[51]; therefore, these studies about cefovecin should not be extrapolated to ornamental species. This finding is similar to what reported in reptiles[52,53] and primates,[54–56] with shorter half-lives than in domestic carnivores.

To minimize the use of antibiotics in aquaculture, alternatives are being studied, including prophylactic immune-stimulant treatments. There is increasing evidence regarding the effects of probiotics and prebiotics on fish immune response.

Evidence-Based Advances in Common Disorders

Carp edema virus

Carp edema virus (CEV) is responsible for viral edema of carp and koi sleepy disease in koi and common carp (C carpio).[57] This poxvirus causes edema and death in young fish.[58] In older animals, it is responsible for lethargy, sunken eyes, skin erosion, fish lying on the bottom of the pond, and death from anoxia.[57] Death most commonly occurs after a stressful event, in spring and autumn with a water temperature ranging from 15°C to 25°C. Until recently, the disease was thought to be restricted to koi in

Japan, where it was discovered 40 years ago.[57] Several imported koi were found infected by CEV in different European countries since 2009,[59–62] and in the United States since 1996.[63,64] In a Polish study, koi and common carps were sampled as part of a surveillance program.[62] Mortality events were observed only in the koi. A large proportion (45%) of the common carp farms were nonetheless positive for the virus, although this species is also susceptible to the virus. This suggests that fish carrying the CEV are more widely spread than previously reported. Another recent discovery is the ability of the virus to cause disease at temperature ranging from 7°C to 15°C.[60,61] Three genetic lineages have been documented in Europe so far.[62] Based on the sequencing of partial 4a gene sequence, 2 genogroups have been described. Genogroup II has been documented mainly in koi imported from Israel and Japan to Europe, but also in common carps in Poland. Genogroup I has been retrieved from common carp in United Kingdom and Poland. The observed genetic diversity suggests that introduction of the virus into the European carp population might not be recent, and/or could have arisen from multiple introduction events.

Given its clinical signs, CEV should be included in the differential diagnosis of koi herpesvirus disease and other mass mortality events, especially during spring and autumn. Definitive diagnosis requires polymerase chain reaction. Salt has been proposed as a treatment alleviating clinical signs.[57] Further studies are warranted to better document the geographic spread, epidemiology, and genetic diversity of CEV.

Chytrid fungi in crustaceans

Chytridiomycosis is a widespread disease in free-ranging and captive amphibians worldwide. This fungus has been extensively researched because it is responsible for amphibian die offs and species extinctions. Two studies have recently demonstrated that *Batrachochytrium dendrobatidis* (Bd) can infect crayfish (*Procambarus* sp, *Orconectes* sp).[65,66] Bd is able to complete its life cycle in the digestive tract of crayfish.[66] In addition, McMahon and coworkers[66] observed gill recession and increased mortality in crayfish exposed to Bd or to water in which Bd was removed by filtration. This suggests that Bd produces water-borne factors that are pathogenic for crayfish. Crayfish can also harbor Bd for several month and act as a reservoir.[66] This indicates that crayfish trade may play a role in the spread of Bd. Studies of others freshwater crustaceans would be warranted to determine which species can host Bd or other potentially harmful fungi.

Fish nutrition: example of advances in seahorse nutrition

Nutritional deficiencies associated with poor reproductive performance of captive specimens are among common fish disorders. Some aspects of seahorse (*Hippocampus* spp.) nutrition have been investigated by randomized trials over the past 5 years. Seahorses have been shown to absorb dietary carotenoids and supplementation with carotenoids leads to a brighter yellow color.[67] Although no effect of carotenoids was found on seahorse survival or growth rate, commercial supplements often contain carotenoids.[67] In addition, deficiencies in polyunsaturated fatty acids have been shown to impact juvenile growth, brood size, number of broods, and egg size in seahorses, although egg viability was not affected.[68,69] One of the parameters of interest is the ratio among two Ω-3 fatty acids, the docosahexaenoic acid to eicosapentaenoic acid ratio.[70] The favored storage form could be docosahexaenoic acid, whereas eicosapentaenoic acid is used as a source of energy.[71] A dietary ratio of greater than 1 has been recommended, similar to the 1.3 ratio measured in eggs obtained from wild-caught long-snouted seahorses (*Hippocampus guttulatus*).[72] In captivity, polyunsaturated fatty acids are provided to seahorses through the gut-loading of preys, mostly brine shrimp and mysis. The final product thus has a different docosahexaenoic acid to eicosapentaenoic acid ratio compared with the supplement. In an attempt to find the most appropriate ratio, experimental studies comparing the effects of various supplementation recipes have been conducted (**Table 3**).

Current Controversies and Clinical Topics Requiring Additional Evidence

Gas bubble disease: the example of seahorses

Gas bubble disease (GBD), a common disease of seahorses,[75] most likely regroups several diseases under a single name. In juveniles, the ingestion of air bubbles has been proposed as a cause of GBD.[76] The etiology of GBD in adults has not been established formally, but hypotheses include dissolved gases supersaturation, gas bubble ingestion,[76] infection by gas-producing bacteria, or metabolic issues owing to nutritional imbalances.[70] Supersaturation is defined by dissolved gases being higher than the atmospheric pressure, and can occur owing to inappropriate life support system, injection of pressurized gas into a system (from a deep water source for instance), or photosynthesis, among others.[77] Acetazolamide, a carbonic anhydrase inhibitor, is sometimes used as a treatment of GBD.[75] After injection of acetazolamide, carbon dioxide excretion is reduced and blood carbon dioxide concentration increases in rainbow trout.[78] However, the pharmacokinetic and safety of acetazolamide have not been investigated. This therapy is extrapolated from the treatment of piscine ocular oxygen secretion syndrome, a condition where carbonic anhydrase

Table 3
Selected studies documenting the effect of various polyunsaturated fatty acids supplements in seahorses

Type of Evidence	DHA:EPA Ratio[a]	Outcome	Reference
Randomized trial	2.5 in the supplement	Higher survival rate of juveniles when gut-loading *Artemia* with Chlorella algae than with DHA-Selco (100% mortality with supplement vs 40% mortality with algae).	Palma,[73] 2011
Nonrandomized, controlled trial	2	With a concentration of 13.5 μL/L of polyunsaturated fatty acids, antioxidant enzymes were stimulated. Higher concentration resulted in saturation of antioxidant enzymes and could cause oxidative stress.	Yin and Tang,[74] 2012
Randomized trial	0.96–1.96	Overinflation of the swim bladder in juveniles fed the diet of enriched brine shrimp with a 0.96 ratio (0% survival), vs 100% survival when feeding copepodes with a 1.96 ratio.	Palma et al,[70] 2014
Randomized trial	0.6–0.8	No significant difference in growth among groups. Hepatic lipid storage.	Segade,[71] in press

Abbreviations: DHA, docosahexaenoic acid; EPA, eicosapentaenoic acid.
[a] Ratio of final diet distributed to seahorse unless specified otherwise.

activity has been shown to increase in the ocular choroid, causing gas bubbles in the choroid rete of fish.[79] Conversely, in case of dissolved gas supersaturation, carbonic anhydrase activity is reduced in fish lens.[80] The pathophysiology of GBD has not been elucidated and use of acetazolamide is, therefore, very controversial in this case. Of note, nitrogen is the most common gas implicated in supersaturation problems in aquatic environments.[77] Thus, treatment with carbonic anhydrase would be useless if GBD in seahorses is in fact owing to nitrogen supersaturation. Prevention of GBD in juveniles relies on side illumination of the aquarium,[76] restraining the access to the water surface before 2 months of age,[76] providing sufficient light intensity (500–1500 lux in *Hippocampus erectus* and 2000 lux in *Hippocampus kuda*) and adequate temperature (26°C–29°C in *H erectus* and 29°C in *H kuda*).[81,82] More research is ongoing to expand knowledge about the etiology, prevention, and treatment of GBD, especially in adult seahorses.

Sea star wasting disease and densovirus
Sea star wasting disease has been responsible for large-scale sea star die-offs in multiple locations and species since 2013.[83] The etiologic agent is suspected to be a virus, most likely the sea star–associated Densovirus.[83] Because sea star–associated Densovirus is not detected in every sea star displaying clinical signs and some unaffected sea star carry the virus with a lower load, the link between the virus and the disease is not demonstrated based on Koch postulates.[83,84] Repeated sampling of sea star–associated Densovirus–positive sea stars revealed a very high rate of false-negative results (62%–89%).[83] This might explain the presence of clinically abnormal but polymerase chain reaction–negative sea stars. In addition, sea stars have an open vascular system, which could explain the detection of the virus in nonclinical animals. So far, transmission trials have been performed with tissue isolated from diseased sea stars.[83] Culture–inoculation–reisolation experiments might be required to discard remaining doubts about the etiology of sea star wasting disease, but the virus has not been propagated in cell culture to date. More studies are needed to better understand this disease.

Antinociception in fish and aquatic invertebrates
The debate about the ability of fish and invertebrates to feel pain is ongoing.[85,86] Fish and at least some invertebrates are able to learn and develop complex avoidance behaviors when faced with noxious stimuli.[86,87] Although there is increasing evidence that nociception is widespread among aquatic animals, they may not possess the anatomic features and ability to consciously feel pain, because they lack a neocortex, which is needed for conscious integration.[85] Antinociception in fish and invertebrates is still in its infancy, but research efforts have recently increased on this matter. The development of validated models to measure clinically relevant antinociception in fish is needed. Numerous studies rely on acetic acid injections, heat, or electric stimuli, which may not provide relevant information regarding perioperative antinociception.[88] Clinically relevant models include minimum anesthetic concentration depression models associated with physical noxious stimuli, and surgery.[89–92] Pharmacokinetic, pharmacodynamic, and safety studies have been conducted for a limited number of drugs and species (**Table 4**). Of note, the impact of the site of injection on pharmacokinetics has not been evaluated and some studies report a caudal injection site.[37,89,92]

Extrapolation of treatment regimen from aquaculture or research species might not be adequate. The metabolism and excretion of drugs might be especially different in freshwater, marine, or anadromous/catadromous species. Information on strictly marine species is especially scarce.

Table 4
Selected studies documenting the effects of analgesic molecules in fish

Drug	Species	Dosage	Study Types/ Noxious Stimuli	Signs Monitored	Effects	Reference
Buprenorphine	Rainbow trout	0.01–0.1 mg/kg IM	Acetic acid injection	Feeding, ventilation rate, activity	No effect on feeding or activity	Mettam et al,[88] 2011
Buprenorphine	Zebrafish (Danio rerio) larvae	0.1 mg/L (bath)	Acetic acid (bath)	Locomotor activity	Decrease of locomotor response to acetic acid	Steenbergen and Bardine[93] 2014
Butorphanol	Chain Dogfish (Scyliorhinus retifer)	0.5–5 mg/kg IM	Needle insertion	MAC reduction	No MAC reduction	Davis et al,[90] 2016
Butorphanol	Goldfish (Carassius auratus)	0.1–0.4 mg/kg IM	Needle insertion	MAC reduction	Only the lowest dose reduces MAC	Ward et al,[89] 2012
Butorphanol	Koi	0.4 mg/kg IM	Surgery	Behavior, biochemistry	Mild behavioral sparing effect	Harms et al,[91] 2015
Butorphanol	Koi	10 mg/kg IM	Surgery	Behavior and feeding	Decreased respiratory rate, apparent analgesic effect. Buoyancy problems	Baker et al,[92] 2013
Carprofen	Rainbow trout	1–5 mg/kg IM	Acetic acid injection	Feeding, ventilation rate, activity	Improved feeding but not activity at 2.5 and 5 mg/kg	Mettam et al,[88] 2011
Ketoprofen	Chain Dogfish	1–4 mg/kg IM	Needle insertion	MAC reduction	No MAC reduction	Davis et al,[90] 2006
Ketoprofen	Goldfish	0.5–2 mg/kg IM	Needle insertion	MAC reduction	All doses reduce MAC	Ward et al,[89] 2012
Ketoprofen	Koi	2 mg/kg IM	Surgery	Behavior, biochemistry	Lower increase in creatine kinase	Harms et al,[91] 2005
Lidocaine	Rainbow trout	3–20 mg/kg locally	Acetic acid injection	Feeding, ventilation rate, activity	Antinociception between 6 and 20 mg/kg	Mettam et al,[88] 2011

Drug	Species	Dose	Study	Measure	Finding	Reference
Medetomidine	Goldfish	0.01–0.025 mg/kg IM	Needle insertion	MAC reduction	Only the highest dose reduces MAC	Ward et al,[89] 2012
Meloxicam	Goldfish	5 mg/kg IM	Toxicity study		No toxicity observed	Larouche,[94] 2015
Meloxicam	Nile tilapia	1 mg/kg IM	PK study	Plasma concentration	Short half-life, frequent administration required	Fredholm et al,[37] 2016
Morphine	Atlantic Salmon (Salmo salar)	100 mg/kg IM	PK study	Plasma concentrations	Half-life: 13.5 h	Nordgreen et al,[95] 2009
Morphine	Goldfish	50 mg/kg IM	Heat	Thermal threshold modification	No increase in thermal threshold	Nordgreen et al,[96] 2009
Morphine	Goldfish	30 mg/kg IM	Electric shock	ASR	Naloxone decreased the voltage threshold to induce ASR	Ehrensing et I,[97] 1982
Morphine	Goldfish	10–40 mg/kg IM	Needle insertion	MAC reduction	All doses reduce MAC	Ward et al,[89] 2012
Morphine	Goldfish	40 mg/kg IM	PK study	Plasma concentrations	Half-life: 12.5 h	Nordgreen et al,[95] 2009
Morphine	Goldfish	0.12–48 mg/L bath	Absorption study	Plasma concentrations	Plasma concentration was <1% of that in water	Newby et al,[98] 2009
Morphine	Goldfish	40 mg/kg IC	PK; acetic acid	Plasma concentration, rubbing behavior	Half-life: 37 h; decrease in rubbing behavior	Newby et al,[98] 2009
Morphine	Koi	5 mg/kg IM	Surgery	Behavior and feeding	Apparent analgesic effect; bouts of excessive activity	Baker et al,[92] 2013
Morphine	Rainbow trout	3000 mg/kg IM	Acetic acid	Feeding	Improved feeding	Sneddon,[99] 2003
Morphine	Rainbow trout	40 mg/kg IP	PK	Plasma concentrations	Morphine half-life: 18.3 h M3G half-life: 107 h	Newby et al,[100] 2008
Tramadol	Common Carp	2.6–26 mg/kg IM	Electric shock	ASR	Dose-dependent increase in ASR	Chervova and Lapshin,[101] 2011

Abbreviations: ASR, agitated swimming response; IC, intracoelomic; IM, intramuscular; M3G, morphine-3-beta-D-glucuronide; MAC, minimum anesthetic concentration; PK, pharmacokinetic study.

New Ideas

Oncologic treatments

Very a few case reports are available regarding use of chemotherapy in fish.[15,102,103] Because metabolism of chemotherapeutic drugs is mostly unknown in fish, it is also unknown whether active metabolites are excreted in the water and subsequently recycled though the filtration system, potentially resulting in owner and conspecific exposure. Therefore, studies are needed to assess residues after fish treatment.

Radiation therapy has also been investigated in zebrafish used as models for human neoplasms.[104] To the authors knowledge, peer-reviewed reports documenting the clinical applications of radiation therapy in fish are still lacking with the exception of a single case report describing the use of monthly megavoltage radiation therapy at 8 Gy in the same goldfish affected with a recurring myxoma of the face.[103] No clinical effect was observed and the fish was ultimately euthanized. Protocols for the irradiation of soft tissue masses still need to be developed and evaluated in piscine patients.

Fish euthanasia ethics

Euthanasia in fish has not been studied thoroughly. The dosages of tricaine methane-sulfonate, barbiturates, or T-61 ensuring a rapid and irreversible loss of brain functions have not been established. In addition, dosages are expected to be different depending on the species. In the absence of evidence-based information, the use of physical measures might be recommended to ensure that an irresponsive animal is really dead (for example, brain pithing, decapitation, bleeding, or freezing).

SUMMARY

Because of the large diversity in species, diseases, water conditions and temperatures, considerable efforts are still required to gather sufficient knowledge to reach evidence-based medicine standards in fish and aquatic animals under human care.

REFERENCES

1. Groff JM. Neoplasia in fishes. Vet Clin North Am Exot Anim Pract 2004;7:705–56.
2. Claver JA, Quaglia AIE. Comparative morphology, development and function of blood cells in non-mammalian vertebrates. J Exot Pet Med 2009;18:87–97.
3. Gardner IA, Burnley T, Caraguel C. Improvements are needed in reporting of accuracy studies for diagnostic tests used for detection of finfish pathogens. J Aquat Anim Health 2014;26:203–9.
4. DiVincenti L, Priest H, Walker KJ, et al. Comparison of select hematology and serum chemistry analytes between wild-caught and aquarium-housed lake sturgeon (Acipenser fulvescens). J Zoo Wildl Med 2013;44:957–64.
5. Fallah FJ, Khara H, Rohi JD, et al. Hematological parameters associated with parasitism in pike, Esox lucius caught from Anzali wetland. J Parasit Dis 2015;39:245–8.
6. Lu J, Lu H, Cao G. Hematological and histological changes in Prussian carp Carassius gibelio infected with Cyprinid Herpesvirus 2. J Aquat Anim Health 2016;28:150–60.
7. Calhoun DM, Schaffer PA, Gregory JR, et al. Experimental infections of bluegill with the trematode Ribeiroia ondatrae (Digenea: Cathaemasiidae): histopathology and hematological response. J Aquat Anim Health 2015;27:185–91.
8. Tao Z, Bullard SA, Arias CR. Diversity of bacteria cultured from the blood of lesser electric rays caught in the northern gulf of Mexico. J Aquat Anim Health 2014;26:225–32.

9. Nhu TQ, Park SB, Kim SW, et al. MALDI-TOF MS-based identification of *Edward-siella ictaluri* isolated from Vietnamese striped catfish (Pangasius hypophthalmus). J Vet Sci 2015.

10. Olate VR, Nachtigall FM, Santos LS, et al. Fast detection of *Piscirickettsia salmonis* in *Salmo salar* serum through MALDI-TOF-MS profiling. J Mass Spectrom 2016;51:200–6.

11. Neville SA, Lecordier A, Ziochos H, et al. Utility of matrix-assisted laser desorption ionization-time of flight mass spectrometry following introduction for routine laboratory bacterial identification. J Clin Microbiol 2011;49:2980–4.

12. The UniProt Consortium. UniProt: a hub for protein information. Nucleic Acids Res 2015;43:D204–12.

13. Lewbart GA, Spodnick G, Barlow N, et al. Surgical removal of an undifferentiated abdominal sarcoma from a koi carp (*Cyprinus carpio*). Vet Rec 1998; 143:556–8.

14. Magi GE, Renzoni G, Piccionello AP, et al. Primary ocular chondrosarcoma in a discus (*Symphisodon aequifasciatus*). J Zoo Wildl Med 2013;44:225–31.

15. Vergneau-Grosset C, Summa N, Rodriguez CO Jr, et al. Excision and subsequent treatment of a leiomyoma from the periventiduct of a koi (*Cyprinus carpio koi*). J Exot Pet Med 2016;25:194–202.

16. Fang W, Li G, Zhou S, et al. Pharmacokinetics and tissue distribution of thiamphenicol and florfenicol in Pacific white shrimp *Litopenaeus vannamei* in freshwater following oral administration. J Aquat Anim Health 2013;25:83–9.

17. Phillips BE, Harms CA, Lewbart GA, et al. Population pharmacokinetics of enrofloxacin and its metabolite ciprofloxacin in the green sea urchin (*Strongylocentrotus droebachiensis*) following intracoelomic and immersion administration. J Zoo Wildl Med 2016;47:175–86.

18. Liang JP, Li J, Li JT, et al. Accumulation and elimination of enrofloxacin and its metabolite ciprofloxacin in the ridgetail white prawn *Exopalaemon carinicauda* following medicated feed and bath administration. J Vet Pharmacol Ther 2014;37:508–14.

19. Chang ZQ, Gao AX, Li J, et al. The effect of temperature and salinity on the elimination of enrofloxacin in the Manila clam *Ruditapes philippinarum*. J Aquat Anim Health 2012;24:17–21.

20. Pionnier N, Falco A, Miest JJ, et al. Hoole D Feeding common carp Cyprinus carpio with β-glucan supplemented diet stimulates C-reactive protein and complement immune acute phase responses following PAMPs injection. Fish Shellfish Immunol 2014;39:285–95.

21. Aramli MS, Golshahi K, Nazari RM, et al. Effect of freezing rate on motility, adenosine triphosphate content and fertilizability in beluga sturgeon (*Huso huso*) spermatozoa. Cryobiology 2015;70:170–4.

22. Zhang J, Liu Y, Tian L, et al. Effects of dietary mannan oligosaccharide on growth performance, gut morphology and stress tolerance of juvenile Pacific white shrimp, *Litopenaeus vannamei*. Fish Shellfish Immunol 2012;33:1027–32.

23. Shahsavani D, Baghshani H, Alishahi E. Efficacy of allicin in decreasing lead (Pb) accumulation in selected tissues of lead-exposed common carp (*Cyprinus carpio*). Biol Trace Elem Res 2011;142:572–80.

24. Vaseeharan B, Prasad GS, Ramasamy P, et al. Antibacterial activity of *Allium sativum* against multidrug-resistant *Vibrio harveyi* isolated from black gill-diseased *Fenneropenaeus indicus*. Aquacult Int 2011;19:531–9.

25. Dotta G, de Andrade JI, Tavares Goncalves EL, et al. Leukocyte phagocytosis and lysozyme activity in Nile tilapia fed supplemented diet with natural extracts of propolis and *Aloe barbadensis*. Fish Shellfish Immunol 2014;39:280–4.

26. Dotta G, Brum A, Jeronimo GT, et al. Effect of dietary supplementation with propolis and *Aloe barbadensis* extracts on hematological parameters and parasitism in Nile tilapia. Rev Bras Parasitol Vet 2015;24:66–71.

27. Dotta G, Ledic-Neto J, Goncalves EL, et al. Acute inflammation and hematological response in Nile tilapia fed supplemented diet with natural extracts of propolis and *Aloe barbadensis*. Braz J Biol 2015;75:491–6.

28. Bae J-Y, Park GH, Lee J-Y, et al. Effects of dietary propolis supplementation on growth performance, immune responses, disease resistance and body composition of juvenile eel, Anguilla japonica. Aquacult Int 2012;20:513–23.

29. Deng J, An Q, Bi B, et al. Effect of ethanolic extract of propolis on growth performance and plasma biochemical parameters of rainbow trout (*Oncorhynchus mykiss*). Fish Physiol Biochem 2011;37:959–67.

30. Beyraghdar Kashkooli O, Ebrahimi Dorcheh E, Mahboobi-Soofiani N, et al. Long-term effects of propolis on serum biochemical parameters of rainbow trout (*Oncorhynchus mykiss*). Ecotoxicol Environ Saf 2011;74:315–8.

31. Yonar ME, Yonar SM, Pala A, et al. Trichlorfon-induced haematological and biochemical changes in *Cyprinus carpio*: ameliorative effect of propolis. Dis Aquat Org 2015;114:209–16.

32. El-Asely AM, Abbass AA, Austin B. Honey bee pollen improves growth, immunity and protection of Nile tilapia (*Oreochromis niloticus*) against infection with *Aeromonas hydrophila*. Fish Shellfish Immunol 2014;40:500–6.

33. Adel M, Pourgholam R, Zorriehzahra J, et al. Hemato - immunological and biochemical parameters, skin antibacterial activity, and survival in rainbow trout (*Oncorhynchus mykiss*) following the diet supplemented with *Mentha piperita* against Yersinia ruckeri. Fish Shellfish Immunol 2016;55:267–73.

34. Adel M, Safari R, Pourgholam R, et al. Dietary peppermint (*Mentha piperita*) extracts promote growth performance and increase the main humoral immune parameters (both at mucosal and systemic level) of Caspian brown trout (*Salmo trutta caspius* Kessler, 1877). Fish Shellfish Immunol 2015;47:623–9.

35. Grosset C, Weber ES 3rd, Gehring R, et al. Evaluation of an extended-release formulation of ceftiofur crystalline-free acid in koi (*Cyprinus carpio*). J Vet Pharmacol Ther 2015;38:606–15.

36. Rigos GKP, Papandroulakis N. Single intramuscular administration of long-acting oxytetracycline in grouper (*Epinephelus marginatus*). Turk J Vet Anim Sci 2010;34:441–5.

37. Fredholm D, Mylniczenko N, KuKanich B. Pharmacokinetic evaluation of meloxicam after intravenous and intramuscular administration in Nile tilapia (*Oreochromis niloticus*). J Zoo Wildl Med 2016;47:736–42.

38. Zhu X, Liu S, Bai Y, et al. Pharmacokinetics of cefquinome in tilapia (*Oreochromis niloticus*) after a single intramuscular or intraperitoneal administration. J Vet Pharmacol Ther 2015;38:601–5.

39. Yanong RPE, Curtis EW, Simmons R, et al. Pharmacokinetic studies of florfenicol in koi carp and threespot gourami *Trichogaster trichopterus* after oral and intramuscular treatment. J Aquat Anim Health 2011;17:129–37.

40. Miller RA, Pelsor FR, Kane AS, et al. Oxytetracycline pharmacokinetics in rainbow trout during and after an orally administered medicated feed regimen. J Aquat Anim Health 2012;24:121–8.

41. Gaunt PS, Langston C, Wrzesinski C, et al. Multidose pharmacokinetics of orally administered florfenicol in the channel catfish (Ictalurus punctatus). J Vet Pharmacol Ther 2013;36:502–6.

42. Xie X, Zhao Y, Yang X, et al. Comparison of praziquantel pharmacokinetics and tissue distribution in fresh and brackish water cultured grass carp (*Ctenopharyngodon idellus*) after oral administration of single bolus. BMC Vet Res 2015; 11:84.

43. Allender MC, Kastura M, George R, et al. Bioencapsulation of metronidazole in adult brine shrimp (*Artemia* sp.). J Zoo Wildl Med 2011;42:241–6.

44. Basti D, Bouchard D, Lichtenwalner A. Safety of florfenicol in the adult lobster (*Homarus americanus*). J Zoo Wildl Med 2011;42:131–3.

45. Churgin SM, Musgrave KE, Cox SK, et al. Pharmacokinetics of subcutaneous versus intramuscular administration of ceftiofur crystalline-free acid to bearded dragons (*Pogona vitticeps*). Am J Vet Res 2014;75:453–9.

46. Goswami OB, Jain SP, Khanna SS. Studies on the visceral venous system of some Teleosts. Proc Indian Acad Sci - Section B 1970;72:194–200.

47. Harder W. Anatomie der Fische. Stuttgart (Germany): Schweizerbart'sche Verlagsbuchhandlung; 1975 [in German].

48. Stoskopf M. Anatomy. In: Stoskopf MK, editor. Fish medicine. Apex (NC): Saunders; 1993. p. 2–30.

49. Garcia-Parraga D, Rodriguez JM, Alvaro T, et al. Preliminary study of cefovecin (Convenia®) pharmacokinetics in several aquatic species. In Proceedings Symp Euro Assoc Aquatic Mammals. 2010.

50. Steeil J, Schumacher J, Georges RH, et al. Pharmacokinetics of cefovecin (Convenia®) in white bamboo sharks (*Chiloscyllium plagiosum*), and Atlantic Horseshoe Crabs (Limulus polyphemus). In Proceedings 44th annual conference of the International Association for Aquatic Animal Medicine 2013.

51. Stegemann MR, Sherington J, Blanchflower S. Pharmacokinetics and pharmacodynamics of cefovecin in dogs. J Vet Parmacol Ther 2006;29:501–11.

52. Thuesen LR, Bertelsen MF, Brimer L, et al. Selected pharmacokinetic parameters for cefovecin in hens and green iguanas. J Vet Pharmacol Ther 2009;32: 613–7.

53. Nardini G, Barbarossa A, Dall'Occo A, et al. Pharmacokinetics of cefovecin sodium after subcutaneous administration to Hermann's tortoises (*Testudo hermanni*). Am J Vet Res 2014;75:918–23.

54. Raabe BM, Lovaglio J, Grover GS, et al. Pharmacokinetics of cefovecin in cynomolgus macaques (*Macaca fascicularis*), olive baboons (*Papio anubis*), and rhesus macaques (*Macaca mulatta*). J Am Assoc Lab Anim Sci 2011;50: 389–95.

55. Bakker J, Thuesen LR, Braskamp G, et al. Single subcutaneous dosing of cefovecin in rhesus monkeys (*Macaca mulatta*): a pharmacokinetic study. J Vet Pharmacol Ther 2011;34:464–8.

56. Papp R, Popovic A, Kelly N, et al. Pharmacokinetics of Cefovecin in squirrel monkey (*Saimiri sciureus*), rhesus macaques (*Macaca mulatta*), and cynomolgus macaques (*Macaca fascicularis*). J Am Assoc Lab Anim Sci 2010;49:805–8.

57. Miyazaki T, Isshiki T, Katsuyuki H. Histopathological and electron microscopy studies on sleepy disease of koi Cyprinus carpio koi in Japan. Dis Aquat Org 2005;65:197–207.

58. Ono S-I, Nagai A, Sugai NA. Histopathological study on juvenile color carp, Cyprinus carpio, showing edema. Fish Pathol 1986;21:167–75.

59. Haenen O, Way K, Stone D, et al. 'Koi Sleepy Disease' found for the first time in koi carps in the Netherlands. Tijdschr Diergeneeskd 2014;139:26–9 [in Dutch].

60. Way K, Stone D. Emergence of carp edema virus-like (CEV-like) disease in the UK. CEFAS Finfish News 2013;15:32–4.

61. Lewisch E, Gorgoglione B, Way K, et al. Carp edema virus/koi sleepy disease: an emerging disease in Central-East Europe. Transbound Emerg Dis 2015;62: 6–12.

62. Matras M, Borzym E, Stone D, et al. Carp edema virus in Polish aquaculture–evidence of significant sequence divergence and a new lineage in common carp Cyprinus carpio (L.). J Fish Dis 2016;40(3):319–25.

63. Hedrick RP, Antonio DB, Munn RJ. Poxvirus like agent associated with epizootic mortality in juvenile koi (Cyprinus carpio). FHS Newsletter 1997;25:1–3.

64. Waltzek TB, Gotesman M, Steckler N, et al. Overview of DNA viruses impacting ornamental aquaculture. In Proceedings International Symposium on Aquatic Animal Health. 2014.

65. Brannelly LA, McMahon TA, Hinton M, et al. Batrachochytrium dendrobatidis in natural and farmed Louisiana crayfish populations: prevalence and implications. Dis Aquat Org 2015;112:229–35.

66. McMahon TA, Brannelly LA, Chatfield MW, et al. Chytrid fungus Batrachochytrium dendrobatidis has nonamphibian hosts and releases chemicals that cause pathology in the absence of infection. Proc Natl Acad Sci 2013;110: 210–5.

67. Segade A, Robaina F, Otero-Ferrer F, et al. Effects of the diet on seahorse (Hippocampus hippocampus) growth, body colour and biochemical composition. Aquacult Nutr 2015;21:807–13.

68. Saavedra M, Masdeu M, Hale P, et al. Dietary fatty acid enrichment increases egg size and quality of yellow seahorse Hippocampus kuda. Anim Reprod Sci 2014;145:54–61.

69. Palma J, Andrade JP. Growth, reproductive performances, and brood quality of long snout seahorse, Hippocampus guttulatus, fed enriched shrimp diets. J World Aquacult Soc 2012;43:802–13.

70. Palma J, Bureau DP, Andrade JP. The effect of diet on ontogenic development of the digestive tract in juvenile reared long snout seahorse Hippocampus guttulatus. Fish Physiol Biochem 2014;40:739–50.

71. Segade A, Robaina F, Novelli B, et al. Effect of the diet on lipid composition and liver histology of short snout seahorse Hippocampus hippocampus. Aquacult Nutrition 2016;22(6):1312–9.

72. Faleiro F, Narciso L. Lipid dynamics during early development of Hippocampus guttulatus seahorses: searching for clues on fatty acid requirements. Aquaculture 2010;137:56–64.

73. Palma J. Effect of different Artemia enrichments and feeding protocol for rearing juvenile long snout seahorse, Hippocampus guttulatus. Aquaculture 2011;318: 439–43.

74. Yin F, Tang B. Lipid metabolic response, peroxidation, and antioxidant defence status of juvenile lined seahorse, Hippocampus erectus, fed with highly unsaturated fatty acids enriched Artemia nauplii. J World Aquacult Soc 2012;43: 716–26.

75. Koldewey H. Syngnathid husbandry in public aquariums. Londres (United Kingdom): Zoological Society of London and Project Seahorse; 2005.

76. Woods CM. Improving initial survival in cultured seahorses, Hippocampus abdominalis Leeson, 1827 (Teleostei: Syngnathidae). Aquaculture 2000;190:377–88.

77. Noga E. Gas supersaturation (gas bubble disease (GBD)). In: Noga E, editor. Fish disease: diagnosis and treatment. 2nd edition. Ames (IA): Wiley-Blackwell; 2010. p. 107–9.

78. Dimberg K. Inhibition of carbonic anhydrase in vivo in the freshwater-adapted rainbow trout: differential effects of acetazolamide and metazolamide on blood CO_2 levels. Comp Biochem Physiol Part A Physiol 1988;91:253–8.

79. Williams D, Hopcroft T, Pantel U, et al. Levels of choroidal body carbonic anhydrase activity and glycogen in farmed halibut. Vet J 1998;156:223–9.

80. Gültepe N, Ateş O, Hisar O, et al. Carbonic anhydrase activities from the rainbow trout lens correspond to the development of acute gas bubble disease. J Aquat Anim Health 2011;23:134–9.

81. Zhang Y, Qin G, Lin J, et al. Growth, survivorship, air-bubble disease, and attachment of feeble juvenile seahorses, *Hippocampus kuda* (Bleeker, 1852). J World Aquacult Soc 2015;46:292–300.

82. Lin Q, Lin J, Huang L. Effects of light intensity, stocking density and temperature on the air-bubble disease, survivorship and growth of early juvenile seahorse *Hippocampus erectus* Perry, 1810. Aquacult Res 2010;42:91–8.

83. Hewson I, Button JB, Gudenkauf BM, et al. Densovirus associated with sea-star wasting disease and mass mortality. Proc Natl Acad Sci 2014;111:17278–83.

84. DelSesto CJ. Assessing the pathogenic cause of Sea Star Wasting Disease in Asterias forbesi along the east coast of the United States, 2015. Master's Thesis, University of Rhode Island. Available at: http://digitalcommons.uri.edu/cgi/viewcontent.cgi?article=1801&context=theses. Accessed November 23, 2016.

85. Rose J, Arlinghaus R, Cooke SJ, et al. Can fish really feel pain? Fish 2014;15:97–133.

86. Sneddon LU. Pain in aquatic animals. J Exp Biol 2015;218:967–76.

87. Elwood RW. Pain and suffering in invertebrates? ILAR J 2011;52:175–84.

88. Mettam J, Oulton L, McCrohan C, et al. The efficacy of three types of analgesic drugs in reducing pain in the rainbow trout, *Oncorhynchus mykiss*. Appl Anim Behav Sci 2011;133:265–74.

89. Ward J, McCartney S, Chinnadurai S, et al. Development of a minimum-anesthetic-concentration depression model to study the effects of various analgesics in goldfish (*Carassius auratus*). J Zoo Wildl Med 2012;43:214–22.

90. Davis MR, Mylniczenko N, Storms T, et al. Evaluation of intramuscular ketoprofen and butorphanol as analgesics in chain dogfish (*Scyliorhinus retifer*). Zoo Biol 2006;25:491–500.

91. Harms CA, Lewbart GA, Swanson CR, et al. Behavioral and clinical pathology changes in koi carp (*Cyprinus carpio*) subjected to anesthesia and surgery with and without intra-operative analgesics. Comp Med 2005;55:221–6.

92. Baker TR, Baker BB, Johnson SM, et al. Comparative analgesic efficacy of morphine sulfate and butorphanol tartrate in koi (*Cyprinus carpio*) undergoing unilateral gonadectomy. J Am Vet Med Assoc 2013;243:882–90.

93. Steenbergen PJ, Bardine N. Antinociceptive effects of buprenorphine in zebrafish larvae: an alternative for rodent models to study pain and nociception? Appl Anim Behav Sci 2014;152:92–9.

94. Larouche C. Evaluation of toxic effects of meloxicam intramuscular injection in goldfish (Carassius auratus auratus). In Proceedings 47th Annual Conference of the American Association of Zoo Veterinarians. 2015;58.

95. Nordgreen J, Kolsrud HH, Ranheim B, et al. Pharmacokinetics of morphine after intramuscular injection in common goldfish *Carassius auratus* and Atlantic salmon *Salmo salar*. Dis Aquat Org 2009;88:55–63.

96. Nordgreen J, Garner JP, Janczak AM, et al. Thermonociception in fish: effects of two different doses of morphine on thermal threshold and post-test behaviour in goldfish (*Carassius auratus*). Appl Anim Behav Sci 2009;119:101–7.

97. Ehrensing RH, Michell GF, Kastin AJ. Similar antagonism of morphine analgesia by MIF-1 and naloxone in *Carassius auratus*. Pharmacol Biochem Behav 1982; 17:757–61.

98. Newby N, Wilkie M, Stevens E. Morphine uptake, disposition, and analgesic efficacy in the common goldfish (*Carassius auratus*). Can J Zool 2009;87:388–99.

99. Sneddon LU. The evidence for pain in fish: the use of morphine as an analgesic. Appl Anim Behav Sci 2003;83:153–62.

100. Newby N, Robinson J, Vachon P, et al. Pharmacokinetics of morphine and its metabolites in freshwater rainbow trout (*Oncorhynchus mykiss*). J Vet Pharmacol Ther 2008;31:117–27.

101. Chervova L, Lapshin D. Behavioral control of the efficiency of pharmacological anesthesia in fish. J Ichthyol 2011;51:1126–32.

102. Love NE, Lewbart GA. Pet fish radiography: technique and case history reports. Vet Radiol Ultrasound 1997;38:24–9.

103. Stevens B, Vergneau-Grosset C, Rodriguez C, et al. Treatment of a facial myxoma in a goldfish (Carassius auratus) with intralesional bleomycin chemotherapy and radiation therapy. In Proceedings 47th annual conference of the International Association for Aquatic Animal Medicine, 2016.

104. Epperly MW, Bahary N, Quader M, et al. The zebrafish- *Danio rerio* - is a useful model for measuring the effects of small-molecule mitigators of late effects of ionizing irradiation. In Vivo 2012;26:889–97.

Evidence-Based Advances in Reptile Medicine

Mark A. Mitchell, DVM, MS, PhD, DECZM (Herpetology)*, Sean M. Perry, DVM

KEYWORDS

- Evidence-based • Diagnosis • Disease • Pathogen • Reptile • Statistics
- Therapeutic

KEY POINTS

- Inclusion body disease, a plague in snake collections, has been found to be associated with the presence of arenavirus in affected snakes.
- Ranavirus is highly pathogenic to red-eared sliders (*Trachemys scripta elegans*), and experimentally infected animals suffer significant mortalities from this pathogen.
- Corn snakes (*Pantherophis guttatus*) and ball pythons (*Python regius*) respond differently to ultraviolet B exposure.
- Osmolalities in reptiles can be highly variable and should be determined on a species-by-species basis.
- Positive pressure ventilation can be used to manage respiratory depression in sea turtles.

INTRODUCTION

The first herpetological medicine society, the Association of Reptile and Amphibian Veterinarians (ARAV), has been in existence for more than 25 years (originated 1991). This professional association initially produced the Bulletin of the ARAV (BARAV) to disseminate scientific material to members. This continued for 10 years, at which time the ARAV transitioned into an official journal, the *Journal of Herpetological Medicine and Surgery* (JHMS), with volume 10 issue 1. In both cases, the ARAV sought to serve as a repository for peer-reviewed, evidence-based knowledge. Early on, much of the literature produced in the BARAV and JHMS was based on case reports and brief communications. Although these types of materials can serve as important initial sources of knowledge for clinicians, they are limited to single cases and descriptive material. Over time, the JHMS has expanded to include cross-sectional studies, case-control studies, and experimental or interventional studies

Disclosure Statement: The authors have nothing to disclose.
Department of Veterinary Clinical Sciences, Louisiana State University, School of Veterinary Medicine, Skip Bertman Drive, Baton Rouge, LA 70803, USA
* Corresponding author.
E-mail address: mmitchell@lsu.edu

that provide evidence-based knowledge. The *Journal of Zoological and Wildlife Medicine* (JZWM) and the *Journal of Exotic Pet Medicine* (JEPM) are other nondomestic species journals that routinely publish on herpetological medicine too; they too often provide a mixture of hypothesis-driven research articles, brief communications, and case reports.

A primary reason that there is limited evidence-based research available for reptiles is because of the low number of specialists working in the field. The growth of the evidence-based medicine in most specialties can be tied to the increasing number of diplomates associated with the specialty, especially when these individuals are in academic institutions where there is an expectation to produce scholarship. In the United States, there are currently less than 6 individuals with specialty certification in reptile medicine in academic environments. However, this is not what should define how prolific evidence-based medicine is for a specialty. All veterinarians working in a field should consider themselves clinician scientists and feel an obligation to their profession to produce scholarship. Case-control studies, cross-sectional studies, and clinical trials can often be accomplished using available patients and limited resources. Collaboration between specialists and institutions can provide more robust studies and data sets to provide the herpetologic medicine community with solid evidence to develop educated diagnostic and therapeutic plans. Evidence-based knowledge in reptile medicine will not grow until the veterinarians practicing in the field heed the call to contribute to its development.

EVIDENCE-BASED ADVANCES IN DIAGNOSTICS

Veterinarians rely on clinical pathology data to assess the physiologic status of their patients. This type of data can provide important insight into the current state of an animal and help to guide treatment. However, this type of data is not without its shortcomings. To interpret the results of hematologic and biochemistry data, it is important to have species-specific reference intervals for comparison and know that the specific methods used to analyze the sample were validated for that species. Unfortunately, this has not been done for very many reptiles, and with more than 10,080 species in the class,[1] it is not likely to occur at any point in the future. Therefore, when the opportunity does arise to evaluate these types of questions for a particular species, it can be used as a reference for others.

Proteins are important constituents found in the blood. There are many different types of proteins, including albumin and the alpha, beta, and gamma globulins, to name a few. Chemistry analyzers typically measure total protein and albumin concentrations, and use the difference between these 2 values to calculate the globulin concentrations. Albumin is an important colloidal protein that serves as a carrier of other compounds in the blood (ie, calcium) and helps to maintain oncotic pressure. Bromocresol green dye binding is a common method used by biochemistry analyzers for measuring albumin concentrations in the blood of reptiles. However, this method is not without potential complications. Albumin, and protein binding in general, can vary between species based on several factors, such as the actual concentration of albumin and the other globulins. Dye binding itself in reptiles may lead to inaccurate results.[2] In order to determine the potential for misclassification of a biochemical parameter, it is essential to design studies that allow for validation. In the case of albumin, protein electrophoresis can be used for comparison. Ceccarelli and colleagues[3] designed a prospective study utilizing agreement analysis to screen for bias between testing methods. Historically, correlation analysis might be used for these types of studies; however, this type of analysis would be inappropriate. Data can be highly correlated but not in agreement. Serum samples collected from 32 Hermann tortoises (*Testudo hermanni*) were processed accordingly and divided for testing. Ten of these animals were clinically ill. Samples were analyzed using the colorimetric method for bromocresol dye binding and electrophoresis. As noted earlier, for this type of study to add value to the evidence-based literature, the statistical analyses needed to be done correctly. Concordance was assessed using Bland-Altman plots, and potential constant and proportional errors were evaluated using the Passing-Bablok method.[3] The results of the study showed that a systematic error was found when reviewing the Bland-Altman plots for the diseased animals, with higher values recorded using the bromocresol green dye binding method. Misinterpreting these results may lead a veterinarian to think an animal is dehydrated or not realize that a patient is hypoalbuminemic and in need of colloidal supplementation. This type of study reinforces why it is important for veterinarians to not "fear statistics." To truly gain knowledge from this study, it is important to understand how the statistical analysis was done. This remains a limitation for many clinicians, especially in the reptile specialty.

The authors of the previous study recognized that to truly build on evidence-based knowledge, it would be important to establish reference intervals for interpreting the protein electrophoresis results of Hermann tortoises.[4] Again, to establish reference intervals requires some knowledge of statistics. The American Society of Veterinary Clinical Pathologists Quality Assurance and Laboratory Standards Committee established Guidelines for the Determination of Reference Intervals in Veterinary Species in 2012.[5] These guidelines have served as an invaluable reference for clinician scientists designing studies focused on establishing reference intervals. The guidelines educate individuals as to how important sample size is to establishing reference intervals, the different methods for assessing the distribution of the data, how to screen data for outliers, and how to analyze the data using appropriate statistical methods.[5] Developing an understanding of these methods is as important as how a sample is collected and processed, but are often instead just an afterthought. In the follow-up study on Hermann tortoises, the sample size was small ($n = 22$), which is a common limitation seen in the reptile literature, but the authors assessed the data for outliers and confirmed the Gaussian distribution of the data using the recommendations for data $20<n<40$.[5] Acknowledging the distribution is especially important for how data are reported. It is not uncommon for measures of central tendency to be reported incorrectly. For example, while the mean, median, and mode are similar for normally distributed data, they are not with non-normally distributed data. When the latter is true, the best measure of central tendency is the median. Reporting the mean and standard deviation in these cases is incorrect and can confuse the reader. In the Hermann tortoise study, there were no significant differences in the protein fractions identified in the electrophoresis, including albumin (mean ± standard deviation [SD], 2.45 ± 0.61 g/dL; minimum-maximum, 0.93–3.22), alpha globulins (mean ± SD, 1.06 ± 0.38 g/dL; minimum-maximum, 0.37–1.75), beta globulins (mean ± SD, 0.89 ± 0.40 g/dL; minimum-maximum, 0.31–1.80), and gamma globulins (mean ± SD, 0.24 ± 0.09 g/dL; minimum-maximum, 0.12–0.42), by sex, except for the albumin to globulin ratio (females: mean ± SD, 1.25 ± 0.19; minimum-maximum, 0.89–1.48; males: mean ± SD, 0.97 ± 0.15; minimum-maximum, 0.80–1.23).[5] The establishment of well-defined reference intervals is important to increasing the sensitivity and specificity of clinical pathology data, as it will allow one to minimize the likelihood of drawing the wrong conclusions (false-positive or false-negative) about the physiologic state of patients. The 2 studies discussed here should serve as examples as to how clinician scientists can use data already available (eg,

Hermann tortoises) to generate evidence-based knowledge to help refine clinical skills.

Although the previous studies are the most common type of contributions to generating new evidence-based knowledge for clinical pathology data, there remains a dearth of research identifying the potential sources of biochemistries in the tissues of reptiles. To date, only 5 studies have evaluated tissue enzyme activity in reptiles, including yellow rat snakes (*Pantherophis obsoletus quadrivittatus*),[6] green iguanas (*Iguana iguana*),[7] loggerhead sea turtles (*Caretta carreta*),[8] American alligators (*Alligator mississippiensis*),[9] and Kemp's ridley sea turtles (*Lepidochelys kempii*).[10] Interpreting the results of plasma or serum enzyme data without knowledge as to where the enzyme originated from is difficult, and can often lead to misclassification of a disease or the organ system affected by a disease process. In the authors' experience, this is frequently done with aspartate aminotransferase (AST). It is not uncommon for AST to be considered important to the liver, although the aforementioned studies do not suggest it is found in high concentrations in the liver.[7–10] The most recent articles noted[8–10] deserve special mention, because they represent what can be done by any clinician scientist regardless of his or her practice type (eg, academia, zoologic institution, general practice). These 3 cases represent opportunistic sampling in which animals were being sacrificed or were available because of a stranding event. These types of cross-sectional studies can provide important initial insight into specific hypotheses of interest. They also set the groundwork for prospective randomized trials. In this case, this might include randomized clinical trials to compare enzyme activities between study subjects based on a drug trial or specific disease. Although the sample sizes for these studies were small (alligators, n = 6[9]; loggerhead sea turtles, n = 5[8]; Kemp's ridley sea turtles, n = 13[10]), statistical methods were used and maximized the value of the data beyond purely descriptive statistics. In the alligators, several important findings were reported, including AST concentrations in the liver and alanine aminotransferase (ALT) concentrations in the kidney.[9] This study again showed that AST activity is not necessarily specific to the liver, with similar concentrations found in the kidney. Interestingly, ALT activity was high in the kidney, more than 15-fold to the next tissue (skeletal muscle) and 60-fold higher than liver, which is a site-specific location for this enzyme in people and many mammals. In the Kemp's ridley sea turtles, AST, creatine kinase (CK), and lactate dehydrogenase (LDH) were found in multiple tissues; however, analogous to previous studies, the highest concentrations were found in skeletal and cardiac muscles.[10] Also similar to the other studies, enzymes were found in multiple tissues, but activities were low.[10] These types of studies suggest that there is variability between species and reinforces why it is important to pursue this type of research on a species-by-species basis to expand evidence-based knowledge.

EVIDENCE-BASED ADVANCES IN THERAPEUTICS
Rehydrating Reptiles

Inappropriate husbandry, poor nutrition, and disease are common causes for dehydration in reptiles.[11,12] Rehydration should be done while considering the physiologic state of the patient, including osmolality. Unfortunately, there has long been confusing anecdotal messages being published regarding the osmolality of reptiles.[11,12] In addition, it is common practice for clinicians to select fluids for rehydration based on convenience and fluid availability rather than considering the osmolality of the patient. Common fluids used in veterinary medicine include Lactated Ringer solution (273 mOsm/L), 0.9% NaCl (308 mOsm/L), and 5% dextrose (252 mOsm/L). Best practices for rehydrating a reptile should include the osmolality of a patient, the fluid being selected to rehydrate the patient, and the method for determining the osmolality. Recent clinical investigational studies on bearded dragons (*Pogona vitticeps*) and corn snakes (*Pantherophis guttatus*) are examples of reports of differences in osmolality between different reptiles (bearded dragons: mean = 295.4 mOsm/kg; corn snakes: mean = 344.5 mOsm/kg) and a need for calculating an osmolality of a reptile patient to ensure best practice when replenishing fluids.[11,12] The studies used a freezing point osmometer and formulae with different potential biochemistry parameters to determine osmolalities of these species. Agreement analysis was used to determine which formula provided the best agreement with the measured osmolality. The study confirmed that a high degree of agreement could be achieved by using species-specific calculations in the absence of a freezing point osmometer (bearded dragons: [1.85 (sodium + potassium)]; corn snakes: [2 × (sodium + potassium)] + [glucose/18]).[11,12]

Novel Forms of Treatment

Salmonella subspecies are important zoonotic pathogens harbored by reptiles. Concerns for the prevalence of *Salmonella* subspecies in some species of reptiles, such as chelonians less than 10.4 cm, have led to interstate regulations prohibiting the sale of these animals in the United States.[13,14] Historically, treatment of *Salmonella* subspecies in reptiles was done using antibiotics, including chelonians.[15,16] This has led to concerns for antibiotic resistance and increased public risk.[17,18] Identifying novel treatments, and testing them using appropriately designed studies, is needed to affirm the value of new remedies and reduce the risk to human caretakers of reptiles. An experimental study was performed to determine the value of various nonantibiotics for reducing or eliminating *Salmonella* from turtle eggs. Previous studies assessing the effectiveness of antibiotics for treating turtle eggs did not consider the difference in prevalence in *Salmonella* species within nests.[17–19] However, this can significantly impact the outcome. Thus, in the current study, eggs within nests were randomly assigned to treatments. The results of the study indeed showed that the combination of polyhexamethylene biguanide and bleach using a negative pressure system could significantly decrease the odds (odds ratio: 0.2, 95% confidence interval [CI]: 0.1–0.2) of *Salmonella* subspecies in the hatchlings.[19] As antibiotic resistance continues to rise in clinical cases and environmental samples, studies evaluating nonantibiotic treatments for reptiles, and other species, should be pursued.

Positive pressure ventilation is commonly performed in reptiles during anesthetic events to help reduce or minimize adverse effects associated with apnea. Although commonly considered as an important component of a standard operating procedure in reptile anesthesia, it can also be used as a treatment in cases where bradypnea and apnea are a concern. The idea of using positive pressure ventilation to manage medical, and not surgical/anesthetic, reptile cases is novel. Cold-stunned turtles are a common finding in the northeastern United States during the late fall.[20,21] Turtles that do not migrate south often develop life-threatening hypothermia and respiratory depression. A recent retrospective study evaluated the value of mechanical positive pressure ventilation in cold-stunned sea turtles to determine whether this treatment/procedure could be used to improve prognosis and survival.[22] Recruitment of the turtles included cases with complete medical records and no known ventilator complications. Twenty-nine sea turtles out of 48 original cases were selected for the retrospective review, including 21 Kemp's ridley (*L kempii*), 4 loggerhead (*Caretta caretta*), and 4 green turtles (*Chelonia mydas*). Most (n = 20, 68.9%) of the turtles were successfully extubated from the mechanical ventilation, while 7 (24.1%) died during ventilation, and 2 (7%) were euthanized during treatment. Most of the extubated turtles (n = 11, 55%) were weaned from the mechanical ventilator and survived over 24 hours; however, only 20% (n = 4) of turtles survived to release. Ultimately, this study showed that positive pressure ventilation could be used to manage moribund, cold-stunned sea turtles. Although the results of this study suggest that the success rate of positive pressure mechanical ventilation is low, the genetic importance of each threatened or endangered sea turtle to its species is immeasurable. Retrospective clinical studies such as this represent the type of historical studies that veterinarians can contribute to their specialty, regardless of their practice type. This type of study also serves to remind how important it is to maintain high-quality medical records. Nearly 40% of the available cases could not be used, limiting the power of the study. Another limitation of this type of retrospective study was that animals presented in different stages of hypothermia and thus physiologic states. A prospective clinical trial could help alleviate many of the shortcomings with this type of study, and it will be important for specialists in the field to perform these types of studies to increase evidence-based knowledge.

EVIDENCE-BASED ADVANCES IN COMMON DISORDERS
Secondary Nutritional Hyperparathyroidism/Hypovitaminosis D

Secondary nutritional hyperparathyroidism remains an important disease in captive reptiles.[23] Affected animals routinely present for anorexia, weakness, muscle tremors, pathologic fractures, and seizures. The disease has been tied to inappropriate nutrition, including low calcium or vitamin D in the diet and high phosphorus in the diet, as well as husbandry deficiencies, including a lack of exposure to ultraviolet B (UVB) radiation.[23–25] Much of the evidence-based knowledge of this disease is limited to understanding of the role of circulating 25-hydroxyvitamin D concentrations in animals. Although initial studies focused on lizards, more recent studies have focused on chelonians and snakes.[24] The classic study design used for these trials is to randomly assign animals to treatment groups and expose them to UVB radiation, while not supplementing the control group. As might be expected with such a large group of species, there are certainly differences noted between and within groups and species, respectively.

Chelonians represent a diverse group of animals, and within this group it is possible to find herbivorous, omnivorous, and carnivorous species. Therefore, it might be expected that there will be differences in vitamin D metabolism within this group. The first study to evaluate the role of UVB on chelonians used an omnivorous species, the red-eared slider (*Trachemys scripta elegans*).[24] A randomized clinical trial was used to determine whether UVB exposure had an effect on circulating 25-hydroxyvitamin D concentrations in the turtles. Twelve, unsexed yearling turtles were used for the study, and the animals had just emerged from winter brumation so they had not eaten food for over 2 months. Animals were randomly assigned to one of two groups (treatment: exposed to UVB light; control: not exposed to UVB light) using a random number generator. The study was performed over 30 days. The turtles exposed to UVB for 30 days showed a significant rise in 25-hydroxyvitamin D concentrations (treatment group: baseline = 10.7 ± 3.4 nmol/L, 30 days = 71.7 ± 46.9; control group: baseline = 11.2 ± 4.3 nmol/L, 30 days = 31.4 ± 13.2). In addition to proving that UVB exposure increased the circulating 25-hydroxyvitamin D concentrations in red-eared sliders, the findings also suggested that this species of turtle derives vitamin D through their diet, as the difference in 25-hydroxyvitamin D concentrations in the control group also significantly increased over the course of the study. This was not unexpected, as the animals were fasted during their winter aestivation. A follow-up experimental trial evaluating 3 different forms of UVB exposure (natural sunlight, mercury-vapor bulb, fluorescent bulb) in Hermann tortoises (T hermanni) found interesting results.[26] Eighteen animals were used in the study, and these animals were randomly assigned to one of the three treatment groups. Blood samples were collected at baseline (20 days after exposure to sunlight following brumation) and 35 days following exposure to the assigned treatment. Interestingly, the 25-hydroxy-vitamin D concentrations decreased in both the fluorescent tube group (day 0: 313.7 ± 109.5 nmol/L, day 35: 134.4 ± 51.4) and self-ballasted mercury vapor group (day 0: 368.0 ± 119.3 nmol/L, day 35: 155.7 ± 80.7), whereas it remained stable in animals exposed to natural sunlight (day 0: 387.7 ± 114.5 nmol/L, day 35: 411.5 ± 189.7).[26] This result is interesting, because in lizards, a decay or decline in vitamin D has been noted in animals not provided UVB exposure, but the half-life is longer than 35 days (rhinoceros iguana [Cyclura cornuta]: 69 day half-life).[27] These differences reinforce that temporal studies are needed to further refine understanding of vitamin D metabolism in reptiles, and thus understanding of nutritional diseases (eg, secondary nutritional hyperparathyroidism). Further, the results of the Hermann tortoise study, combined with the red-eared slider study, should reinforce to clinician scientists that grouping or categorizing reptiles based on basic similarities such as being chelonians may lead to erroneous conclusions. It is important to recognize that each species is unique, and it should serve as a reminder that there is a need to continue to develop evidence-based knowledge to ensure best care for patients.

Snakes are an interesting group to consider for study, because secondary nutritional hyperparathyroidism has not been an important disease in these reptiles due to their carnivorous lifestyles. However, vitamin D deficiency can extend beyond secondary nutritional hyperparathyroidism because of its role in cardiovascular health, immune function, and endocrine health, among other functions.[28] In snakes, there have been 2 studies done evaluating the role of UVB exposure on circulating 25-hydroxyvitamin concentrations, with very different results.[25,29] Acierno and colleagues[25] used corn snakes (Pantherophis guttatus) for their study, while Hedley and Eatwell[29] used ball pythons (Python regius). In the corn snake study, only males were used because of a limited sample size (n = 12), while in the ball python study, 14 animals were used; 6 females were in the UVB exposure group, and 5 males and 3 females were in the control group. The corn snakes exposed to UVB for 28 days showed a significant rise in 25-hydroxyvitamin D concentrations (treatment group: baseline = 63 ± 36.9 nmol/L, 28 days = 196 ± 16.7; control group: baseline = 57.3 ± 45.6 nmol/L, 28 days = 57.2 ± 15.3), while the ball pythons exposed to 70 days of UVB did not (treatment group [all females]: baseline = 197 ± 35 nmol/L, 70 days = 203.5 ± 13.8; control group [5 males, 3 females]: baseline = 77.7 ± 41.5 nmol/L, 70 days = 83 ± 41.9). The differences noted between these studies suggest that species differences exist, but that sex may also play a role. It is important when designing a study, especially with a small sample size, to focus on the primary independent variable or risk factor of interest. In these studies, exposure to UVB serves this role, and sex, as a secondary variable, should only be evaluated if sufficient power (ie, >0.80 power, because there is an appropriate sample size) is available to minimize the likelihood of a type II error (ie, accepting the null hypothesis when it is not true).

Infectious Diseases

Ranaviruses are members of the Family Iridovirus and have had a major impact on amphibian populations.[30,31] Recently, ranavirus has also been found to become a problem in reptiles.[32,33] Although the ability to diagnose viruses and other pathogens in reptiles has increased with the advent of molecular diagnostic testing, a major deficiency in evidence-based knowledge is a lack of understanding of the epidemiology of these novel viruses. Fortunately, evidence-based epidemiologic investigations have been initiated to develop an understanding of ranavirus infections in box turtles (*Terrapene carolina carolina*). Any diagnostic test used to assess the disease status of an animal should be validated before being applied. Prior to initiating any studies assessing the ranavirus status of box turtles, a reverse-transcriptase polymerase chain reaction (RT-PCR) assay was developed.[34] The assay was validated using standard positive and negative controls, confirming its value. Following the development of the RT-PCR assay, a cross-sectional study was done to gain an understanding of the prevalence of disease.[35] These types of studies are excellent starting points, because they allow one to estimate the impact of the disease. Interestingly, the prevalence of ranavirus in the 606 box turtles sampled from 5 different states was low (1.5%, 95% CI: 0.8%–2.9%).[35] On first glance, this might suggest that the disease has a low impact on box turtles; however, epidemiologic investigations require a global assessment, and a follow-up pathogenesis study suggests that the prevalence might be low because of the high mortality associated with infection.[36] Affected animals developed significant vasculitis and died or were euthanized within 30 days of infection. Environmental temperature was not found to have a significant impact on the mortality rates between infected turtles, but a trend found in the data suggested that it may play a role in the pathogenesis. Limited sample size, and thus a lower power than desired, were reasons given for the potential lack of significance between treatment groups at different temperatures. Because ranaviruses are stenothermal, follow-up studies with higher sample sizes were recommended. Physiologic responses identified in infected turtles can also be used to help assess prognosis or guide clinicians while other diagnostics are pending. Hematologic and biochemistry testing are commonly used in reptiles to assess their physiologic response to potential pathogens. A randomized clinical trial was done as part of the previous epidemiologic investigations to determine whether experimental ranavirus infection has an effect on hematologic and biochemistry parameters in red-eared slider turtles.[37] Total solids were significantly decreased ($P = .034$) over time in infected turtles (preinoculation sample: 3.8 g/dL, terminal sample: 3.1 g/dL), which was consistent with the findings of the pathogenesis study where severe vasculitis was observed.[36,37] Differences in the white blood cell count at different time points were also noted. Infected turtles housed at 22°C showed an elevation in white blood cell counts between days 18 and 22, while infected turtles housed at 28°C showed increases in white blood cell counts between days 8 and 11.[37] The earlier elevation in white blood cell counts noted in the turtles housed in warmer temperatures was likely associated with the turtles' higher metabolic rate and immune function. It was interesting to note that major changes in hematology and biochemistry patterns were not noted between infected and noninfected turtles. The authors suggested that this was likely due to the rapid progression of the disease and the ability of the virus to elude the immune system. Overall, the compilation of these studies represents the types of epidemiologic investigations that are needed to characterize host-pathogen-environment interactions in reptiles.

As epidemiologists, the authors routinely joke with their colleagues studying infectious diseases. Although the authors find identifying new pathogens (eg, viruses) valuable, in many cases these results represent no more new information than a case report or case series. It is essential that this knowledge be expanded to include the epidemiology associated with that pathogen. Similar to the example provided earlier with ranavirus, it is important to validate the methods used to diagnose or screen for a particular pathogen, apply the test to affected and unaffected populations, develop an understanding of the pathogenesis of the disease, and develop novel therapeutics. One of the pathogens that this is starting to happen with, but needs to be expounded upon, is the disease historically known as inclusion body disease (IBD). IBD is a disease that has long caused issues for veterinarians. This disease has been diagnosed in both boids and pythons, and, historically, there have not been any sensitive and noninvasive ante-mortem diagnostic tests (other than necropsy or biopsy and histopathology) or treatments available.[38–40] IBD has been attributed to a retrovirus and a 68-kd protein representing a nonviral intracytoplasmic inclusion.[39,40] However, recently, Stenglein and colleagues[41] used metagenomics to screen samples from IBD-positive snakes (annulated tree boa [*Corallus annulatus*], boa constrictor [*Boa constrictor*], Dumeril boa [*Boa dumerili*]) and found that 6 of 8 were positive for arenavirus, while 0 of 18 control snakes were negative for the virus. It was also interesting to note that the virus was divergent from currently understood mammalian lineages. This has been further reinforced in other reports too, including confirmation of IBD snakes being arenavirus positive in The Netherlands.[42] Once this association between the arenavirus pathogen and IBD intracytoplasmic inclusion has been confirmed, it is important to identify additional methods for diagnosis and specific studies to fulfill Koch's postulate to confirm that the virus is the causative agent of IBD. Chang and colleagues[43] designed an antibody specific for the 68-kd protein, now known as the nucleoprotein (NP) of reptarenavirus, for use in immunoassays. Immunohistochemical staining of paraffin-embedded tissues using IBD-positive and -negative samples revealed a moderate sensitivity (83%) and exceptional specificity (100%).[43] This suggests that there would be no false positives using this method, which can help minimize the likelihood of misclassifying a positive snake. These researchers followed this up by estimating the prevalence of this disease in snakes in the United States and using a validated monoclonal anti-NP antibody assay to screen samples.[44] One hundred thirty-one boas and pythons representing 28 different collections were screened. Positive snakes were confirmed by the presence of the classic eosinophilic intracytoplasmic inclusions in the blood cells. The prevalence in this cross-sectional study was 19% (95% CI: 12.4%–25.8%), suggesting that this disease is not uncommon in snakes and may go unnoticed. Further reinforcing this theory was that most affected boa constrictors (n = 22; 87%) were clinically normal. The authors were able to use the positive blood samples to measure the level of agreement between that diagnostic and an RT-PCR, immunohistochemistry using their monoclonal antibody, and Western blots using their monoclonal antibody in boas. In all 3 cases, the authors found excellent agreement between the standard and the newly developed assays for boas (RT-PCR: kappa = 0.92; Western blots: kappa = 0.89; immunohistochemistry: kappa = 0.92). There remain to be studies fulfilling Koch's postulate and potential treatments for this disease; however, a great deal of growth has happened in evidence-based knowledge with this disease in a short time considering that the arenavirus-IBD association was only first identified in 2012, and the disease has been known for more than 30 years.

CURRENT CONTROVERSIES

One could argue that much of what is practiced in reptile medicine is associated with some controversy, because it is subjective in nature rather than objective. This primarily is the result of evidence-based knowledge being more descriptive than quantitative. A specific recent example of a controversy:

- Is there a need for UVB exposure in crepuscular/nocturnal reptiles? The author and colleagues have performed 3 UVB exposure studies in leopard geckos (*Eublepharis macularius*).[45–47] During discussions at the annual conference of the ARAV, some attendees raised concerns for the need for UVB in these types of species; however, based on the randomized experimental study designs used for the studies, it was obvious that the leopard geckos increased their 25-hydroxyvitamin D concentrations significantly after being exposed to UVB light. Additional studies are needed to further refine what an increase in 25-hydroxyvitamin D concentrations represents for leopard geckos; however, this should not only be for these nocturnal species, but all species showing this type of response.

NEW IDEAS

As noted earlier in this article, UVB radiation is generally seen as a benefit to reptiles because of how it impacts their vitamin D homeostasis. However, while UVB is known to produce positive effects in reptiles, it is not without its potential adverse effects. A recent case report that included a cross-sectional survey from 2 reptile pathologists suggested that UVB exposure may contribute to the development of squamous cell carcinoma (SCC) in bearded dragons (*Pogona viticeps*).[48] In the survey, 12 SCC cases were identified, representing 6% of the bearded dragon cancer cases reported at the pathologists' facilities over 10 years. Most of the lesions were on the head (10/12, 83.3%) and associated with the mucocutaneous junctions (11/12, 91.6%). Because these sites for SCC are similar to those reported for other animals and people as an adverse effect to ultraviolet radiation,[49,50] it is possible that current husbandry recommendations may predispose some dragons to cancer. Following up this report with a case-control study would be an excellent start to increasing evidence-based knowledge. Because this disease is apparently rare (<10%), a longitudinal study, such as a cohort study, or an experimental study is not suggested, because it may take too long for the animals to develop the disease; additionally, researchers would have to determine a toxic level of UVB. The case-control study could be retrospective and allow a clinician scientist to screen cases with SCC matched to noncases of SCC to determine what independent factors may predict or prevent SCC formation.

Mycoplasma spp are a group of bacteria that have long perplexed veterinarians, because they are difficult to isolate and can be insidious. Most evidence-based knowledge regarding this pathogen is associated with tortoises.[51] In this group of reptiles, it is not uncommon for animals to develop respiratory tract infections. More recently, *Mycoplasma* spp have been reported in snakes too.[52–54] This is an important finding, because it represents what might be an undiagnosed condition. The lesions commonly identified in chelonians with mycoplasmosis can include upper and lower respiratory tract infections; these types of lesions are often identified in snakes too but not associated with a specific pathogen. To date, there have been 3 reports of *Mycoplasma* spp in snakes.[52–54] In the first case report, tracheitis and pneumonia were reported in a Burmese python (*Python molurus bivittatus*).[52] In the second case report, *Mycoplasma* spp was again isolated from a snake with pneumonia,[53] and in the third case report, *Mycoplasma* spp were isolated from 3 carpet pythons (*Morelia spilota*) with stomatitis.[54] These 3 case reports suggest that additional study is needed to further characterize the role of *Mycoplasma* spp in the pathogenesis of respiratory disease in snakes. Similar to the previous discussions on ranavirus and arenavirus, a well-planned epidemiologic investigation that includes isolating the organism and/or validating an assay(s) for diagnosis, applying the assay(s) to determine the prevalence or incidence of disease in snakes, and performing experimental studies to characterize the pathogenesis and novel treatments is needed.

SUMMARY

As noted earlier in the introduction, reptile medicine is at a crossroads where it is important that it turns from a specialty that remains primarily descriptive to one based on evidence-based knowledge. Although case reports and case series provide important first notices of novel findings, they are limited in their scope and application. Cross-sectional studies, likewise, while important, are limited in providing answers to specific variable testing with a temporal application. It is essential for the specialty to expand into case-control studies, cohort studies, and experimental/intervention studies that enable broader investigational opportunities. This is starting, but more is needed. In reviewing the JHMS over the past 5 years, 35 articles were case reports, and 51 articles were original studies. If all of those representing the specialty contribute to this advancement, significant growth in evidence-based knowledge will be achieved.

REFERENCES

1. Uetz P. Species numbers. Available at: http://www.reptile-database.org/db-info/SpeciesStat.html. Accessed April 2, 2017.
2. Muller K, Brunnberg L. Determination of plasma albumin concentration in healthy and diseased turtles: comparison of protein electrophoresis and the bromocresol green dye-binding method. Vet Clin Pathol 2010;39(1):79–82.
3. Ceccarelli R, Macrelli M, Fiorucci L. Determination of serum albumin concentrations in healthy and diseased Hermann's tortoises (*Testudo hermanni*): a comparison using electrophoresis and the bromocresol green dye-binding method. J Herp Med Surg 2013;23(1–2):20–4.
4. Fiorucci L, Ceccarelli M, Macrelli R, et al. Protein electrophoresis in Hermann's tortoises (*Testudo hermanni*): a first step in reference value determination. J Herp Med Surg 2013;23(1–2):15–9.
5. Friedrichs KR, Harr KE, Freeman KP, et al. ASVCP reference interval guidelines: determination of de novo reference intervals in veterinary species and other related topics. Vet Clin Pathol 2012;41(4):441–53.
6. Ramsay EC, Dotson TK. Tissue and serum enzyme activities in the yellow rat snake (*Elaphe obsoleta quadrivittatus*). Am J Vet Res 1995;56(4):423–8.
7. Wagner RA, Wetzel R. Tissue and plasma enzyme activities in the juvenile green iguanas (*Iguana iguana*). Am J Vet Res 1999;60(2):201–3.
8. Anderson EA, Socha VL, Gardner J, et al. Tissue enzyme activities in the loggerhead sea turtle (*Caretta caretta*). J Zoo Wildl Med 2013;44(1):62–9.
9. Bogan JE, Mitchell MA. Characterizing tissue enzyme activities in the American alligator (*Alligator mississippiensis*). J Herp Med Surg 2014;24(3–4):77–81.
10. Petrosky KY, Knoll JS, Innis C. Tissue enzyme activities in Kemp's ridley turtles (*Lepidochelys kempii*). J Zoo Wildl Med 2015;46(3):637–40.
11. Dallwig RK, Mitchell MA, Acierno MJ. Determination of plasma osmolality and agreement between measured and calculated values in healthy adult bearded dragons (*Pogona vitticeps*). J Herp Med Surg 2010;20(2–3):69–73.
12. Sanchez-Migallon Guzman D, Mitchell MA, Acierno MJ. Determination of plasma osmolality and agreement between measured and calculated values in captive

male corn snakes (*Pantherophis guttatus guttatus*). J Herp Med Surg 2011;21(1): 16–9.

13. Ackman DM, Drabkin P, Birkhead G, et al. Reptile-associated salmonellosis in New York state. Pediatr Infect Dis J 1995;14:955–9.

14. Wells EV, Boulton M, Hall W, et al. Reptile-associated salmonellosis in preschool aged children in Michigan, January 2001-June 2003. Clin Infect Dis 2004;39: 687–91.

15. Siebling RJ, Neal PM, Granberry WD. Evaluation of methods for the isolation of *Salmonella* and *Arizona* organisms from pet turtles treated with antimicrobial agents. Appl Microbiol 1975;29:240–5.

16. Siebling RJ, Caruso D, Neuman S. Eradication of *Salmonella* and *Arizona* species from turtle hatchlings produced from eggs treated on commercial turtle farms. Appl Environ Microbiol 1984;47:658–62.

17. D'Aoust JY, Daley E, Crozier M, et al. Pet turtles: a continuing international threat to public health. Am J Epidemiol 1990;132:233–8.

18. Shane SM, Gilbert R, Harrington KS. *Salmonella* colonization in commercial pet turtles (*Pseudemys scripta elegans*). Epidemiol Infect 1990;105:307–15.

19. Mitchell MA, Adamson T, Singleton CB, et al. Evaluating the efficacy if Clorox® and Baquacil® against *Salmonella* sp. in red-eared slider (*Trachemys scripta elegans*) eggs and hatchlings. Am J Vet Res 2007;68(2):158–64.

20. Innis C, Nyaoke AC, Williams CR, et al. Pathologic and parasitologic findings of cold-stunned Kemp's ridley sea turtles (*Lepidochelys kempii*) stranded on Cape Cod, Massachusetts, 2001-2006. J Wildl Dis 2009;45(3):594–610.

21. Innis CJ, Ravich JB, Tlusty MF, et al. Hematologic and plasma biochemical findings in cold-stunned Kemp's ridley turtles: 176 cases (2001-2005). J Am Vet Med Assoc 2009;235(4):426–32.

22. Spielvogel CF, King L, Cavin JM, et al. Use of positive pressure ventilation in cold-stunned sea turtles: 29 cases (2008-2014). J Herp Med Surg, in press.

23. Mans C, Braun J. Update on common nutritional disorders of captive reptiles. Vet Clin North Am Exot Anim Pract 2014;17(3):369–95.

24. Acierno MJ, Mitchell MA, Roundtree MK, et al. Effects of ultraviolet radiation on 25-hydroxyvitamin D_3 synthesis in red-eared slider turtles (*Trachemys scripta elegans*). Am J Vet Res 2006;67(12):2046–9.

25. Acierno MJ, Mitchell MA, Zachariah TT, et al. Effects of ultraviolet radiation on plasma 25-hydroxyvitamin D_3 concentrations in corn snakes (*Elaphe guttata*). Am J Vet Res 2008;69(2):294–7.

26. Selleri P, Di Girolamo N. Plasma 25-hydroxyvitamin D(3) concentrations in Hermann's tortoises (*Testudo hermanni*) exposed to natural sunlight and two artificial ultraviolet radiation sources. Am J Vet Res 2012;73(11):1781–6.

27. Ferguson GW, Gehrmann WH, Bradley KA, et al. Summer and winter seasonal changes in vitamin D status of captive rhinoceros iguanas (*Cyclura cornuta*). J Herp Med Surg 2015;25(3–4):128–36.

28. Watson MK, Stern AW, Labelle AL, et al. Evaluating the clinical and physiological effects of long term ultraviolet B radiation on guinea pigs (*Cavia porcellus*). PLoS One 2014;9(12):e114413.

29. Hedley J, Eatwell K. The effects of UV light on calcium metabolism in ball pythons (*Python regius*). Vet Rec 2013;173(14):345.

30. Daszak P, Berger L, Cunningham AA, et al. Emerging infectious diseases and amphibian population declines. Emerg Infect Dis 2009;5:735–48.

31. Green DE, Converse KA, Schrader AK. Epizootiology of sixty-four amphibian morbidity and mortality events in the USA, 1996-2001. Ann N Y Acad Sci 2002; 969:323–39.
32. De Voe RK, Geissler K, Elmore S, et al. Ranavirus-associated morbidity and mortality in a group of captive eastern box turtles (*Terrapene carolina carolina*). J Zoo Wildl Med 2004;35:534–43.
33. Johnson AJ, Pessier AP, Wellehan JFX, et al. Ranavirus infection of free-ranging and captive box turtles and tortoises in the United States. J Wildl Dis 2008;44: 851–63.
34. Allender MC, Bunick D, Mitchell MA. Development and validation of a TaqMan quantitative PCR for detection of frog virus 3 in eastern box turtles (*Terrapene carolina carolina*). J Virol Methods 2013;188:121–5.
35. Allender MC, Mitchell MA, McRuer D, et al. Prevalence, clinical signs, and natural history characteristics of frog virus 3-like infections in Eastern box turtles (*Terrapene carolina carolina*). Herp Conserv Biol 2013;8(2):308–20.
36. Allender MC, Mitchell MA, Torres T, et al. Pathogenicity of frog virus 3-like virus in red-eared slider turtles (*Trachemys scripta elegans*) at two environmental temperatures. J Comp Pathol 2013;149:356–67.
37. Allender MC, Mitchell MA. Hematologic response to experimental infections of frog virus 3-like virus in red eared sliders (*Trachemys scripta elegans*). J Herp Med Surg 2013;23(1–2):25–31.
38. Carlisle-Nowak MS, Sullivan N, Carrigan M, et al. Inclusion body disease in two captive Australian pythons (*Morelia spilota variegata* and *Morelia spilota spilota*). Aust Vet J 1998;76(2):98–100.
39. Jacobson ER, Orós J, Tucker SJ, et al. Partial characterization of retroviruses from boid snakes with inclusion body disease. Am J Vet Res 2001;62(2):217–24.
40. Wozniak E, McBride J, DeNardo D, et al. Isolation and characterization of an antigenically distinct 68-kd protein from nonviral intracytoplasmic inclusions in boa constrictors chronically infected with the inclusion body disease virus (IBDV: Retroviridae). Vet Pathol 2000;37(5):449–59.
41. Stenglein MD, Sanders C, Kistler AL, et al. Identification, characterization, and in vitro culture of highly divergent arenaviruses from boa constrictors and annulated tree boas: candidate etiological agents for snake inclusion body disease. MBio 2012;3(4):e00180-12.
42. Bodewes R, Kik MJ, Raj VS, et al. Detection of novel divergent arenaviruses in boid snakes with inclusion body disease in The Netherlands. Vet J 2016;218: 13–8.
43. Chang LW, Fu A, Wozniak E, et al. Immunohistochemical detection of a unique protein within cells of snakes having inclusion body disease, a world-wide disease seen in members of the families Boidae and Pythonidae. PLoS One 2013; 8(12):e82916.
44. Chang L, Fu D, Stenglein MD, et al. Detection and prevalence of boid inclusion body disease in collections of boas and pythons using immunological assays. Vet J 2016;218:13–8.
45. Wangen K, Kirschenbaum J, Mitchell MA. Measuring 25-hydroxyvitamin D levels in leopard geckos exposed to commercial ultraviolet lights. Proc Assoc Rept Amphib Vet 2013;42.
46. Johnson JG, Mitchell MA, Joslyn S, et al. Effect of ultraviolet B radiation on bone density in leopard geckos (Eublepharis macularius). Proc Assoc Rept Amphib Vet 2014;137.

47. Gould A, Molitor L, Rockwell K, et al. Evaluating the clinical effects of short dura- tion ultraviolet B radiation exposure in leopard geckos (Eublepharis macularius). Proc Assoc Rept Amphib Vet 2015; 529.

48. Hannon DE, Garner MM, Reavill DR. Squamous cell carcinomas in inland bearded dragons (*Pogona vitticeps*). J Herp Med Surg 2011;21(4):101–6.

49. Dorn CR, Taylor DO, Schneider R. Sunlight exposure and risk of developing cuta- neous and oral squamous cell carcinomas in white cats. J Natl Cancer Inst 1972; 46:1073–8.

50. Gallagher RP, Lee TK. Adverse effects of ultraviolet radiation: a brief review. Prog Biophys Mol Biol 2006;92:119–31.

51. Jacobson ER, Brown MB, Wendland LD, et al. Mycoplasmosis and upper respi- ratory tract disease of tortoises: a review and update. Vet J 2014;201(3):257–64.

52. Penner JD, Jacobson ER, Brown DR, et al. A novel *Mycoplasma* sp. Associated with proliferative tracheitis and pneumonia in a Burmese python (*Python molurus bivittatus*). J Comp Pathol 1997;117(3):283–8.

53. Schmidt V, Marschang RE, Abbas MD, et al. Detection of pathogens in *Boidae* and *Pythonidae* with and without respiratory disease. Vet Rec 2013;172(9):236.

54. Marschang RE, Heckers KO, Dietz J. Detection of a *Mycoplasma* sp. In a python (*Morelia spilota*) with stomatitis. J Herp Med Surg 2016;26(3–4):90–3.

Evidence-Based Rabbit Housing and Nutrition

Marcus Clauss, MSc, Dr med vet, DECVCN*,
Jean-Michel Hatt, MSc, Dr med vet, DACZM, DECZM (Avian)

KEYWORDS

- Rabbit • Husbandry • Housing • Enrichment • Water • Nutrition • Diet • Hay

KEY POINTS

- Rabbits should not be kept individually, but as pairs or groups.
- Rabbits are housed in various ways; opportunity to hide, hop, and run should be provided.
- Rabbits should be offered water ad libitum from open dish drinker systems.
- Rabbits should be offered hay ad libitum together with a restricted amount of high-fiber pellets and a regular, consistent provision of green leafy vegetables.

There is a large body of literature on the husbandry and nutrition of rabbits used in commercial meat production systems and in laboratory settings, with more limited information directly gained in pet rabbits. For example, a recent 313-page monograph on rabbit nutrition contains a 20-page article on pet rabbits,[1] and a recent review thesis on rabbit welfare[2] identified approximately 150 studies in production or laboratory rabbits versus nine studies in pet rabbits. The large body of literature on production rabbits is being made available to the pet veterinary community by various reviews that also include such information,[3–9] but it should be kept in mind that this information is mostly gained by comparing various conditions that all represent deviations from what could be considered optimal. Requirements demonstrated in laboratory or production rabbits should be considered minimum standards that should be surpassed in pet rabbit husbandry; additional requirements apply to pet rabbits that are linked to their expected longer lifespan.

Wild rabbits are crepuscular herbivores that live in extensive burrow systems in large social groups, are exposed to distinct seasonal changes in climate and resource ability, and are subject to intense predation. Domestic rabbits have been bred for lives under different conditions, but in contrast to most other domestic animals, domestic rabbit welfare is typically assessed by comparison with the wild.[10] In performing

The authors have nothing to disclose.
Clinic for Zoo Animals, Exotic Pets and Wildlife, Vetsuisse Faculty, University of Zurich, Winterthurerstrasse 260, Zurich 8057, Switzerland
* Corresponding author.
E-mail address: mclauss@vetclinics.uzh.ch

such comparisons, the socioeconomic relevance of maintaining rabbits as production and laboratory animals may justify larger deviations from ideal conditions than may seem acceptable for pet animals kept for recreational purposes. Furthermore, conditions in the wild need not necessarily represent the ideal state for individuals (such as predation, interspecific competition, resource scarcity, and intraspecific aggression for the losing individuals), and concepts for how the absence of such aspects in well-managed domestic animals may compensate for other shortcomings are rarely presented. A notable exception is a review that relates an apparent lack of benefits of group housing in commercial breeding rabbit does to the absence of predation, which the authors suggest as a major driver for group-living in wild rabbit does.[11]

Additionally, one should be aware that rabbit welfare research has focused on aspects that are addressed with a degree of feasibility, such as diet, cage size and design, enrichment, or sociality, whereas aspects that are logistically challenging to mend, such as the opportunity to perform burrowing behavior, have received less attention. Certain deviations from wild conditions are (mainly without experimental evidence but based on common understanding) considered not problematic, such as the change of the daily routine of pet rabbits from a crepuscular/nocturnal to a diurnal lifestyle, or the provision of dried forages as a substitute for forages ingested in the wild.

In compiling this review on evidence-based guidelines for rabbit housing and nutrition, we report mainly facts based on research, but given the lack of studies for pet rabbits, we also mention aspects related to common sense and speculation.

HOUSING
Climate

The rabbit's thermal comfort zone is around 20°C, with posture changes directed at heat conservation at 10°C and at heat dissipation at 30°C.[12] Optimum climatic conditions for rabbits are 13°C to 20°C and 55% to 65% relative humidity.[13] It is important to protect rabbits against overheating, such as by lack of shade and ventilation. The rabbit's average lethal ambient temperature is given as 42.8°C.[13] Providing rabbits with shelter that provides protection from draught and heat convection and humidity typically allows housing them outside at ambient temperatures below their optimal climatic conditions, because the animals can provide their own microclimate.

Space and Structure

Several studies have demonstrated that compared with stacked, standard laboratory cages, keeping rabbits in different systems can increase their welfare. Components that contribute to this effect are increased space, variation in cage height, multiple raised platforms used as an elevated resting space or a hiding opportunity under which the animal will sit, flooring different from a wire mesh, keeping cages at ground level, offering straw bedding, and offering gnawing material.[2,13] Note, for example, that the provision of dens, or "house" structures, has not been investigated in this respect, but is considered to provide even more of a hiding opportunity than a platform. For pet rabbits, the unstructured, single-level, grid-floored, and small plastic cages previously recommended in this journal seem outdated[14]; instead, a multilevel, structured enclosure with a designated clean, protected, and dry hiding spot that provides sufficient space for all animals, should be provided. The Rabbit Welfare Association recommends at least a 3 m × 2.5 m enclosure for a pair of pet rabbits.[15] Depending on the character of the animals, providing more than one shelter may be beneficial to allow animals that prefer to hide from each other to do so.

Pet rabbits are kept in a large variety of housing systems, from small cages used to breed show animals to animals roaming freely in their owners' garden or house.[16–19] That rabbits can be trained to use litter boxes for urination facilitates the latter option.[8] Cages bought as pet supply are typically smaller than cages made by the owners themselves.[16] There is evidence from a questionnaire survey on pet rabbits that animals with more access to space show less stereotypies,[17] and pet rabbits are more active when offered larger pens.[18,20] Rabbits should be kept in such a way that they can perform not only a slow hopping locomotion, but also short runs from time to time, ideally in outdoor enclosures where they can also dig. Care should be taken to ensure rabbits cannot dig their way out of the enclosure. In our view, there is no evidence that allows ranking different housing systems, such as a large garden enclosure with an opportunity for digging burrows and a structured multilevel shelter compared with having litter-trained rabbits roam freely in a part of the owner's living space (with a designated hiding and resting area, and potentially even leash walks). However, keeping rabbits as pets while just meeting minimum space requirements for production or laboratory animals, although potentially within a legal framework, cannot be considered adequate.

Sociality

The welfare of rabbits is typically improved if they are kept together with other rabbits.[2,21] To stress this point, explaining to clients that laboratory rabbits actively choose the company of conspecifics when given a choice[22–24] is helpful. The presence of a conspecific typically induces more locomotion, which can even lead to beneficial effects on bone structure[2] and possibly has prophylactic effects against urinary sludge forming uroliths.[25] Although keeping rabbits as solitary animals is legal in most countries, and in particular the management of breeding bucks in other ways is problematic in breeding systems, pet rabbits should at least be kept in pairs, and gonadectomy is indicated to mix sexes in nonbreeding pairs. Nevertheless, the compatibility of partner animals must be guaranteed by close initial surveillance to avoid injuries caused by aggression.

Enrichment

In studies with production rabbits, the provision of a platform, of gnawing material, and of hay has been considered enrichment.[2] For pet rabbits, these measures should be considered standard good practice. For rabbits, enrichment items that represent food are typically more efficient than nonfood items (toys),[26] which stresses the relevance of the feeding regime. The main mode of interaction with toys is chewing,[22,27] and toy use is reduced with increasing forage feeding.[28] Similar to the positive effects of providing hay (discussed in nutrition section), providing chewing sticks in a commercial rabbit production setting reduced the number of ear injuries inflicted on cage mates.[29] Providing a basket or box structure filled with hay is supposed to act as a surrogate outlet not only of chewing but also of digging behavior[8]; offering hay in hayracks can induce rabbits to use a digging motion first to remove the food from the racks before ingestion.[30] Large plastic tubs with soil can be supplied to allow some digging.[15]

Mirrors have a positive effect on rabbits, potentially as a substitute for social contacts,[31,32] but should not be used to justify keeping a single individual animal. Rabbits apparently accept tunnel structures well.[15] Other specific nonfood enrichment for pet rabbits may include the careful interaction with humans, walking on a leash,[8] and sporadic access to larger areas (eg, larger garden enclosures secured against escape and predation).

Other Aspects of Housing

As many animals with a flight response, rabbits are susceptible to sudden loud, star-tling noises.[13] Regular handling of production and pet rabbits reduces fearfulness.[2,20] Regular, gentle handling can therefore be recommended for pet rabbits. However, specific guidelines as to how rabbits are to be handled or carried should be followed,[9] including the understanding that lifting rabbits up from the ground on the owner's arm can trigger fear of height in the animals.[8] Rabbits can be clicker-trained using positive reinforcement.[8]

Rabbits prefer clean bedding material, such as straw, to the absence of bedding material; however, when given the choice, they prefer no bedding to soiled bedding material.[33] Therefore, a regular change of this material should be a matter of course.

When putting together a new group of rabbits, the animals should be under surveil-lance. In contrast to the general recommendation that new animals should be intro-duced to each other in surroundings unfamiliar to all of them (ie, a new or introduction pen), a recent study in female commercial breeding rabbits showed a lower incidence of inflicted wounds when animals were added to a group in the group's habitual enclosure as compared with an identical, disinfected enclosure new to both parties.[34] In our opinion, multiple hiding places are important for introduc-tions. However, for two unfamiliar pet rabbits, placing them together in a bathtub (where the awkward footing makes them less likely to act aggressively) has also been recommended,[8] although the very same surface conditions might also entail the danger of injuries caused by slipping.

WATER PROVISION

Pet rabbits should always have access to drinking water ad libitum. Restricting water access to only certain time periods leads to a reduced daily water intake.[35–38] To stress the relevance of drinking water provision, the observation that a 2-kg rabbit typically drinks as much as a 10-kg dog is readily used.[39] When given a choice be-tween open dish drinkers and nipple drinkers, rabbits show a clear preference for the open dishes[38]; this is probably linked to the three times higher water intake rate from open dishes.[38] Water intake tends to be lower from nipple drinkers,[38,40,41] and in group-kept rabbits, one study observed higher levels of aggression when water was provided in nipple drinkers as compared with open dishes.[40] To guarantee an optimal hydration and possibly also a prophylaxis against urolithiasis, open dish drink-ing systems should be used. Note that there are open dish systems with a storage bot-tle that combine some benefits of nipple drinkers (storage; less space use) and open dishes (allowing more appropriate drinking behavior). It should be noted that although it is generally believed that a suboptimal water provision can be a contributing factor to urolithiasis, epidemiologic or experimental studies investigating this concept are lacking.

NUTRITION
Digestive Tract Physiology

Rabbits have ever-growing incisors and cheek teeth, a simple stomach, and a com-plex caecum and colon where microbial fermentation takes place, and where a spe-cific mechanism separates indigestible fibrous substances from microbial matter; the latter is selectively retained in the caecum and excreted periodically as ceco-trophs, which are directly reingested from the anus,[42] and typically not observed by rabbit owners. The major function of the coprophagic or cecotrophic behavior is considered to be the prevention of the loss of microbial protein. It has been observed that at increasing dietary levels of protein or starch, rabbits do not consume their cecotrophs completely,[25,43,44] which is typically considered an indication that the diet should be adjusted. Potentially, the report of impacted cecotrophs by rabbits owners, the condition most frequently reported in a survey on pet rabbits,[16] indicates that such diet adjustments are warranted. Alternatively, other conditions, such as obesity, might prevent the proper ingestion of cecotrophs. Cecotroph impaction is particularly problematic as a starting point for myasis.

General Recommendations

The natural diet of rabbits consists of a variety of grasses, forbs, herbs, and leaves.[45–47] A long-standing feeding recommendation for pet rabbits is to feed hay ad libitum with a certain amount of leafy green vegetables and a high-fiber pelleted feed.[3,14,48,49] Specifically, the use of fruits, grains, bread, low-fiber pelleted feeds, and muesli mixes or rabbit mixes that contain a variety of these items is discouraged.[7,42,50] In contrast to these recommendations, such feeds are still often used in pet rabbit husbandry.[16,51–53] The evidence in favor of the diet of hay, green leafy vegetables, and high-fiber pellets is not based on experiments in which the recommended diet was directly assessed against other potentially reasonable diets, but is based on several results of studies that evaluated certain aspects of rabbit diets, and on common sense. The purpose of this diet is to use the benefits of hay as a staple fiber-rich and laborious-to-chew diet item; ensure a minimum of energy and trace element provision with a pelleted/extruded compound feed; provide extra water and vitamin intake and behavioral enrichment with the green leafy vegetables; and avoid the ingestion of energy-dense, high starch/sugar diet items by excluding fruits, grains, bread, low-fiber pelleted feeds, muesli or cereal mixes, and corresponding treats.

The advice to monitor body weight and body condition should always be part of nutritional recommendations. For most households, weighing a pet rabbit regularly poses little logistical challenge. Additionally, body condition scores[3,54] and ratios linking body weight to linear body measurements[54] exist that facilitate an evaluation of an individual rabbit's condition.

The Relevance of a High-Fiber Diet

Production rabbits are typically fed diets higher in fiber, and hence lower in easily digestible nutrients, than other monogastric production animals.[55] The presence of indigestible fiber is considered a prerequisite for the normal functioning of the colonic separation mechanism.[42] In production rabbits, it was shown that increasing the level of dietary fiber reduced the incidence of diarrhea and associated mortality,[56,57] most likely because in low-fiber diets, easily digestible material reaches the site of microbial fermentation[58] and leads to an unfavorable change in the microbiome composition, and because a lack of fiber reduces colonic motility.

Measurements of the natural diet of rabbits indicate levels of crude fiber (CF) of 25% to 30% (in dry matter), and levels of neutral detergent fiber (NDF) of 50% to 60%.[47,59] By contrast, a survey of complete feeds for production rabbits in Switzerland indicated a mean CF of 15% (range, 13%–18%) and a mean NDF of 38% (range, 34%–41%; Marcus Clauss, personal observation, 2008), which corresponds to typical recommendations for intensively reared production rabbits.[55] Interestingly, a survey of complete feeds marketed for pet rabbits in Switzerland indicated a similar mean CF of 15% (range, 8%–21%) and mean NDF of 37% (range, 26%–47%; Marcus Clauss, personal observation, 2008), suggesting that pet rabbit feeds had been formulated to resemble production rabbit feeds, not the natural diet. A survey on pet rabbit feeds in Italy in

2009 revealed a similar range of CF (8%–20%) and NDF (20%–42%),[60] and a survey on pet rabbit feeds in Spain in 2014 a CF range of 10% to 29%.[61] Telephonic inquiry with Swiss producers about the initial release of individual products in their portfolio indicated that the higher-fiber brands were the ones more recently released (Marcus Clauss, personal observation, 2008), indicating that these companies responded to an increasing awareness of the relevance of dietary fiber for rabbits. This inquiry seems to match a subjective impression that there is a general trend among pet food producers to not necessarily exclude low-fiber products from their portfolios, but to add new high-fiber products. In the only large-scale long-term study on the health of pet (dwarf) rabbits, a medium-fiber pelleted diet (CF 16%) fed ad libitum without access to hay not only led to obesity but to the exclusion of many animals because of problems related to intestinal dysbacteriosis.[62] Although studies that identify recommendable fiber levels for pet rabbits are missing, veterinarians should encourage rabbit owners to use feeds of at least 20% CF.

Forage Feeding

Dried forages (hays) are an essential component and a recommended staple item of feeding regimes for pet rabbits.[6,7,42,63] Surveys reveal that most pet rabbits are fed hay,[16,19,51,52] but veterinarians should verify this information with individual owners, because these surveys also still indicate a low proportion of owners who do not feed hay.

Actually, rabbits can be kept on forage-only diets; they also survive on such diets in the wild. Studies have demonstrated repeatedly that it does not seem problematic to maintain rabbits on forage-only diets,[64–68] or pelleted diets that are based on forage.[65,68–74] Given a lower digestive efficiency in rabbits compared with other herbivorous small mammals, such as guinea pigs,[64] the early second cut hay (with lower levels of fiber) may be more adequate for rabbits than late cuts (with higher levels of fiber). The main reason why the supplementation of forage with an additional artificial diet is often recommended is to prevent problems that could arise from a lack of a specific nutrient in the forage, in particular trace minerals. In theory, this could also be prevented by providing a variety of forages that do not all originate from the same location. Note that this provision of forage variety should not result in a series of short-term diet changes, but be implemented as simultaneous feeding. If, however, as is more often the case, the animals receive forage from just one batch for longer period of time, supplying a pelleted/extruded feed (high in fiber) that is balanced in its mineral and vitamin content, at amounts of one tablespoon per kilogram of animal, is usually recommended.[7] Given their natural occurrence in hays, additional provision of calcium and vitamin D should, in theory, not be necessary in hay-based diets.

Basically any hay offered ab libitum to rabbits already represents a heterogeneous food source on which the animals can exercise selective feeding behavior, choosing the more digestible plant parts and refusing the less digestible ones.[64] Rabbits have been shown to prefer alfalfa hay cut in the afternoon over hay from the same field cut in the morning, possibly because of the higher sugar levels after a period of sunlight,[75] and to be able to distinguish between plants of different protein content.[76,77] Choosing hay from pastures with a larger variety of plants (as opposed to a grass monoculture) increases the opportunity for selective feeding, and offering more than one hay could increase it even more. Although it may seem plausible that increasing the variety of plant material, and hence the opportunity for selective feeding, might represent a benefit for the animals, studies that actually document a beneficial effect of such regimes are lacking. In some cases of rabbit owners who express their affection for their animals by providing a variety of fruits and grains, refocusing the engagement on the provision of a variety of forages may be a successful strategy.

In choosing a forage, guidelines for the assessment of its hygienic and nutritive status[6] should be followed. Because rabbits do not digest fiber as well as many other herbivores[64] (but nevertheless require it), hays of higher nutritive status (typically, aromatic smelling hay that are, in the case of grass hays, soft to the touch) should be used.[6]

Veterinarians advising their clients can use a list of arguments to explain the need for forage provision.

- The high importance of forages for rabbits is reflected in legislation; for example, in Switzerland, the provision of hay is obligatory when keeping rabbits.
- The nutrient and mineral composition of hay, with high levels of fiber and a positive calcium to phosphorus ratio, is typically ideal for rabbits.[6]
- The ingestion of hay is more laborious for rabbits than most other diet items[78]; additionally, because of its low energy content, rabbits need to consume a higher amount of hay compared with more energy-dense diet items to meet their requirements.[25,41,57,79] This keeps the animals occupied with a natural behavior for longer periods of time,[30] and therefore
  - Leads to a general enrichment effect as demonstrated for the use of hays in production rabbits[2];
  - Reduces not only the wounding of cagemates,[80,81] but also excessive grooming and fur-chewing,[30,80,81] thus reducing the amount of hair in the stomach[82] and hence the risk for the formation of trichobezoars;
  - Reduces chewing on other objects including bedding, thus preventing the ingestion of such materials[30];
  - Reduces the risk of obesity, even when offered ad libitum[67,69,71,72];
  - Leads, because of the higher amount of chewing movements associated with the longer intake period, to a high level of tooth wear appropriate for rabbits.[65,83]
- The ingestion of hay is associated with a high water intake in rabbits that exceeds that observed on other dry diet items ingested at the same amount of dry matter,[25,41,79] leading to less concentrated urine on hay compared with other dry diets,[41] which is prophylactic against urolithiasis.

Fresh Food: Green Leafy Vegetables Versus Fruits

The incentive to use fresh diet items originates from their high palatability for rabbits, from their water content, and from their content of vitamins.[84] Apart from either allowing rabbits to feed for themselves in outside enclosures, offering them freshly plucked grass and herbs, or even growing small patches of grass in plastic containers that are placed as enrichment items in their enclosures,[4] green leafy vegetables are typically recommended. A list of appropriate green leafy vegetables is found in an previous contribution to this journal,[14] with restrictions for high-oxalate items, such as spinach, kale, or cabbage. The main reason of recommending green leafy vegetables, but not the feeding of fruits or other vegetables, is the high sugar content in these latter items.[85] Additionally, the latter contain little calcium and unfavorable calcium to phosphorus ratios.[84]

Offering rabbits fresh diet items leads to an increased overall water intake and more diluted urine,[41,86] and thus is prophylactic against urolithiasis.

Pelleted/Extruded Complete Feeds Versus "Rabbit Mixes"

The major difference between pelleted or extruded complete feeds and grain mixes, muesli, and cereal mixes or rabbit mixes is that the former diets provide all nutrients in every diet item (piece), so that a selective intake of certain diet components is not possible. By contrast, mixes are composed of a variety of diet items, and animals are known to selectively ingest certain of these items while avoiding others. Therefore, even if the total mix might be balanced in terms of nutrients, the portion actually ingested may not be so. In mix diets, the pelleted components (that guarantee mineral balance) are typically the least preferred part and are often not ingested,[16,50,79] which may lead to mineral imbalances, in particular calcium deficiency.[50] The possibility to select for high-energy diet items offered by mixes results in high weight gain and obesity on such diets.[67]

The persistence of mix diets for pet rabbits is probably founded in the perceived attractiveness of these diets for rabbit owners. In a survey of potential rabbit owners, an association between the plan to feed mix diets and the tendency to ascribe anthropocentric emotions to the animals was found,[53] supporting the notion that an anthropocentric approach may lead to the perception of mix diets as adequate. When we presented our lecture on rabbit feeding to an important Swiss retailer to promote the cessation of selling mix diets for rabbits, the reaction was that irrespective of the physiologic arguments, these diets were such an important source of income because of their popularity that they would not be removed from the portfolio (Jean-Michel Hatt and Marcus Clauss, personal observation, 2006).

It must be noted that also pelleted or extruded complete diets of high fiber content, when fed ad libitum, may lead to excessive weight gains.[25,67] Therefore, until a fiber threshold is determined above which these feeds can be fed safely ad libitum, the recommendation to restrict the amount of these feeds makes sense.

To date, there are no studies on the relative merits of pelleted versus extruded complete diets. Extruded diets have the potential (selling) advantage that they can be complete feeds where every piece contains the same nutrients, and visually diverse mixes of shapes and colors that satisfy the human tendency to favor a muesli look. Given that extruded diets are typically harder than pelleted diets[87,88] and also retain their consistency when chewed into smaller pieces in contrast to pellets that tend to crumble, extruded diets may be more favorable in terms of enhancing tooth wear. However, this remains to be investigated.

Specific Issues Related to Rabbit Nutrition

Diet transitions

Although it is generally recommended to perform gradual diet changes, we are not aware of specific studies that have addressed the issue. In a study where a large variety of diet items was fed to rabbits with grass hay at a minimum of 10% of the dietary intake, a 2-day transition period for the changing of diets did not cause problems.[41] It is generally believed that abrupt diet changes are particularly dangerous with respect to fresh feed, as when a large amount of vegetables is introduced abruptly into the diet, or when animals are put from a winter hay diet without transition and temporal restrictions onto a grass pasture. Similarly, the abrupt offering of large amounts of grain-based pelleted feeds or muesli and cereal mixes may be problematic.

Tooth wear and overgrowth

Lack of abrasion, an unbalanced calcium to phosphorus ratio, and genetic predisposition have been repeatedly discussed as reasons for dental problems in pet rabbits. Tooth growth in rabbits typically compensates for wear, irrespective of the degree of wear.[65,83,89] Tooth wear on incisors is increased with increasing hay intake (compared with pellets/extrudates or mix diets)[65,83,89]; tooth wear on cheek teeth increases with increasing diet abrasiveness.[65] No study has produced evidence so far that there is a minimum of tooth growth that leads, if insufficient abrasion takes place, to dental abnormalities. In a study that did not investigate tooth wear but long-term health effects of liquid diets, in which laboratory rabbits were fed a liquid diet for a whole year without the deliberate supplementation of gnawing opportunities,[90] no problems with dental overgrowth were observed (Mickey Latour, personal communication, 2017). Mix diets were associated with dental disease in one survey.[16] Because most of these animals also received hay, the problem seems less likely to lie in the lack of chewing action than in the imbalanced mineral provision caused by selective feeding on mix diets. Therefore, the concept seems plausible that calcium/phosphorus imbalances caused by diet or lack of access to UV light result in poor bone and tooth formation, that lead to malpositioning and hence overgrowth.[50,91] However, dental abnormalities have been produced in two studies with either a pelleted complete diet[62] or a muesli mix,[83] fed without access to hay in both cases. Although the calcium/phosphorus of the ingested diets were as recommended[83] or can be assumed to have followed recommendations,[62] dental abnormalities developed, which suggests a relevance of hay feeding for dental health. However, given that one of these studies was performed with dwarf rabbits,[62] and that a genetic predisposition for dental anomalies is suspected in brachycephalic rabbit breeds,[92,93] further work is required to ascertain the cause for dental abnormalities in rabbits. The degree to which the provision of gnawing material not primarily provided for ingestion (gnawing sticks, chewing blocks, wood) affects tooth wear and growth has, to our knowledge, not been investigated.

Calcium metabolism and urolithiasis

In contrast to carnivores, primates, or ruminants, but similar to many rodents, perissodactyls, or elephants, rabbits absorb more calcium from the gut than they require and excrete surplus via urine.[68] The calcium concentration in urine depends on the calcium level of the diet and on the water intake.[41] It has been proposed that avoiding feeds high in calcium, such as legume (eg, alfalfa) hays, can help prevent urolith formation in rabbits.[94,95] However, because wild rabbits consume high proportions of legumes in their natural diet,[45,96] one might suspect that the animals are adapted to the calcium levels in legume forage. Our failure to trigger urolith formation when feeding rabbits with alfalfa only for 25 weeks despite demonstrated high levels of sludge in the bladder and urine[25] seems to confirm this view. Notably, the presence of sludge was not associated with negative clinical symptoms. In that study, rabbits were kept in large groups (ie, animals were comparatively active) with open dish drinkers. Although avoiding high dietary calcium levels is prophylactic, we suggest that water intake (as ensured by using open dishes and additionally feeding fresh items, such as grass or green leafy vegetables regularly) and exercise are important additional prophylactic measures to prevent urolith formation.

Obesity

Obesity is not rare in pet rabbits,[3,16,54,97] and is most probably caused by a combination of lack of exercise and feeding of energy-dense diets. Obesity has been linked to a variety of health problems, such as myasis, urinary scalding, urolithiasis caused by inactivity, or pododermatitis,[3,98] although epidemiologic studies testing for these links in pet rabbits are rare.[99]

REFERENCES

1. Lowe JA. Pet rabbit feeding and nutrition. In: de Blas C, Wiseman J, editors. Nutrition of the rabbit. Wallingford (CT): CAB International; 2010. p. 294–313.
2. Roelofs S. Domestic rabbit welfare. Welfare issues surrounding a multi-purpose animal [MSc Thesis]. Utrecht (The Netherlands): University of Utrecht; 2016.

3. Stapleton N. The chubby bunny: a closer look at obesity in the pet rabbit. Vet Nurse 2014;5:312–9.
4. Stapleton N. There's no such thing as a free meal: environmental enrichment for rabbits. Vet Nurse 2015;6:228–33.
5. Stapleton N. Stranger danger: the importance and perils of companionship in rabbits. Vet Nurse 2016;7:206–12.
6. Clauss M. Clinical technique: feeding hay to rabbits and rodents. J Exot Pet Med 2012;21:80–6.
7. Irlbeck NA. How to feed the rabbit (*Oryctolagus cuniculus*) gastrointestinal tract. J Anim Sci 2001;79:343–6.
8. Crowell-Davis SL. Behavior problems in pet rabbits. J Exot Pet Med 2007;16: 38–44.
9. Bradbury AG, Dickens GJE. Appropriate handling of pet rabbits: a literature review. J Small Anim Pract 2016;57:503–9.
10. Trocino A, Xiccato G. Animal welfare in reared rabbits: a review with emphasis on housing systems. World Rabbit Sci 2006;14:77–93.
11. Szendrö Z, McNitt JI. Housing of rabbit does: group and individual systems: a review. Livestock Sci 2012;150:1–10.
12. McEwen GN, Heath JE. Resting metabolism and thermoregulation in the unrestrained rabbit. J Appl Physiol 1973;35:884–6.
13. Marai IFM, Rashwan AA. Rabbits behavioural response to climatic and managerial conditions: a review. Archiv für Tierzucht 2004;47:469–82.
14. Bradley T. Rabbit care and husbandry. Veterinary Clin North Am Exot Anim Pract 2004;7:299–313.
15. Speight C. Environmental enrichment for pet rabbits: how can the RVN help educate owners? Vet Nurs J 2016;31:144.
16. Mullan SM, Main DCJ. Survey of the husbandry, health and welfare of 102 pet rabbits. Vet Rec 2006;159:103–9.
17. Normando S, Gelli D. Behavioral complaints and owners' satisfaction in rabbits, mustelids, and rodents kept as pets. J Vet Behav Clin Appl Res 2011;6:337–42.
18. Dixon LM, Hardiman JR, Cooper JJ. The effects of spatial restriction on the behavior of rabbits (*Oryctolagus cuniculus*). J Vet Behav Clin Appl Res 2010;5: 302–8.
19. Rooney NJ, Blackwell EJ, Mullan SM, et al. The current state of welfare, housing and husbandry of the English pet rabbit population. BMC Res Notes 2014;7:942.
20. Mullan SM, Main DCJ. Behaviour and personality of pet rabbits and their interactions with their owners. Vet Rec 2007;160:516–20.
21. Verga M, Luzi F, Carenzi C. Effects of husbandry and management systems on physiology and behaviour of farmed and laboratory rabbits. Horm Behav 2007; 52:122–9.
22. Huls WL, Brooks DL, Bean-Knudsen D. Response of adult New Zealand white rabbits to enrichment objects and paired housing. Lab Anim Sci 1991;41:609–12.
23. Chu LR, Garner JP, Mench JA. A behavioral comparison of New Zealand White rabbits (*Oryctolagus cuniculus*) housed individually or in pairs in conventional laboratory cages. Appl Anim Behav Sci 2004;85:121–39.
24. Seaman SC, Waran NK, Mason G, et al. Animal economics: assessing the motivation of female laboratory rabbits to reach a platform, social contact and food. Anim Behav 2008;75:31–42.
25. Clauss M, Burger B, Liesegang A, et al. Influence of diet on calcium metabolism, tissue calcification and urinary sludge in rabbits (*Oryctolagus cuniculus*). J Anim Physiol Anim Nutr 2012;96:798–807.

26. Harris LD, Custer LB, Soranaka ET, et al. Evaluation of objects and food for environmental enrichment of NZW rabbits. J Am Assoc Lab Anim Sci 2001;40:27–30.
27. Poggiagliolmi S, Crowell-Davis SL, Alworth LC, et al. Environmental enrichment of New Zealand White rabbits living in laboratory cages. J Vet Behav Clin Appl Res 2011;6:343–50.
28. Lang C, Weirich C, Hoy S. Frequency of occupation with different objects by growing rabbits under various conditions. J Agric Sci Technology A 2011;1: 833–41.
29. Princz Z, Dalle Zotte A, Radnai I, et al. Behaviour of growing rabbits under various housing conditions. Appl Anim Behav Sci 2008;111:342–56.
30. Prebble JL, Langford FM, Shaw DJ, et al. The effect of four different feeding regimes on rabbit behaviour. Appl Anim Behav Sci 2015;169:86–92.
31. Dalle Zotte A, Princz Z, Matics Z, et al. Rabbit preference for cages and pens with or without mirrors. Appl Anim Behav Sci 2009;116:273–8.
32. Edgar JL, Seaman SC. The effect of mirrors on the behaviour of singly housed male and female laboratory rabbits. Anim Welfare 2010;19:461–71.
33. Morisse JP, Boilletot E, Martrenchar A. Preference testing in intensively kept meat production rabbits for straw on wire grid floor. Appl Anim Behav Sci 1999;64: 71–80.
34. Graf S, Bigler L, Failing K, et al. Regrouping rabbit does in a familiar or novel pen: effects on agonistic behaviour, injuries and core body temperature. Appl Anim Behav Sci 2011;135:121–7.
35. Ben Rayana A, Ben Hamouda M, Bergaoui R. Effect of water restriction times of 2 and 4 hours per day on performances of growing rabbits. Paper presented at: 9th World Rabbit Congress. Verona (Italy), June 10–13, 2008.
36. Lebas F, Delaveau A. Influence de la restriction du temps d'accès à la boisson sur la consommation alimentaire et la croissance du lapin. Ann Zootech 1975; 24:311–3.
37. Prud'hon M, Chérubin M, Carles Y, et al. Effets de différents niveaux de restriction hydrique sur l'ingestion d'aliments solides par le lapin. Ann Zootech 1975;24: 299–310.
38. Tschudin A, Clauss M, Codron D, et al. Preference of rabbits for drinking from open dishes versus nipple drinkers. Vet Rec 2011;168:190.
39. Cizek LJ. Relationship between food and water ingestion in the rabbit. Am J Physiol 1961;201:557–66.
40. El-Mahdy MR, Karousa MM. Social behaviour, growth performance and carcass traits in growing New Zealand white rabbits as affected by iodine treated water, water source and watering system. Egypt J Rabbit Sci 1995;5:65–76.
41. Tschudin A, Clauss M, Codron D, et al. Water intake in domestic rabbits (*Oryctolagus cuniculus*) from open dishes and nipple drinkers under different water and feeding regimes. J Anim Physiol Anim Nutr 2011;95:499–511.
42. Rees Davies R, Rees Davies JAE. Rabbit gastrointestinal physiology. Veterinary Clin North Am Exot Anim Pract 2003;6:139–53.
43. Fekete S, Bokori J. The effect of the fiber and protein level of the ration upon the cecotrophy of rabbit. J Appl Rabbit Res 1985;8:68–71.
44. Dillmann K. Untersuchungen an Kaninchen zu verdauungsphysiologischen Auswirkungen unterschiedlicher Stärke- und Rohfasergehalte im Mischfutter unter Berücksichtigung futtermitteltechnologischer Einflüsse [Dissertation thesis]. Hannover (Germany): TiHo Hannover; 2013.

45. Katona K, Biro Z, Hahn I, et al. Competition between European hare and European rabbit in a lowland area, Hungary: a long-term ecological study in the period of rabbit extinction. Folia Zoologica 2004;53:255–68.
46. Marques C, Mathias ML. The diet of the European wild rabbit, Oryctolagus cuniculus (L.), on different coastal habitats of central Portugal. Mammalia 2001;65: 437–49.
47. Thompson HV, King CM. The European rabbit, the history and biology of a successful colonizer. Oxford (England): Oxford Science Publications; 1994.
48. Kupersmith DS. A practical overview of small mammal nutrition. Semin Avian Exot Pet Med 1998;7:141–7.
49. Jenkins JR. Feeding recommendations for the house rabbit. Veterinary Clin North Am Exot Anim Pract 1999;2:143–51.
50. Harcourt-Brown FM. Calcium deficiency, diet and dental disease in pet rabbits. Vet Rec 1996;139(23):567–71. Available at: http://www.ncbi.nlm.nih.gov/entrez/query.fcgi?cmd=Retrieve&db=PubMed&dopt=Citation&list_uids=8972070.
51. Tschudin A, Clauss M, Hatt JM. Umfrage zur Fütterung und Tränke von Kaninchen (Oryctolagus cuniculi) in der Schweiz 2008/2009. Schweizer Archiv für Tierheilkunde 2011;153:134–8.
52. Schepers F, Koene P, Beerda B. Welfare assessment in pet rabbits. Anim Welfare 2009;18:477–85.
53. Edgar JL, Mullan SM. Knowledge and attitudes of 52 UK pet rabbit owners at the point of sale. Vet Rec 2011;168:353.
54. Sweet H, Pearson AJ, Watson PJ, et al. A novel zoometric index for assessing body composition in adult rabbits. Vet Rec 2013;173:369.
55. De Blas JC. Nutritional impact on health and performance in intensively reared rabbits. Animal 2013;7(Suppl 1):102–11.
56. Gidenne T. Fibres in rabbit feeding for digestive troubles prevention: respective role of low-digested and digestible fibre. Livestock Prod Sci 2003;81:105–17.
57. Gidenne T. Dietary fibres in the nutrition of the growing rabbit and recommendations to preserve digestive health: a review. Animal 2015;9:227–42.
58. Gidenne T, Jehl N, Lapanouse A, et al. Inter-relationship of microbial activity, digestion and gut health in the rabbit: effect of substituting fibre by starch in diets having a high proportion of rapidly fermentable polysaccharides. Br J Nutr 2004; 92:95–104.
59. Wallage-Drees JM, Deinum B. Quality of the diet selected by wild rabbits (Oryctolagus cuniculus) in autumn and winter. Neth J Zoolog 1985;36:438–48.
60. Ricci R, Sartori A, Palagiano C, et al. Study on the nutrient adequacy of feeds for pet rabbits available in the Italian market. World Rabbit Sci 2010;18:131–7.
61. Molina J, Martorell J, Hervera M, et al. Preliminary study: fibre content in pet rabbit diets, crude fibre versus total dietary fibre. J Anim Physiol Anim Nutr 2015; 99(S1):23–8.
62. Dalle Zotte A, Sartori A. Evaluation of performance and health status of dwarf rabbits from weaning to maturity. Proceeding of the 10th World Rabbit Congress. Sharm El-Sheikh, Egypt, September 3–6, 2012.
63. Harrenstien L. Gastrointestinal diseases of pet rabbits. Semin Avian Exot Pet Med 1999;8:83–9.
64. Franz R, Kreuzer M, Hummel J, et al. Intake, selection, digesta retention, digestion and gut fill of two coprophageous species, rabbits (Oryctolagus cuniculus) and guinea pigs (Cavia porcellus), on a hay-only diet. J Anim Physiol Anim Nutr 2011;95:564–70.

65. Müller J, Clauss M, Codron D, et al. Growth and wear of incisor and cheek teeth in domestic rabbits (*Oryctolagus cuniculus*) fed diets of different abrasiveness. J Exp Zoolog A 2014;321:283–98.
66. Lebas F. Reflections on rabbit nutrition with a special emphasis on feed ingredients utilization. Proceedings of the 8th World Rabbit Congress. Puebla, Mexico, September 7-10, 2004.
67. Prebble JL, Shaw DJ, Meredith AL. Bodyweight and body condition score in rabbits on four different feeding regimes. J Small Anim Pract 2015;56:207–12.
68. Hagen KB, Tschudin A, Liesegang A, et al. Organic matter and macromineral digestibility in domestic rabbits (*Oryctolagus cuniculus*) as compared to other hindgut fermenters. J Anim Physiol Anim Nutr 2015;99:1197–209.
69. Fernandez-Carmona J, Bernat F, Cervera C, et al. High Lucerne diets for growing rabbits. World Rabbit Sci 1998;6:237–40.
70. Ferreira WM, Herrera ADPN, Scapinello C, et al. Apparent digestibility of nutrients of simplified diets based on forages for growing rabbits. Arq Bras Med Vet Zootecnia 2007;59:451–8.
71. Fernandez-Carmona J, Cervera C, Moya J, et al. Feeding ryegrass hay to growing rabbits, a note. World Rabbit Sci 2001;9:95–9.
72. Leiber F, Meier JS, Burger B, et al. Significance of coprophagy for the fatty acid profile in body tissues of rabbits fed different diets. Lipids 2008;43:853–65.
73. de Faria HG, Motta Ferreira W, Scapinello C, et al. Effect of the use of simplified diets based on forages on digestibility and performance of New Zealand rabbits. Revista Brasileira de Zootecnia 2008;37:1797–801.
74. Wolf P, Zumbrock B, Kamphues J. Breed dependent influences on relative size of intestinal tract as well as composition of its chyme in rabbits. Züchtungskunde 2010;82:165–75.
75. Mayland H, Gregorini P, Mertens D, et al. Diurnal changes in forage quality and their effects on animal preference, intake, and performance. Proceedings of the 35th California Alfalfa Symposium. Visalia, CA. UC Cooperative Extension, University of California, Davis. December 12–14, 2005.
76. Bakker ES, Reiffers RC, Olff H, et al. Experimental manipulation of predation risk and food quality: effect on grazing behaviour in a central-place foraging herbivore. Oecologia 2005;146:157–67.
77. Somers N, D'Haese B, Bossuyt B, et al. Food quality affects diet preference of rabbits: experimental evidence. Belgian J Zoolog 2008;138:170–6.
78. Schröder A. Vergleichende Untersuchungen zur Futteraufnahme von Zwergkaninchen, Meerschweinchen und Chinchilla bei Angebot unterschiedlich konfektionierter Einzel- und Mischfuttermittel [Dissertation thesis]. Hannover (Germany): TiHo Hannover; 2000.
79. Prebble JL, Meredith AL. Food and water intake and selective feeding in rabbits on four feeding regimes. J Anim Physiol Anim Nutr 2014;98:991–1000.
80. Berthelsen H, Hansen LT. The effect of hay on the behaviour of caged rabbits (*Oryctolagus cuniculus*). Anim Welfare 1999;8(2):149–57.
81. Lidfors L. Behavioural effects of environmental enrichment for individually caged rabbits. Appl Anim Behav Sci 1997;52:157–69.
82. Beynen AC, Mulder A, Nieuwenkamp AE, et al. Loose grass hay as a supplement to a pelleted diet reduces fur chewing in rabbits. J Anim Physiol Anim Nutr 1992;68:226–34.
83. Meredith AL, Prebble JL, Shaw DJ. Impact of diet on incisor growth and attrition and the development of dental disease in pet rabbits. J Small Anim Pract 2015;56(6):377–82.

84. Souci SW, Fachmann W, Kraut H. Food composition and nutrition tables. 4th edition. Stuttgart (Germany): Wissenschaftliche Verlagsgesellschaft; 1989.

85. Schwitzer C, Polowinsky SY, Solman C. Fruits as foods: common misconceptions about frugivory. In: Clauss M, Fidgett AL, Hatt JM, et al, editors. Zoo animal nutrition IV. Fürth (Germany): Filander Verlag; 2009. p. 131–68.

86. Wolf P, Bucher L, Kamphues J. The feed-, energy- and water intake in dwarf rabbits under feeding conditions of companion pets in the field. Kleintierpraxis 1999; 44:263–80.

87. Tran QD, van Lin CGJM, Hendriks WH, et al. Lysine reactivity and starch gelatinization in extruded and pelleted canine diets. Anim Feed Sci Technology 2007;138:162–8.

88. Van der Poel AFB, Fransen HMP, Bosch MW. Effect of expander conditioning and/or pelleting of a diet containing tapioca, pea and soybean meal on the total tract digestibility in growing pigs. Anim Feed Sci Technology 1997;66:289–95.

89. Wolf P, Kamphues J. Untersuchungen zu Fütterungseinflüssen auf die Entwicklung der Incisivi bei Kaninchen, Chinchilla und Ratte. Kleintierpraxis 1996; 41:723–32.

90. Latour MA, Hopkins D, Kitchens T, et al. Effects of feeding a liquid diet for one year to New Zealand white rabbits. Comp Med 1998;48:67–70.

91. Harcourt-Brown FM, Baker SJ. Parathyroid hormone, haematological and biochemical parameters in relation to dental disease and husbandry in rabbits. J Small Anim Pract 2001;42(3):130–6. Available at: http://www.ncbi.nlm.nih.gov/entrez/query.fcgi?cmd=Retrieve&db=PubMed&dopt=Citation&list_uids=11303855.

92. Crossley DA. Clinical aspects of lagomorph dental anatomy: the rabbit *(Oryctolagus cuniculus)*. J Vet Dent 1995;12:137–40.

93. Stucki F, Bartels T, Steiger A. Assessment of animal welfare aspects in extreme breeds of rabbits, poultry and pigeons. Schweizer Archiv für Tierheilkunde 2008;150:227–34.

94. Eckermann-Ross C. Hormonal regulation and calcium metabolism in the rabbit. Veterinary Clin North Am Exot Anim Pract 2008;11:139–52.

95. Kamphues J. Harnsteine bei kleinen Heimtieren. Paper presented at: Fortbildungsveranstaltung "Praxisrelevante Fragen zur Ernährung kleiner Heimtiere". Hannover, October 02, 1999.

96. Alves J, Vingada J, Rodrigues P. The wild rabbit (*Oryctolagus cuniculus*) diet on a sand dune area in central Portugal: a contribution towards management. Wildl Biol Pract 2006;2:63–71.

97. Courcier EA, Mellor DJ, Pendlebury E, et al. Preliminary investigation to establish prevalence and risk factors for being overweight in pet rabbits in Great Britain. Vet Rec 2012;171:197.

98. Sánchez JP, de La Fuente LF, Rosell JM. Health and body condition of lactating females on rabbit farms. J Anim Sci 2012;90:2353–61.

99. Mancinelli E, Keeble E, Richardson J, et al. Husbandry risk factors associated with hock pododermatitis in UK pet rabbits (*Oryctolagus cuniculus*). Vet Rec 2014;174:429.

Evidence-Based Reptile Housing and Nutrition

Dennis Oonincx, BEc, MSc, PhD[a],*, Jeroen van Leeuwen, MSc, PhD[b]

KEYWORDS

- Reptiles • Vitamin D • Ultraviolet light • Nutrition • Welfare • Enrichment

KEY POINTS

- Meeting the husbandry requirements of a reptile should be done on a species-specific basis.
- Field data on diets and microclimate provide an indication on husbandry requirements.
- Providing ultraviolet light via suitable lamps seems beneficial for most species.
- Providing a varied diet seems beneficial for most species.
- Providing several microclimates per enclosure seems beneficial for most species.

INTRODUCTION

The class of reptiles contains approximately 10,000 extant species.[1] Whereas large differences in ecology occur, there are also communalities. This article aims to describe these communalities and translate these to general guidelines for housing and feeding reptiles based on peer-reviewed publications. Species-specific guidelines are beyond the scope of this article owing to the aforementioned ecological diversity. It is important that species-specific information is gathered for the proper care of a species.

HOUSING AND LIGHTING

Visible light (400–700 nm) has several effects on reptile behavior. First, light intensity is used as an indication of temperature; higher intensities are associated with higher temperatures. This has been shown for basking species, such as anoles and turtles, but also in the nocturnal tokay gecko.[2–5] Light during the night can, however, suppress activity, as was shown in adult prairie rattlesnakes.[6]

Disclosure Statement: The authors have nothing to disclose.
[a] Laboratory of Entomology, Plant Sciences Group, Wageningen University, Droevendaalsesteeg 1, 6708PB Wageningen, The Netherlands; [b] Biometris, Plant Sciences Group, Wageningen University, Droevendaalsesteeg 1, 6708PB Wageningen, The Netherlands
* Corresponding author.
E-mail address: dennisoonincx@gmail.com

Vet Clin Exot Anim 20 (2017) 885–898
http://dx.doi.org/10.1016/j.cvex.2017.04.004
1094-9194/17/© 2017 Elsevier Inc. All rights reserved.

Many reptile species have a circadian rhythm (measured as melatonin level).[7] Photoperiod differences affect phase, amplitude, and duration of this rhythm. In Hermann's tortoises, annual changes in melatonin rhythms occur under natural conditions, with maximal amplitude in summer and their complete disappearance in winter.[8] Although timing of daily activity is often coupled to photoperiod,[9] the link to the reproduction cycle in reptiles is unclear. In fence lizards, ambient temperatures drive the reproductive cycle, not changes in photoperiod.[10] Effects of photoperiodic changes on the well-being of reptiles in captivity warrant further investigations.

Whereas humans can only see visible light, some reptiles are able to also see within the ultraviolet range (290–400 nm).[11–13] The femoral gland secretions of desert iguanas absorb ultraviolet A (UVA) light, which allows detection by conspecifics.[13] Furthermore, in that species and in Yarrow's spiny lizards, social interactions increase when a source of ultraviolet light is provided.[14] This suggests that these species have visual sensitivity within the UVA range. Similarly, red-eared sliders, 2 gecko species, and several chameleon and anole species have UV receptors and, therefore, see within the UVA range.[15,16] The anoles use this for intraspecific communication via dewlap recognition.[12,17] This suggests that, for reptiles, the presence of UVA has an effect on social interactions.

The relevance of ultraviolet B (UVB) light (290–320 nm) for the health and welfare of a variety of reptile species has received much attention. UVB facilitates the conversion of 7-dehydrocholesterol in the skin to vitamin D. Vitamin D is best known as a regulator of Ca and P metabolism in vertebrates, but can exert many more actions.[18] Vitamin D deficiency is frequently encountered in captive reptiles and leads to a complex of diseases, collectively called metabolic bone disease.[19,20] Maternal vitamin D deficiency can lead to hatching failure of fully developed embryos.[21] Vitamin D–deficient specimens may not show clinical signs of deficiency such as tetany.[22] Especially in nocturnal and crepuscular species clinical signs of vitamin D deficiency are rare. However, a lack of clinical deficiency symptoms does not exclude effects on health and welfare. Therefore, further studies are needed to evaluate the effect of vitamin D level on parameters, such as mortality, welfare, and reproduction. Vitamin D status is best evaluated based on vitamin D metabolite (25OHD) levels. It can take several weeks of UVB exposure before metabolite levels increase,[23] whereas these remain stable for several months without UVB exposure in adult, nonproductive, bearded dragons.[24] Similarly, Komodo dragons exposed to direct sun for 150 days per year can maintain a stable vitamin D status throughout the year.[25] Dietary provision of vitamin D in high dosages is effective in some species,[26] but in bearded dragons, Komodo dragons, and panther chameleons, exposure to UVB seems to be the primary method to attain a sufficient vitamin D status.[21,22,27] A variety of snakes, lizards, tortoises, and turtles, including crepuscular and nocturnal species, synthesize vitamin D via UVB exposure.[22,26–37] Certain species (panther chameleons and Jamaican anoles) increase their UVB exposure when they have a low dietary vitamin D intake.[38,39] Similarly, vitamin D–deficient bearded dragons actively bask when provided with a light source emitting UV radiation.[23] Whether this means that UVB is detected visually, or that the behavior is due to UVA is unknown. There are indications that nocturnal and crepuscular species synthesize vitamin D more efficiently than diurnal species.[31] This, together with the fact that it is not uncommon to come across nocturnal species during the daytime, might mean that minimal UVB exposure provides them with sufficient vitamin D.[40] Therefore, the required UV intensity differs between species owing to their ecology. Recently, a selection of snake and lizard species was allocated to 1 of 4 UV zones based on their ecology.[41,42] These zones correspond with a range within the UV index, which is a scale for the potency of UV radiation. It provides a guideline regarding which

UV exposure is suitable for a species. In general, exposure to direct sunshine is considered optimal; however, good UV lamps can also strongly increase vitamin D status.[11,22,43] The use of improper lamps, however, either with an output that is too high or that contains shortwave UVB (<290 nm), can result in basal cell generation, epidermal necrosis, and keratoconjunctivitis.[44] Furthermore, during the first hours of use, the UV output of many UVB lamps is far higher, and potentially dangerous, than after a period of 100 hours.[44] Therefore, it is advisable to only expose animals to UV lamps after such a period.

HOUSING AND ENVIRONMENTAL ENRICHMENT

Evidence-based minimal enclosure size requirements are available for only a small number of species. For instance hatchlings of alligators, Nile-, freshwater-, and salt-water crocodiles and broad-snouted caimans, have been studied.[45–47] These are considered economically relevant and therefore farmed in groups. Increased densities lead to intraspecific dominance, whereas lower densities increase antagonistic behavior. Both can result in depressed or skewed growth rates.[45,46] Also, soft-shelled turtles grow slower at a higher stocking density.[48] This is linked to increased activity and increased immune function (as measure of stress). In contrast, density, growth rate, and corticosterone levels are not correlated in zoo-kept juvenile tuataras,[49] whereas leopard geckos grow quicker when housed individually.[50] Besides absolute pen size, hiding places play a role by enabling the animals to avoid fighting.[46] As such, materials to hide in, or under, increase the effective size of an enclosure. Such retreats are forms of environmental enrichment.[51] In addition, thermal gradients, accommodation of circadian rhythms, varied diets, and different ways of offering diets are methods of providing enrichment. These methods aim to increase activity and fitness, and provide mental stimulation, which reduces stress levels.[52] Enrichment studies, therefore, should take behavioral aspects together with neural, endocrine, reproductive, metabolic, psychological, phylogenetic, and ecological factors,[53] because no single measure corresponds directly with an animal's welfare state.[54] Whereas in the seventies it was considered "wrong to introduce soil, moss or living plants into a reptilian vivarium,"[55] nowadays more natural settings are associated with positive effects on reptile well-being. The provision of a burrowing substrate, branches for climbing, and offering live prey improves the problem-solving ability of rat snakes.[56] Box turtles offered mulch, paper shredding, and a hide box have lower stress levels, based on lower heterophil to lymphocyte ratios.[57] They also spent less time trying to escape than turtles with only a paper substrate. Tree runners become more active when provided with scattered insects in a complex environment, than by insects slowly released from a device.[52] Probably this is due to high predictability of slowly released insects, compared with randomly scattered insects. Whether environmental enrichment is effective depends on the form, but also the species for which it is applied. For instance, an elevated basking platform does not have an effect on behavior, growth, survival, or corticosterone levels in Eastern fence lizards.[58] However, green iguanas without climbing opportunities have elevated corticosterone metabolite levels.[59] Furthermore, Nile soft-shelled turtles[60] and sea turtles[61,62] showed interest in playing with an object, whereas this was not the case for leopard geckos. Especially large reptile species, such as monitors, tortoises, and crocodilians, can learn and solve problems.[51] This might also apply to small species such as anoles and skinks, but has not yet been sufficiently studied. The effects of environmental enrichment on reptiles are slowly receiving more scholarly interest. Currently, it remains to be determined whether enrichment holds additive value for the well-being of captive reptiles.

Most reptile species are best kept individually or in pairs. Generally, males are territorial and fight when placed together, but also females placed together show antagonistic behavior. Most reptile species are solitary, although social organization also occurs. Some skinks species live in monogamous pairs or even family groups, as do armadillo lizards.[63–65] Hatchling crocodilians are gregarious and protected by their parents for up to 2.5 months.[46,66] However, even for social species, there is no evidence that social interactions improve their well-being in captivity.

HOUSING AND TEMPERATURE

Reptiles are ectothermic animals; behavioral and physiologic processes, such as mating, feeding, and digesting, depend on temperature. Therefore, they require specific ambient temperatures for optimal functioning. A temperature gradient around their preferred body temperature allows them to regulate their body temperature within a narrow range. For example, leopard geckos grow faster when provided with a temperature gradient compared with constant temperatures.[67] Preferred body temperatures are highly species specific. The ambient temperatures within a species natural range can provide a first indication. However, the microclimate in their ecological niche can differ greatly. For example, temperature ranges for subterrestrial species are much narrower than for terrestrial or climbing species within the same location. In addition, preferred body temperatures during the day and night may differ with the diel activity pattern of the species. For example, body temperatures of nocturnal geckos in Australia are lower at night than during the day. However, when provided with a temperature gradient in captivity, their preferred temperature during the day and at night is the same.[68] This pattern is the same for leopard geckos,[67] but tokay geckos prefer higher temperatures at night.[2] In contrast, most diurnal reptiles, including skinks, lacertids, and iguanids, prefer lower temperatures during the night.[68] For semiaquatic species, such as terrapins, alligators, and crocodiles, both a dry basking spot and a proper water temperature are important for thermoregulation.[69,70] For nontropical species, also seasonal temperature fluctuations are of importance. For example, temperatures too warm to stay dormant, but too cold to stay active decrease energy reserves and hence body mass in vipers.[71] Therefore, optimal temperatures during both active and inactive periods are important.

Furthermore, temperature affects the growth rate and maturation of reptiles. Turtles and tortoises grow quicker and mature earlier at higher temperatures.[72–74] In nature, where predators occur, this is likely to positively impact fitness.[69] However, in captivity high ambient temperature are associated with increased carapacial scute pyramiding in leopard and spurred tortoises.[75] Excessive temperatures are more detrimental, and lead to more stress or even death, than too low temperatures. This has been shown for juvenile saltwater crocodiles that showed an increase in corticosterone level and deaths at a water temperature 4°C higher than their optimal temperature of 32°C.[76] Incubation temperatures determine sex in many reptile species, both egg-laying and live-bearing. Moreover, hatchling size and coloration, and posthatching growth and behavior can be affected.[74,77–79] Excessive incubation temperatures are more likely to lead to physical abnormalities than too low incubation temperatures.[80,81]

Corticosterone levels are an indicator for temperature-related stress because it is induced at inappropriate temperatures. However, corticosterone levels can also be induced by higher activity and stress independent of temperature.[82] Furthermore, corticosterone levels increase owing to handling or deprived housing conditions.[45,59,83] Other factors, such as time of day, season, stage of gestation,[84] and variation between individuals play a role as well.[59,85] Hence, corticosterone only serves as a proper stress indicator when sufficient, species-specific reference values are available.

EVIDENCE-BASED INFORMATION ON DISEASES RELATED TO HOUSING CONDITIONS

Housing conditions can lead to several diseases. As mentioned, incorrect ultraviolet lighting causes serious problems such as basal cell generation, epidermal necrosis, and keratoconjunctivitis.[44] Incorrect application of heating sources, for example, surface heating instead of radiation, can lead to loosening of ventral scales in tortoises, and necrotic ventral dermatitis in snakes.[86] Too low humidity leads to dysecdysis in many reptile species[86] and pyramiding in spurred, and possibly other tortoises.[87] Excessive humidity can lead to dermatitis.[88] Last, lizards that try to escape a cage and repeatedly run into transparent cage walls will suffer from nose lesions.[89] Water dragons and other iguanids in particular are prone to this condition.

NUTRITION
Evidence-Based Information on Nutrition

Whether an animal receives the nutrients it requires depends on (1) the composition of the provided feed items, (2) which of these are accepted, (3) to what extend these are digested, and (4) the nutrient requirements of the consuming animal. However, little is known about the nutrient requirements of reptile species or of the digestibility of feed items provided to them. Therefore, a varied diet that allows self-selection of food items relatively rich in a limiting nutrient, or low in an over-abundant nutrient is preferable.[22,90,91] Calcium, a nutrient of concern for many reptile species, can be provided in the form of a bowl with calcium carbonate. Although not all species make use of this, Western fence lizards,[92] leopard geckos, day geckos, and rough knob-tailed geckos accept this form of supplementation well (personal observations).

Several species, for example, tortoises and bearded dragons, grow quicker in captivity than under natural conditions.[22,93,94] This could be because food is not limited, which allows optimal growth. However, high growth rates are potentially associated with obesity, renal disease, metabolic bone disease, and in tortoises with pyramiding. However, a causal relationship has not been proven.[93]

Dietary constituents can be divided in plant material, such as leafy plants, and fruits, and animal material, such as arthropods, fish, birds, or mammals. Some reptile species are highly specialized toward one of these categories, whereas others consume both plant and animal material. Furthermore, dietary preference can change in an animal as it matures (ontogenetic change). Large carnivores, such as Komodo dragons, shift from other lizards and insects to mammals.[95] But also smaller lizards, primarily herbivorous as adults, sometimes consume insects or other animal material as juveniles.[22,96–98] A similar ontogenetic shift is known in yellow bellied sliders.[99] It seems that omnivorous species prefer animal material if provided with a choice and that juvenile omnivores tend to consume relatively more animal material compared with their adult counterparts.[22,96,100] Probably this is caused by protein being the first limiting nutrient for growth and reproduction. Although dietary classifications are more rigid than diets selected by reptiles, some generalizations can be made.

Herbivorous species

Herbivores often have a requirement for fibers that they digest via endosymbionts. For example, red footed tortoises prefer diets high in fibers, although carrion is eaten first if it is available in nature.[100] In contrast, desert tortoises seem to select foods with higher protein and magnesium contents, whereas they avoid feed high in fiber.[91,101] Its dietary nitrogen requirement is however lower than for instance for a green iguana ($\leq$41 vs 151 mg/kg$^{0.8}$/d). A higher dietary protein content ($\leq$24% vs $\geq$30% dry matter [DM]) facilitates higher growth rates in green iguanas.[102] Also in the wild, this species prefers plants with a high protein content and fiber content up to 33% DM.[103] Plant composition can differ between seasons and consequently so can herbivore diets. For instance, plants preferentially consumed by chuckwallas contain more protein in early spring than in summer (20% vs 14% crude protein on a dry matter basis).[104] Chuckwallas also prefer herbage over grass, possibly due to the lower fiber content (29 vs 65% DM), which makes nutrients more easily available. Fruits and flowers, especially when brightly colored, are regularly preferred over leafy greens and can form a significant portion of the diet in nature.[96,100,104] Dietary ingredients containing high levels of antinutritional factors such as oxalic acid, tannins, or phytate should be offered sparsely, because they can inhibit mineral absorption.[105] More specialized feeders might be able to detect harmful substances, such as antinutritional factors or toxins, via tongue flicking.[106] However, as a general rule it is wise to only provide access to plant material that does not contain any toxins.

Insectivorous species

Most insectivores eat a variety of insect species and spiders in the wild.[94,107] Furthermore, opportunistic insectivores will consume large amounts of seasonally available insects, such as termite alates.[94] Studies that compared the suitability of different insect species as food for insectivores are scarce. Western fence lizards provided with either house crickets or mealworm larvae consumed a higher weight of crickets. However, their weight gain and feed conversion efficiency were higher on mealworms.[92] Although the Western fence lizards provided with mealworms were heavier, they were not longer. Similarly, leopard geckos provided with a fixed weight of either mealworms, house crickets, or a mix of both had a similar length, but the group provided with only mealworms was heavier.[108] Mealworms contain more fat, and therefore more energy, than crickets.[109] This indicates that providing only mealworms to Western fence lizards or leopard geckos leads to more obese animals than providing only crickets or mixed diets.

An advantage of active insect species, such as house crickets, over more passive species, such as mealworms, is that they are often better accepted. Moreover, they are more suitable as environmental enrichment, because they increase insectivore activity and thereby reduce the risk of obesity.[50,52,92] Often the insect species consumed in the wild are not available for captive animals.[94] Furthermore, the composition of wild insects can deviate from commercially produced specimens owing to compositional differences in the insects' diet.[109,110] Wild insects often have a lower fat content and a higher content of carotenoids and omega-3 fatty acids.[111] Insects in general contain low levels of vitamin A because it is not incorporated in the insect body.[21] However, it is suggested that lizards can convert carotenoids to vitamin A.[21] Insects' carotenoid content can be altered, for instance by providing carrots. In migratory locusts, this elevated the carotenoid content, but vitamin A content was not affected.[112] In wild insects, carotenoid concentrations can be high; however, commercial insects are often low in carotenoids owing to their diet.[113] This can lead to hypovitaminosis A, as suggested for a colony of green anoles.[114] In panther chameleons, hypovitaminosis A decreases life span and results in poor egg hatchability.[21] To prevent deficiencies, it is advisable to provide insects with a diet containing high concentrations of limiting nutrients, for instance carotenoids or vitamin E, for 2 or 3 days before feeding them to the insectivore (gut loading).[111] This works better in juvenile insects than adults owing to their larger relative gut content.

Carnivorous species

The diet of carnivorous reptiles often consists of a variety of vertebrate prey such as mice, rats, or 1-day-old chicks. These are often selected based on size and availability. Different species as well as different sizes of 1 species tend to differ in composition. For instance, commercially available mice have a higher dry matter content as they increase in size (19%–33%).[115] In general, the fat content of captive rodents is higher than in wild prey and surpasses carnivore requirements.[116] However, large variation in fat content (9%–30% DM) is possible.[115,116] Also, similarly sized rodents of different species differ in composition; for instance, neonatal rats contain higher vitamin E concentrations than mice or larger rats. Adult mice, in contrast, contain more vitamin A than smaller mice, or rats in general.[116] Concentrations of vitamins and fat in rodents depend, at least to some extent, on the diet provided to the rodents.[117] However, the mineral content of rats and mice seems fairly constant irrespective of size, except for manganese, which is present in higher concentrations in medium and large specimens.[116,118] Hence, the choice of prey affects the nutrient intake of carnivorous species. For instance, a poultry-based diet provides more energy than a rodent-based diet.[95] In Komodo dragons, this difference in diet did not affect growth rates or mineral concentrations in blood plasma.[95] Cholesterol concentrations were higher in the rodent-fed group. Vitamin contents of wild diets and captive diets often differ, especially for fat-soluble vitamins. For instance, the vitamin A and E intake of wild Eastern indigo snakes, which feed on tortoises and other snakes, is higher than those fed with captive-raised rodents.[119] However, the consequences of such differences in dietary intake for reptile health and fertility are unclear.

CURRENT CONTROVERSIES AND CLINICAL TOPICS REQUIRING ADDITIONAL EVIDENCE

People have kept reptiles for decades and this has led to standards and customs in husbandry. Clearly, these standards, often based on anecdotal evidence, are resulting in increased longevity and increased success of captive breeding programs. However, long-term scientific studies are needed to unravel the mechanisms that underlie this anecdotal evidence and determine its value. Questions such as whether the composition of wild diets should be considered as an optimal benchmark, or whether nocturnal or crepuscular species benefit from UVB exposure, are still to be resolved.

NEW IDEAS

The level of calcium supplementation currently being used by most keepers is a mitigation measure to prevent clinical signs of metabolic bone disease. Based on studies in humans, the absorption of calcium without the presence of vitamin D is approximately 10% to 15%, whereas this is increased to 30% to 40% in a vitamin D–sufficient state.[18] A similar effect is known for phosphorus absorption, which increases from 60% to 80%. The Ca:P ratio in insects varies between species; however, in most species it approximates 0.1, whereas a 1:1 ratio is often suggested as a dietary ratio for insectivores.[111] If animals have a sufficient vitamin D status, for instance by appropriate exposure to UVB, the current supplementation regimes might prove unnecessary and possibly hazardous. An important aspect of environmental enrichment that has been little tested so far is the use of olfactory triggering of chemosensory reactive species such as snakes.[56,120]

REFERENCES

1. Uetz P. Reptile database. 2016. Available at: http://www.reptile-database.org/db-info/SpeciesStat.html. Accessed November 17, 2016.
2. Sievert LM, Hutchison VH. Light versus heat: thermoregulatory behavior in a nocturnal lizard (*Gekko gecko*). Herpetologica 1988;44(3):266–73.
3. Hertz PE, Fleishman LJ, Armsby C. The influence of light intensity and temperature on microhabitat selection in two *Anolis* lizards. Funct Ecol 1994;8(6): 720–9.
4. Ruibal R. Thermal relations of five species of tropical lizards. Evolution 1961; 15(1):98–111.
5. Boyer DR. Ecology of the basking habit in turtles. Ecology 1965;46(1–2):99–118.
6. Clarke JA, Chopko JT, Mackessy SP. The effect of moonlight on activity patterns of adult and juvenile prairie rattlesnakes (*Crotalus viridis viridis*). J Herpetol 1996;30(2):192–7.
7. Tosini G, Bertolucci C, Foà A. The circadian system of reptiles: a multioscillatory and multiphotoreceptive system. Physiol Behav 2001;72(4):461–71.
8. Vivien-Roels B, Arendt J, Bradtke J. Circadian and circannual fluctuations of pineal indoleamines (serotonin and melatonin) in *Testudo hermanni* Gmelin (Reptilia, Chelonia): I. Under natural conditions of photoperiod and temperature. Gen Comp Endocrinol 1979;37(2):197–210.
9. Winne C, Keck M. Daily activity patterns of whiptail lizards (Squamata: Teiidae: Aspidoscelis): a proximate response to environmental conditions or an endogenous rhythm? Funct Ecol 2004;18(3):314–21.
10. Marion KR. Reproductive cues for gonadal development in temperate reptiles: temperature and photoperiod effects on the testicular cycle of the lizard Sceloporus undulatus. Herpetologica 1982;38(1):26–39.
11. Adkins E, Driggers T, Ferguson G, et al. Ultraviolet light and reptiles, amphibians. J Herpetol Med Surg 2003;13(4):27–37.
12. Leow ER, Fleishman LJ. Ultraviolet vision in lizards. Nat Int Weekly J Sci 1993; 365(6445):397.
13. Alberts AC. Ultraviolet visual sensitivity in desert iguanas: implications for pheromone detection. Anim Behav 1989;38(1):129–37.
14. Moehn LD. The effect of quality of light on agonistic behavior of iguanid and agamid lizards. J Herpetol 1974;175–83.
15. Tovée MJ. Ultra-violet photoreceptors in the animal kingdom: their distribution and function. Trends Ecol Evol 1995;10(11):455–60.
16. Bowmaker JK, Loew ER, Ott M. The cone photoreceptors and visual pigments of chameleons. J Comp Physiol A Neuroethol Sens Neural Behav Physiol 2005; 191(10):925–32.
17. Leal M. Differences in visual signal design and detectability between allopatric populations of *Anolis* lizards. Am Nat 2004;163(1):26–39.
18. Holick MF. Vitamin D deficiency. N Engl J Med 2007;357(3):266–81.
19. Divers SJ, Mader DR. Reptile medicine and surgery. New York: Elsevier Health Sciences; 2005.
20. Mader DR. Metabolic bone disease in reptiles. Reptiles 2014;22(4):14.
21. Ferguson GW, Jones J, Gehrmann W, et al. Indoor husbandry of the panther chameleon *Chamaeleo [Furcifer] pardalis*: effects of dietary vitamins A and D

and ultraviolet irradiation on pathology and life-history traits. Zoo Biol 1996;15: 279–99.

22. Oonincx DGAB, Stevens Y, van den Borne JJ, et al. Effects of vitamin D_3 supplementation and UVb exposure on the growth and plasma concentration of vitamin D_3 metabolites in juvenile bearded dragons (*Pogona vitticeps*). Comp Biochem Physiol B Biochem Mol Biol 2010;156(2):122–8.

23. Diehl E, Baines FM, Heijboer A, et al. A comparison of UVb lamps in enabling cutaneous vitamin D synthesis in growing bearded dragons. Journal of Animal Physiology and Animal Nutrition, 2017. http://dx.doi.org/10.1111/jpn.12728.

24. Oonincx DGAB, van de Wal MD, Bosch G, et al. Blood vitamin D_3 metabolite concentrations of adult female bearded dragons (*Pogona vitticeps*) remain stable after ceasing UVb exposure. Comp Biochem Physiol B Biochem Mol Biol 2013;165(3):196–200.

25. Gyimesi Z, Burns R. Monitoring of plasma 25-hydroxyvitamin D concentrations in two Komodo dragons, *Varanus komodoensis*: a case study. J Herpetol Med Surg 2002;12(2):4–9.

26. Ferguson GW, Gehrmann WH, Peavy B, et al. Restoring vitamin D in monitor lizards: exploring the efficacy of dietary and UVB sources. J Herpetol Med Surg 2009;19(3):81–8.

27. Gillespie D, Frye FL, Stockham SL, et al. Blood values in wild and captive Komodo dragons (*Varanus komodoensis*). Zoo Biol 2000;19(6):495–509.

28. Acierno MJ, Mitchell MA, Roundtree MK, et al. Effects of ultraviolet radiation on 25-hydroxyvitamin D_3 synthesis in red-eared slider turtles (*Trachemys scripta elegans*). Am J Vet Res 2006;67(12):2046–9.

29. Allen ME, Oftedal OT, Horst RL. Remarkable differences in the response to dietary vitamin D among species of reptiles and primates: is ultraviolet B light essential. Biological effects of light. Atlanta (GA), October 9-11, 1995.

30. Aucone BM, Gehrmann WH, Ferguson GW, et al. Comparison of two artificial ultraviolet light sources used for Chuckwalla, *Sauromalus obesus*, husbandry. J Herpetol Med Surg 2003;13:14–7.

31. Carman EN, Ferguson GW, Gehrmann WH, et al. Photobiosynthetic opportunity and ability for UV-B generated vitamin D synthesis in free-living house geckos (*Hemidactylus turcicus*) and Texas spiny lizards (*Sceloporus olivaceous*). Copeia 2000;(1):245–50.

32. Selleri P, Di Girolamo N. Plasma 25-hydroxyvitamin D_3 concentrations in Hermann's tortoises (*Testudo hermanni*) exposed to natural sunlight and two artificial ultraviolet radiation sources. Am J Vet Res 2012;73(11):1781–6.

33. Acierno MJ, Mitchell MA, Zachariah TT, et al. Effects of ultraviolet radiation on plasma 25-hydroxyvitamin D_3 concentrations in corn snakes (*Elaphe guttata*). Am J Vet Res 2008;69(2):294–7.

34. Wangen K, Kirshenbaum J, Mitchell MA. Measuring 25-hydroxy vitamin D levels in leopard geckos exposed to commercial ultraviolet B lights. Paper presented at: Proceedings of the Association of Reptilian and Amphibian Veterinarians conference. Indianapolis (IN), September 15, 2013.

35. Hibma J. Dietary vitamin D_3 and UV-B exposure effects on green iguana growth rate: is full-spectrum lighting necessary. Bull Chic Herpetol Soc 2004;39(8): 145–50.

36. Hoby S, Wenker C, Robert N, et al. Nutritional metabolic bone disease in juvenile veiled chameleons (*Chamaeleo calyptratus*) and its prevention. J Nutr 2010; 140(11):1923–31.

37. Kroenlein K, Zimmerman SG, Saunders G, et al. Serum vitamin D levels and skeletal and general development of young bearded dragon lizards (*Pogona vitticeps*), under different conditions of UV-B radiation exposure. J Anim Vet Adv 2011;10:229–34.

38. Ferguson GW, Kingeter AJ, Gehrmann WH. Ultraviolet light exposure and response to dietary vitamin D_3 in two Jamaican anoles. J Herpetol 2013;47(4): 524–9.

39. Karsten KB, Ferguson GW, Chen TC, et al. Panther chameleons, *Furcifer pardalis*, behaviorally regulate optimal exposure to UV depending on dietary vitamin D_3 status. Physiol Biochem Zool 2009;82(3):218–25.

40. Jenison G, Nolte J. An ultraviolet-sensitive mechanism in the reptilian parietal eye. Brain Res 1980;194(2):506–10.

41. Ferguson GW, Brinker AM, Gehrmann WH, et al. Voluntary exposure of some western-hemisphere snake and lizard species to ultraviolet-B radiation in the field: how much ultraviolet-B should a lizard or snake receive in captivity? Zoo Biol 2010;29(3):317–34.

42. Baines F, Chattell J, Dale J, et al. How much UV-B does my reptile need? The UV-tool, a guide to the selection of UV lighting for reptiles and amphibians in captivity. J Zoo Aquar Res 2016;4(1):42.

43. Laing CJ, Trube A, Shea GM, et al. The requirement for natural sunlight to prevent vitamin D deficiency in iguanian lizards. J Zoo Wildl Med 2001;32(3):342–8.

44. Gardiner DW, Baines FM, Pandher K. Photodermatitis and Photokeratoconjunctivitis in a ball python (*Python regius*) and a blue-tongue skink (*Tiliqua* spp.). J Zoo Wildl Med 2009;40(4):757–66.

45. Elsey RM, Joanen T, McNease L, et al. Growth rate and plasma corticosterone levels in juvenile alligators maintained at different stocking densities. J Exp Zool 1990;255(1):30–6.

46. Brien ML, Webb GJ, McGuinness KA, et al. Effect of housing density on growth, agonistic behaviour, and activity in hatchling saltwater crocodiles (*Crocodylus porosus*). Appl Anim Behav Sci 2016;184:141–9.

47. Poletta G, Larriera A, Siroski P. Broad snouted caiman (*Caiman latirostris*) growth under different rearing densities. Aquaculture 2008;280(1):264–6.

48. Chen X, Niu C, Pu L. Effects of stocking density on growth and non-specific immune responses in juvenile soft-shelled turtle. *Pelodiscus sinensis* Aquaculture Res 2007;38(13):1380–6.

49. Tyrrell C, Cree A. Plasma corticosterone concentrations in wild and captive juvenile tuatara (*Sphenodon punctatus*). New Zealand J Zoolog 1994;21(4):407–16.

50. Rich CN. Development of a reptile model for assessing environmental contaminants. Stillwater (OK): Oklahoma State University; 1995.

51. Burghardt GM. Environmental enrichment and cognitive complexity in reptiles and amphibians: concepts, review, and implications for captive populations. Appl Anim Behav Sci 2013;147(3):286–98.

52. Januszczak IS, Bryant Z, Tapley B, et al. Is behavioural enrichment always a success? Comparing food presentation strategies in an insectivorous lizard (*Plica plica*). Appl Anim Behav Sci 2016;183:95–103.

53. Burghardt GM, Layne DG. Effects of ontogenetic processes and rearing conditions. In: Warwick C, Frye FL, Murphy JB, editors. Health and welfare of captive reptiles. Dordrecht (The Netherlands): Springer Netherlands; 1995. p. 165–85.

54. Mason G, Mendl M. Why is there no simple way of measuring animal welfare? Anim Welf 1993;2(4):301–19.

55. Jackson OF. An introduction to the housing and treatment of snakes. J Small Anim Pract 1977;18(7):479–91.

56. Almli LM, Burghardt GM. Environmental enrichment alters the behavioral profile of ratsnakes (*Elaphe*). J Appl Anim Welf Sci 2006;9(2):85–109.

57. Case BC, Lewbart GA, Doerr PD. The physiological and behavioural impacts of and preference for an enriched environment in the eastern box turtle (*Terrapene carolina carolina*). Appl Anim Behav Sci 2005;92(4):353–65.

58. Rosier RL, Langkilde T. Does environmental enrichment really matter? A case study using the eastern fence lizard, Sceloporus undulatus. Appl Anim Behav Sci 2011;131(1):71–6.

59. Kalliokoski O, Timm JA, Ibsen IB, et al. Fecal glucocorticoid response to environmental stressors in green iguanas (*Iguana iguana*). Gen Comp Endocrinol 2012;177(1):93–7.

60. Burghardt GM, Ward B, Rosscoe R. Problem of reptile play: environmental enrichment and play behavior in a captive Nile soft-shelled turtle, Trionyx triunguis. Zoo Biol 1996;15(3):223–38.

61. Therrien CL, Gaster L, Cunningham-Smith P, et al. Experimental evaluation of environmental enrichment of sea turtles. Zoo Biol 2007;26(5):407–16.

62. Bashaw MJ, Gibson MD, Schowe DM, et al. Does enrichment improve reptile welfare? Leopard geckos (*Eublepharis macularius*) respond to five types of environmental enrichment. Appl Anim Behav Sci 2016;184:150–60.

63. Bull CM, Cooper SJ, Baghurst BC. Social monogamy and extra-pair fertilization in an Australian lizard, Tiliqua rugosa. Behav Ecol Sociobiol 1998;44(1):63–72.

64. Mouton P, Flemming A, Kanga E. Grouping behaviour, tail-biting behaviour and sexual dimorphism in the armadillo lizard (*Cordylus cataphractus*) from South Africa. J Zool 1999;249(1):1–10.

65. Chapple DG. Ecology, life-history, and behavior in the Australian scincid genus *Egernia*, with comments on the evolution of complex sociality in lizards. Herpetological Monographs 2003;17(1):145–80.

66. Webb GJW, Messel H, Magnusson W. The nesting of Crocodylus porosus in Arnhem Land, Northern Australia. Copeia 1977;1977(2):238–49.

67. Autumn K, De Nardo DF. Behavioral thermoregulation increases growth rate in a nocturnal lizard. J Herpetol 1995;29(2):157–62.

68. Angilletta MJ Jr, Werner YL. Australian geckos do not display diel variation in thermoregulatory behavior. Copeia 1998;1998(3):736–42.

69. Tamplin JW, Moran VF, Riesberg EJ. Response of juvenile diamond-backed terrapins (*Malaclemys terrapin*) to an aquatic thermal gradient. J Therm Biol 2013; 38(7):434–9.

70. Asa CS, London GD, Goellner RR, et al. Thermoregulatory behavior of captive American alligators *(Alligator mississippiensis)*. J Herpetol 1998;191–7.

71. Brischoux F, Dupoué A, Lourdais O, et al. Effects of mild wintering conditions on body mass and corticosterone levels in a temperate reptile, the aspic viper (*Vipera aspis*). Comp Biochem Physiol A Mol Integr Physiol 2016;192:52–6.

72. Ritz J, Griebeler EM, Huber R, et al. Body size development of captive and free-ranging African spurred tortoises (*Geochelone sulcata*): high plasticity in reptilian growth rates. Herpetological J 2010;20(3):213–6.

73. Frazer NB, Greene JL, Gibbons JW. Temporal variation in growth rate and age at maturity of male painted turtles, Chrysemys picta. Am Midl Nat 1993;130(2): 314–24.

74. Rhen T, Lang JW. Temperature during embryonic and juvenile development influences growth in hatchling snapping turtles, Chelydra serpentina. J Therm Biol 1999;24(1):33–41.

75. Heinrich ML, Heinrich KK. Effect of supplemental heat in captive African leopard tortoises (*Stigmochelys pardalis*) and spurred tortoises (*Centrochelys sulcata*) on growth rate and carapacial scute pyramiding. J Exot Pet Med 2016;25(1):18–25.

76. Turton J, Ladds P, Manolis S, et al. Relationship of blood corticosterone, immunoglobulin and haematological values in young crocodiles (*Crocodylus porosus*) to water temperature, clutch of origin and body weight. Aust Vet J 1997;75(2):114–9.

77. Burger J. Incubation temperature has long-term effects on behaviour of young pine snakes (*Pituophis melanoleucus*). Behav Ecol Sociobiol 1989;24(4):201–7.

78. Shine R, Madsen TR, Elphick MJ, et al. The influence of nest temperatures and maternal brooding on hatchling phenotypes in water pythons. Ecology 1997;78(6):1713–21.

79. Robert KA. Temperature-dependent sex determination in the viviparous lizard Eulamprus tympanum. Sydney (NSW): School of Biological Science, The University of Sydney; 2003.

80. Du W-G, Shou L, Liu J-K. The effect of incubation temperature on egg survival, hatchling traits and embryonic use of energy in the blue-tailed skink, *Eumeces elegans*. Anim Biol 2003;53(1):27–36.

81. Ji X, Du W-G. The effects of thermal and hydric environments on hatching success, embryonic use of energy and hatchling traits in a colubrid snake, *Elaphe carinata*. Comp Biochem Physiol A Mol Integr Physiol 2001;129(2–3):461–71.

82. Dupoué A, Brischoux F, Lourdais O, et al. Influence of temperature on the corticosterone stress–response: an experiment in the children's python (*Antaresia childreni*). Gen Comp Endocrinol 2013;193:178–84.

83. Cash WB, Holberton RL, Knight SS. Corticosterone secretion in response to capture and handling in free-living red-eared slider turtles. Gen Comp Endocrinol 1997;108(3):427–33.

84. Woodley SK, Moore MC. Plasma corticosterone response to an acute stressor varies according to reproductive condition in female tree lizards (*Urosaurus ornatus*). Gen Comp Endocrinol 2002;128(2):143–8.

85. Girling J, Cree A. Plasma corticosterone levels are not significantly related to reproductive stage in female common geckos (*Hoplodactylus maculatus*). Gen Comp Endocrinol 1995;100(3):273–81.

86. Divers S. Basic reptile husbandry, history taking and clinical examination. In Pract 1996;18:51–65.

87. Wiesner C, Iben C. Influence of environmental humidity and dietary protein on pyramidal growth of carapaces in African spurred tortoises (*Geochelone sulcata*). J Anim Physiol Anim Nutr 2003;87(1–2):66–74.

88. János D, Imre K, Herman V, et al. A case of blister disease to *Boa constrictor*. Scientific Works. C Series. Vet Med 2012;LVIII(4):88–91.

89. Warwick C, Arena P, Lindley S, et al. Assessing reptile welfare using behavioural criteria. In Pract 2013;35(3):123–31.

90. Richter CP. Total self-regulatory functions in animals and human beings. Harvey Lecture Ser 1943;38(63):1942–3.

91. Tracy CR, Nussear KE, Esque TC, et al. The importance of physiological ecology in conservation biology. Integr Comp Biol 2006;46(6):1191–205.

92. Rich CN, Talent LG. The effects of prey species on food conversion efficiency and growth of an insectivorous lizard. Zoo Biol 2008;27(3):181–7.
93. Ritz J, Hammer C, Clauss M. Body size development of captive and free-ranging leopard tortoises (*Geochelone pardalis*). Zoo Biol 2010;29(4):517–25.
94. Oonincx D, van Leeuwen J, Hendriks W, et al. The diet of free-roaming Australian Central Bearded Dragons (*Pogona vitticeps*). Zoo Biol 2015;34:271–7.
95. Lemm JM, Edwards MS, Grant TD, et al. Comparison of growth and nutritional status of juvenile Komodo monitors (*Varanus komodoensis*) maintained on rodent or poultry-based diets. Zoo Biol 2004;23(3):239–52.
96. Durtsche RD. Ontogenetic plasticity of food habits in the Mexican spiny-tailed iguana, Ctenosaura pectinata. Oecologia 2000;124(2):185–95.
97. Carlos Frederico Duarte R. Ontogenetic shift in the rate of plant consumption in a tropical lizard (*Liolaemus lutzae*). J Herpetol 1998;32(2):274–9.
98. Townsend JH, Slapcinsky J, Krysko KL, et al. Predation of a tree snail *Drymaeus multilineatus* (Gastropoda: Bulimulidae) by Iguana iguana (Reptilia: Iguanidae) on Key Biscayne, Florida. Southeast Nat 2005;4(2):361–4.
99. Bjorndal KA. Diet mixing: nonadditive interactions of diet items in an omnivorous freshwater turtle. Ecology 1991;72(4):1234–41.
100. Moskovits DK, Bjorndal KA. Diet and food preferences of the tortoises *Geochelone carbonaria* and G. denticulata in northwestern Brazil. Herpetologica 1990;207–18.
101. Barboza PS. Nutrient balances and maintenance requirements for nitrogen and energy in desert tortoises (*Xerobates agassizii*) consuming forages. Comp Biochem Physiol A Physiol 1995;112(3):537–45.
102. Donoghue S, Vidal J, Kronfeld D. Growth and morphometrics of green Iguanas (*Iguana iguana*) fed four levels of dietary protein. J Nutr 1998;128(12):2587S–9S.
103. Allen M, Oftedal O, Baer D, Werner D. Nutritional studies with the green iguana. Paper presented at: Proceedings of the Eighth Dr. Scholl Conference on Nutrition in Captive Wild Animals. Chicago (IL), December 8 and 9, 1989.
104. Nagy KA, Shoemaker VH. Energy and nitrogen budgets of the free-living desert lizard *Sauromalus obesus*. Physiol Zool 1975;48(3):252–62.
105. McWilliams DA, Leeson S. Metabolic bone disease in lizards: prevalence and potential for monitoring bone health. Paper presented at: American Zoo and Aquarium Association, Nutrition Advisory Group 2001. Lake Buena Vista (FL), September 19-23, 2001.
106. Schall JJ. Aversion of whiptail lizards (*Cnemidophorus*) to a model alkaloid. Herpetologica 1990;34–9.
107. Rocha C, Vrcibradic D, Van Sluys M. Diet of the lizard *Mabuya agilis* (Sauria; Scincidae) in an insular habitat (Ilha Grande, RJ, Brazil). Braz J Biol 2004;64(1):135–9.
108. Gauthier C, Lesbarreres D. Growth rate variation in captive species: The case of leopard geckos, *Eublepharis macularius*. Herpetol Conserv Biol 2010;5(3):449–55.
109. Oonincx DGAB, van Broekhoven S, van Huis A, et al. Feed conversion, survival and development, and composition of four insect species on diets composed of food by-products. PLoS One 2015;10(12):e0144601.
110. van Broekhoven S, Oonincx DGAB, van Huis A, et al. Growth performance and feed conversion efficiency of three edible mealworm species (Coleoptera: Tenebrionidae) on diets composed of organic by-products. J Insect Physiol 2015;73(0):1–10.

111. Finke MD, Oonincx DG. Insects as food for insectivores. In: Morales-Ramos JA, Rojas MG, Shapiro-Ilan DI, editors. Mass production of beneficial organisms: invertebrates and entomopathogens. London: Academic Press; 2013. p. 583–616.

112. Oonincx DGAB, van der Poel AF. Effects of diet on the chemical composition of migratory locusts (*Locusta migratoria*). Zoo Biol 2011;30:9–16.

113. Oonincx DGAB, Dierenfeld ES. An investigation into the chemical composition of alternative invertebrate prey. Zoo Biol 2012;31(1):40–54.

114. Miller EA, Green SL, Otto GM, et al. Suspected hypovitaminosis A in a colony of captive green anoles (*Anolis carolinensis*). J Am Assoc Lab Anim Sci 2001; 40(2):18–20.

115. Crissey SD, Slifka KA, Lintzenich BA. Whole body cholesterol, fat, and fatty acid concentrations of mice (*Mus domesticus*) used as a food source. J Zoo Wildl Med 1999;30(2):222–7.

116. Dierenfeld ES, Alcorn HL, Jacobsen KL. Nutrient composition of whole vertebrate prey (excluding fish) fed in zoos. Beltsville (MD): US Department of Agriculture, Agricultural Research Service, National Agricultural Library, Animal Welfare Information Center; 2002.

117. Clum NJ, Fitzpatrick MP, Dierenfeld ES. Effects of diet on nutritional content of whole vertebrate prey. Zoo Biol 1996;15(5):525–37.

118. Dierenfeld ES, Fitzpatrick MP, Douglas TC, et al. Mineral concentrations in whole mice and rats used as food. Zoo Biol 1996;15(1):83–8.

119. Dierenfeld ES, Norton TM, Hyslop NL, et al. Nutrient composition of prey items consumed by free-ranging *Drymarchon couperi* (Eastern indigo snakes). Southeast Nat 2015;14(3):551–60.

120. Clark F, King AJ. A critical review of zoo-based olfactory enrichment. Chemical signals in vertebrates 11. New York: Springer; 2008. p. 391–8.

Advancements in Evidence-Based Analgesia in Exotic Animals

Julie A. Balko, VMD*,
Sathya K. Chinnadurai, DVM, MS, DACZM, DACVAA

KEYWORDS

• Analgesia • Avian • NSAID • Opioid • Pain • Reptile • Small mammal

KEY POINTS

- Despite the sparse, yet growing, body of literature regarding analgesic therapy in companion exotic animal species, the recognition and treatment of pain in these animals is of utmost importance.
- Multiple analgesic therapies for exotic animal species are available and often a multimodal, or balanced, approach to pain management will benefit the patient.
- Because there is very large interspecies variability with regard to the pharmacokinetic and pharmacodynamic responses to analgesic drugs, extrapolation of drugs and dosages from similar, yet taxonomically distinct, species, should be practiced with caution.
- Continual reassessment of the individual patient response to analgesic treatment and examination for new or ongoing sources of pain are keys to successful patient management.

INTRODUCTION

The need for timely and appropriate recognition, assessment, and treatment of pain in all veterinary species, including exotic pets, cannot be overstated. Although the assessment of pain perception in nondomestic species is still in its infancy, as reflected by a relatively sparse body of published literature, this does not preclude analgesic management in these species. Furthermore, the inability of animals to communicate the presence, quality, or intensity of pain also should not hamper proper treatment. In fact, the International Society for the Study of Pain recently modified their definition of pain to include the statement that "the inability to communicate verbally does not negate the possibility that an individual is experiencing pain and is in need of appropriate pain-relieving treatment."[1]

Pain recognition in veterinary species is a challenging endeavor and this is especially true for pet exotic animal species. Prey animals will often attempt to elude

The authors have nothing to disclose.
Brookfield Zoo, Chicago Zoological Society, 3300 Golf Road, Brookfield, IL 60513, USA
* Corresponding author.
E-mail address: jbalkovmd@gmail.com

predators by masking outward clinical signs of disease, including pain. This has been objectively identified in laboratory animals, which are reportedly more likely to exhibit clinical signs of pain when an observer is absent from the environment.[2,3] This highlights the considerable importance of meticulous and ongoing assessment of exotic species for signs of pain. Identifiers of pain include both behavioral (eg, changes in activity, appetite, urination and defecation habits, loss of normal behaviors) and physiologic signs (eg, changes in heart rate, respiratory rate, body temperature); recognizing that nonpainful disease states and psychological stressors also can influence these parameters. Although numerous pain scoring systems have been created, no gold standard exists for the assessment of pain in veterinary species. Furthermore, because different species can respond differently to similar noxious stimuli, the development of species-specific algorithms for the assessment of pain is necessary. Likewise, a thorough understanding of normal anatomy, physiology, and behavior for a particular species, and even an individual animal, can aid appropriate pain management.

Preemptive analgesia should be instituted before any painful procedure, unless contraindicated. The benefits of preemptive inhibition of pain pathways have been demonstrated in multiple species.[4,5] Additionally, because pain perception involves multiple processes, in general, administration of a single analgesic agent is often inadequate for complete alleviation of pain; thus, multimodal or combination analgesic therapy is preferred. A balanced analgesic plan can maximize overall drug efficacy while minimizing the potential for individual drug toxicity, and this may be an especially important consideration when treating exotic animal species for which few pharmacokinetic (PK) data on administered analgesic drugs are available.

Because much of the current practice of exotic animal analgesia is based on anecdotal evidence, in many cases, nontraditional therapies may be implemented without objective evidence of effect. Whereas this type of treatment may be advocated in clinical practice according to the belief that "if it may help, then why not try it?" clinicians should consider that such practice risks denying a patient an effective treatment in favor of one with no objective evidence.

There are multiple possible sequelae of undiagnosed or untreated pain, including increased morbidity, increased mortality, or the development of a chronic pain state, all of which can produce a poor quality of life for both the patient and the caretaker. As such, effective, timely analgesic therapy is essential for patient welfare and caretaker satisfaction and should be an integral component of any treatment plan. A dearth of PK and pharmacodynamic (PD) data in exotic animals has resulted in extrapolation from other species, sometimes via very distant phylogenetic connections. However, an increasing body of research regarding analgesic therapy in exotic species has provided clinicians with objective, evidence-based, and (in some cases) species-specific data on which to base clinical analgesic decisions. This article provides an overview of recent advances in evidence-based literature regarding analgesic management in common pet exotic animal species. To assist clinicians, **Table 1** summarizes analgesia protocols for companion exotic animal species, according to currently available published evidence.

ANALGESIC DRUG CATEGORIES
Opioids

Although opioids are often the mainstay of anesthetic and postoperative analgesic management in domestic species, and are indicated for the management of moderate to severe pain, their use in pet exotic species, including birds, reptiles,

Table 1
Analgesia protocols commonly used in exotic animals on the basis of current published evidence

Drug and Species	Key Reference	Species	Study Design	No. of Animals	Dose	Route of Administration	Adverse Effects	Comments
Avians								
Buprenorphine	Ceulemans et al,[10] 2014	American kestrel	Randomized, crossover, PD	12	0.1 mg/kg, 0.3 mg/kg, 0.6 mg/kg	IM	Sedation with 0.6 mg/kg	
Buprenorphine	Gustavsen et al,[11] 2014	American kestrel	PK	13	0.6 mg/kg	IM, IV		94.8% bioavailability IM
Fentanyl	Hoppes et al,[8] 2003	White cockatoo	Controlled, PD	14	0.2 mg/kg	SC	Hyperactivity	Not recommended due to large injection volume
Hydromorphone	Guzman et al,[6] 2013	American kestrel	Randomized, crossover, PD	11	0.1 mg/kg, 0.3 mg/kg, 0.6 mg/kg	IM	Sedation with 0.6 mg/kg	
Hydromorphone	Guzman et al,[7] 2014	American kestrel	PK	12	0.6 mg/kg	IM, IV		Single dose
Meloxicam	Desmarchelier et al,[32] 2012	Domestic pigeon	Randomized, PD	21	0.5 mg/kg, 2.0 mg/kg	IM, repeated doses PO		Postoperative pain model; 0.5 mg/kg ineffective
Meloxicam	Cole et al,[33] 2009	Hispaniolan Amazon parrot	Randomized, crossover, PD	15	0.05 mg/kg, 0.1 mg/kg, 0.5 mg/kg, 1 mg/kg	IM		Arthritis model; ≤0.5 mg/kg was ineffective
Nalbuphine	Guzman et al,[21] 2011	Hispaniolan Amazon parrot	Randomized, crossover, PD	14	12.5 mg/kg, 25 mg/kg, 50 mg/kg	IM		Significantly increased withdrawal threshold with 12.5 mg/kg

(continued on next page)

Table 1
(continued)

Drug and Species	Key Reference	Species	Study Design	No. of Animals	Dose	Route of Administration	Adverse Effects	Comments
Nalbuphine	Keller et al,[22] 2011	Hispaniolan Amazon parrot	PK	8	12.5 mg/kg	IM, IV		Short half-life (<30 min)
Tramadol	Geelen et al,[29] 2013	Hispaniolan Amazon parrot	Randomized, crossover, PD	11	5 mg/kg	IV		Increased withdrawal threshold
Tramadol	Guzman et al,[30] 2012	Hispaniolan Amazon parrot	Randomized, crossover, PD	15 (10, 20 mg/kg), 11 (30 mg/kg)	10 mg/kg, 20 mg/kg, 30 mg/kg	PO		Increased withdrawal threshold with 30 mg/kg
Tramadol	Guzman et al,[31] 2014	American kestrel	Randomized, crossover, PD	12	5 mg/kg, 15 mg/kg, 30 mg/kg	PO		Shorter duration of effect with higher doses
Small mammals								
Buprenorphine–sustained release (SR)	Chum et al,[46] 2014	Rat	Randomized, PD	21	0.3 mg/kg, 1.2 mg/kg, 4.5 mg/kg	SC	Marked sedation with 4.5 mg/kg	Incisional pain model; effective for 48 h (0.3 mg/kg) or 72 h (1.2 mg/kg)
Buprenorphine-SR	Healy et al,[47] 2014	Mouse		36	1.5 mg/kg	SC	Decreased respiratory rate	Significantly increased hot plate and tail-flick latency for 48 h
Buprenorphine-meloxicam	Goldschlager et al,[48] 2013	Rabbit	Randomized, PD	39	0.01 mg/kg–0.1 mg/kg	SC		Postoperative pain model; benefits compared with single analgesic agent
Tramadol	Udegbunam et al,[50] 2015	Rabbit	Randomized, PD	15	10 mg/kg, 20 mg/kg	SC		Postoperative pain model; decreased plasma cortisol concentration

Reptiles and amphibians

Drug	Study	Species	Study type	N	Dose	Route	Findings	Findings
Hydromorphone	Mans et al,[59] 2012	Red-eared slider turtle	Randomized, crossover, PD	17	0.5 mg/kg	SC		Increased thermal withdrawal for 24 h
Morphine	Kinney et al,[57] 2011	Red-eared slider turtle	Randomized, PD	36	2 mg/kg	SC	Decreased feeding, breathing frequency, movement scores	Postoperative pain model; increased thermal withdrawal for 28 h
Tramadol	Baker et al,[62] 2011	Red-eared slider turtle	Crossover, PD	30	5 mg/kg, 10 mg/kg	PO	Less respiratory depression compared with morphine	Increased thermal withdrawal for 4 d
Tramadol	Giorgi et al,[63] 2015	Yellow-bellied slider turtle	Randomized, crossover, PD	19	10 mg/kg	IM		Forelimb or hindlimb; large variability in duration of effect
Tapentadol	Giorgi et al,[67] 2015	Yellow-bellied slider turtle	Randomized, crossover, PD	9	5 mg/kg	IM		Increased thermal withdrawal for 10 h

Abbreviations: IM, intramuscular; IV, intravenous; PD, pharmacodynamic; PK, pharmacokinetic; PO, per os; SC, subcutaneous.

amphibians, and small mammals is less well defined. Few studies have been performed to investigate the number, distribution, and function of opioid receptors in these species; however, research has demonstrated clinical evidence of antinociceptive efficacy. Of note, and as described in this article, studies have also demonstrated vast differences in the PK and PD responses to opioids between species, even those within the same taxa. As such, extrapolation of opioid PK and PD data from one species to another may result in reduced or completely ineffective analgesia and, given the known adverse effects of opioids, may pose a risk to patients. Thus, caution is warranted when applying opioid analgesic data to a species for which no evidence-based data exist. The most common adverse effects of opioid administration include effects on the gastrointestinal (eg, decreased motility, clinical signs of nausea) and respiratory (eg, depression of ventilation) systems; however, these may not all apply to every species.

Of note, tramadol hydrochloride is often grouped with opioids because of its activity at opioid receptors. However, it has demonstrated activity at several other receptors including serotonin, N-methyl-D-aspartate, and alpha-adrenergic, among others. Whereas the parent compound is a weak mu agonist, in mammals, the O-desmethyltramadol (M1) metabolite has much higher affinity for the mu opioid receptor and is presumed to be a greater contributor to its analgesic actions. Although production of tramadol metabolites, including M1, have been reported in avian and nondomestic mammalian species, the eventual downstream effects in these species are unknown. Multiple studies investigating the PK and PD profiles of tramadol in companion exotic animals have recently been published and are described as follows.

Nonsteroidal Anti-inflammatory Drugs

The nonsteroidal anti-inflammatory drugs (NSAIDs) are a class of drugs with anti-inflammatory, analgesic, and antipyretic effects. NSAIDs are indicated for the management of both acute and chronic pain states and are commonly used in nondomestic species, including birds, small mammals, reptiles, and amphibians. However, decisive, evidence-based research supporting their use does not exist for all of the aforementioned species. Pharmacologically, NSAIDs act to inhibit the activity of the enzymes cyclooxygenase-1 (COX-1) and cyclooxygenase-2 (COX-2) to varying degrees with a similar mechanism of action across species. As COX-2 is upregulated in inflammatory states, and because COX-1 is important for the maintenance of many normal, physiologic processes, more recently developed NSAIDs aim to selectively inhibit COX-2 and "spare" COX-1. Adverse effects of NSAIDs include effects on the gastrointestinal, renal, and coagulation systems, among others, and appropriate precautions are advised, even in species in which these adverse effects have not yet been documented.

Local Anesthetics

Local anesthetics block neuronal conduction by reversible inhibition of sodium channels and are frequently used in veterinary species for both local and regional pain control. These agents can be applied topically, infiltrated locally at a surgical site, or used in regional anesthesia (peripheral nerve, epidural, or spinal blockade) and can be a valuable component of a multimodal analgesic protocol. Caution should be exercised with dose calculation, especially when small volumes are indicated, as local anesthetic overdose can lead to major adverse effects, including central nervous system toxicosis, cardiovascular collapse, and death.

ANALGESIC THERAPY: SPECIES-SPECIFIC ADVANCES
Avians

Historically, pure mu opioid receptor agonists have been infrequently used in avian species. Several recent prospective studies have been conducted investigating this class of drugs in birds. Intramuscular administration of hydromorphone to American kestrels (Falco sparverius) at 0.1, 0.3, and 0.6 mg/kg resulted in a dose-responsive thermal antinociceptive effect for at least 6 hours at all doses, with appreciable sedation noted at the highest dose in a subset of birds.[6] The PK of a single dose (0.6 mg/kg) of intramuscular and intravenous hydromorphone was also recently described in this species. Results indicated a high bioavailability and rapid elimination following intramuscular administration with a short terminal half-life and rapid plasma clearance. Plasma hydromorphone concentrations were detectable in 2 of 4 and 3 of 4 birds 6 hours after intramuscular and intravenous administration, respectively, but were undetectable at 9 hours.[7] A 2003 study[8] in white cockatoos (Cacatua spp.) demonstrated no significant change in thermal or electrical withdrawal threshold after intramuscular administration of fentanyl at 0.02 mg/kg. Although the same study reported an antinociceptive effect following subcutaneous administration of fentanyl at a 10-fold higher dose, the large injection volume and associated hyperactivity noted in several birds precluded its recommendation for use.[8] Finally, the PK of a long-acting transdermal fentanyl solution was recently investigated in helmeted guineafowl (Numida meleagris).[9] Results indicated that plasma concentrations higher than previously reported to be analgesic in dogs were maintained for at least 7 days following a single topical dose of 5 mg/kg and no adverse effects were noted.[9] However, until PD data are available, the analgesic effect of this formulation in birds is unknown. Further investigation of the PK of pure mu opioid agonists in avian species is warranted before recommendation for routine use can be made.

Partial mu (buprenorphine) and kappa (butorphanol, nalbuphine) opioid agonists are currently more commonly administered to avian patients. Studies investigating buprenorphine, a partial mu opioid receptor agonist, in birds have demonstrated varied and often species-dependent antinociceptive effects. In American kestrels, the potential analgesic effects of intramuscular buprenorphine have been documented recently; doses of 0.1, 0.3, and 0.6 mg/kg resulted in increased thermal threshold for at least 6 hours, compared with a saline control.[10] Furthermore, there was no significant difference among the 3 doses, aside from mild sedation at the highest dose.[10] The PK of a single dose of intramuscular or intravenous buprenorphine at 0.6 mg/kg were also recently described in kestrels, with high bioavailability (94.8%) following intramuscular administration, and prolonged elimination time compared with other opioids.[11] However, in African gray parrots (Psittacus erithacus spp.), buprenorphine administered intramuscularly at 0.1 mg/kg did not produce an antinociceptive effect[12] and the PK of this dose and administration route revealed that analgesic effects comparable to those reported for humans were maintained for only 2 hours.[13] Thus, although buprenorphine holds potential for treatment of raptors, it may be ineffective in psittacines, and additional research is indicated. No published studies investigating the effects of commercially available sustained release formulations of buprenorphine in avian species are currently available. However, because these formulations have shown great potential in mammalian species, and they offer the benefit of reduced dosing intervals, future investigation regarding their use in birds is warranted.

Butorphanol, a mixed kappa opioid receptor agonist and functional mu opioid receptor antagonist, has traditionally been the most commonly used opioid in avian species. As with other opioid analgesics, variable species efficacy exists, and studies demonstrate that frequent dosing is likely required. Whereas an early study in African gray parrots demonstrated a significant increase in thermal threshold following intramuscular administration,[12] a more recent study in American kestrels found no significant change in thermal threshold following intramuscular butorphanol at 1, 3, and 6 mg/kg. Furthermore, at the highest dose administered in that study (6 mg/kg), mild hyperesthesia or mild hyperalgesia and agitation were noted.[14] The PK of butorphanol have been described in multiple avian species[14–17] and all studies demonstrated the likely need for frequent dosing. Following a 6-mg/kg intramuscular dose of butorphanol in American kestrels, mean terminal half-life was less than 1.5 hours,[14] with similar findings in both red-tailed hawks (Buteo jamaicensis) and great horned owls (Bubo virginianus) following butorphanol 0.5 mg/kg via both the intravenous or intramuscular routes.[15] In Hispaniolan Amazon parrots (Amazona ventralis), the mean terminal half-lives were even shorter at approximately 30 minutes following both intramuscular or intravenous administration using a dose of 5 mg/kg.[16] A similarly short terminal half–life was reported for chickens (Gallus gallus domesticus) administered 2 mg/kg butorphanol intravenously, with plasma concentrations remaining above the minimum effective concentration for analgesia in mammals for approximately 2 hours.[17] Although studies have shown promise with use of a liposome-encapsulated butorphanol formulation[18–20] that is intended to prolong duration of action, no such commercial formulation is currently available.

Nalbuphine hydrochloride, also a mixed kappa opioid receptor agonist and functional mu opioid receptor antagonist similar to butorphanol, is currently infrequently used in veterinary medicine; as such, minimal research has been conducted investigating its effectiveness as an avian analgesic. A study in Hispaniolan Amazon parrots investigated the effects of intramuscular nalbuphine at 12.5, 25.0, and 50.0 mg/kg, and determined that the lowest dose significantly increased thermal withdrawal threshold for up to 3 hours, with no significant changes noted at the higher doses.[21] A PK study in the same species using the lowest dose (12.5 mg/kg) administered either intravenously or intramuscularly, observed excellent bioavailability following intramuscular administration; however, terminal half-lives were short (<30 minutes) following both administration routes.[22] Thus, similar to butorphanol, frequent dosing may be required. Development of a slow-release nalbuphine formulation, nalbuphine decanoate, also has been pursued, with promising preliminary results in avian species.[23,24] However, as for liposome-encapsulated butorphanol, it is not commercially available at present.

Multiple studies investigating the use of tramadol in avian species have recently been published. In red-tailed hawks, orally administered tramadol (11 mg/kg) resulted in plasma concentrations that reached or exceeded concentrations associated with analgesia in humans for at least 4 hours.[25] In Hispaniolan Amazon parrots, a similar oral tramadol dose (10 mg/kg) did not reach plasma levels considered analgesic in humans, whereas a 30 mg/kg dose reached this concentration benchmark for approximately 6 hours after administration.[26] Oral administration of tramadol at 7.5 mg/kg in peafowl demonstrated rapid metabolism of the parent compound, but achieved plasma M1 levels approximately equal to those considered analgesic in humans for 12 to 24 hours.[27] On the basis of results of PK analysis after twice-daily oral tramadol administration (30 mg/kg) in Hispaniolan Amazon parrots, researchers concluded that maintenance of suggested therapeutic plasma levels would likely require dosing every 6 to 8 hours.[28] Administration of 10 mg/kg orally to bald eagles (Haliaeetus leucocephalus) resulted in plasma concentrations in the analgesic range for humans for at least 10 hours in 5 of 6 birds; however, plasma M1 concentrations were achieved at only a single, earlier time point in 2 birds. Recent studies also have investigated the antinociceptive effects of both oral and intravenous tramadol in avian species. A significant increase in the thermal withdrawal threshold was noted in Hispaniolan Amazon parrots at all time points (up to 4 hours) following intravenous administration of 5 mg/kg tramadol, with no sedation or adverse effects noted.[29] Oral administration in Hispaniolan Amazon parrots at 10, 20, and 30 mg/kg produced significant thermal antinociception for up to 6 hours at the highest dose only, with no change observed at the lower doses.[30] Finally, 3 oral doses of tramadol (5, 15, and 30 mg/kg) were investigated in American kestrels. Results demonstrated a significant increase in thermal withdrawal threshold for up to 9 hours, and for up to 3 hours compared with baseline following administration of the lowest dose and the 2 higher doses, respectively, with no adverse effects or changes in agitation-sedation scores noted in any group.[31] Although tramadol holds promise as an analgesic in avian species with no adverse effects yet reported, further research is warranted to determine its appropriate role as part of clinical analgesic therapy.

Meloxicam, a COX-2 selective NSAID, is the most commonly used anti-inflammatory drug in nondomestic companion animals, including birds; however, few PD studies confirming its clinical efficacy in avian species exist. A recent study in domestic pigeons (Columba livia) investigating the efficacy of repeated doses of both a low (0.5 mg/kg) and high (2.0 mg/kg) dose of meloxicam for the treatment of postoperative orthopedic pain determined that the high-dose group had lower postoperative pain scores, increased weight bearing, and faster return to presurgical behaviors compared with the low-dose group.[32] Similarly, in Hispaniolan Amazon parrots with experimentally induced arthritis, significant improvement in weight bearing was observed following administration of intramuscular meloxicam at 1 mg/kg every 12 hours compared with doses of ≤ 0.5 mg/kg.[33] These studies suggest that in psittacine and pigeon species, meloxicam doses of 1 and 2 mg/kg, respectively, may be necessary for analgesic efficacy. The PK of meloxicam via intravenous, intramuscular, and oral routes of administration have recently been described in several species. The mean $\pm$ SD terminal half-life of orally administered meloxicam (1 mg/kg) was 15.8 $\pm$ 8.6 hours[34]; however, this was noted to be less than half in both red-tailed hawks and great horned owls administered oral meloxicam at 0.5 mg/kg.[35] Furthermore, a recent study in African gray parrots demonstrated low bioavailability (28.5%–48.9%) following oral meloxicam administration (1 mg/kg) compared with the intravenous and intramuscular routes.[36] These results highlight the challenges in extrapolating PK data and subsequent dosing strategies to nonstudied species, and the need for caution and close observation for clinical efficacy and adverse effects if such drugs are administered to novel species. A recent study in African gray parrots found no significant change in hematologic or biochemical parameters following twice-daily administration of 0.5 mg/kg meloxicam intramuscularly for 14 days[37]; however, until further research is conducted, the same precautions for NSAID administration in mammals should be practiced with avian species.

Other NSAIDs that have historically been used in avian species include piroxicam, ketoprofen, flunixin meglumine, and carprofen. Aside from a recent PK study in budgerigars (Melopsittacus undulatus) demonstrating a short (<1 hour) half-life of 5 mg/kg flunixin meglumine following intravenous administration,[38] no recent practice-changing research regarding the use of these drugs in avian species has been published.

Local anesthetics have traditionally been underused in avian species as anecdotal evidence implied that birds are more sensitive to the adverse effects of local anesthetics; as such, dosage guidelines for avian species have historically been lower compared with mammals. Although additional safety studies are necessary to determine the validity of this claim, a recent study in chickens reported no adverse cardiovascular effects when birds were administered 6 mg/kg lidocaine intravenously.[39] The PK of a single dose of intravenous lidocaine (2.5 mg/kg) in chickens also has been recently described, with a reported rapid half-life and possible similar mechanism of metabolism and elimination as for mammalian species.[40] Specific local anesthetic techniques also have been reported in avian species, although the extent of efficacy has been mixed. A sciatic femoral nerve block in peregrine falcons (*Falco peregrinus*) produced effective blockade based on intraoperative and postoperative physiologic and behavioral parameters, respectively.[41] In contrast, brachial plexus blockade in both mallard ducks (*Anas platyrhynchos*)[42] and Hispaniolan Amazon parrots[43] failed to produce effective blockade in either species.

Gabapentin, a GABA analog, has been used in the treatment of neuropathic pain in both human and veterinary patients. However, little evidence-based research is available regarding the use of this drug in companion pet exotic species. Although recent PK studies conducted in Hispaniolan Amazon parrots[44] and great horned owls[45] suggested a dosing interval of every 8 hours following oral gabapentin administration, these results are based on effective plasma concentrations reported for humans. Further PD studies are needed before this drug can be recommended as part of a balanced analgesic protocol in birds.

Small Mammals

A long-acting (sustained release) buprenorphine formulation (Buprenorphine-SR) has recently become legally available for veterinary use in species including pet exotic animals (https://www.fda.gov/AnimalVeterinary/DevelopmentApprovalProcess/Minor UseMinorSpecies/ucm125452.htm), and was investigated in rodents. In a rat (*Rattus norvegicus*) model of incisional pain, sustained-release buprenorphine at 0.3 or 1.2 mg/kg increased thermal withdrawal latency for 48 and 72 hours, respectively, with minimal sedation.[46] A similar study in Swiss-Webster mice determined that sustained-release buprenorphine (1.5 mg/kg) resulted in significant antinociception for 48 hours.[47] The benefit of reduced dosing frequency makes sustained-release formulations a desirable option; thus, further investigation in additional exotic animal species is warranted.

The effects of multimodal analgesic therapy with combination buprenorphine-meloxicam (0.01–0.1 mg/kg subcutaneous once daily) compared with buprenorphine (0.03 mg/kg subcutaneous twice daily) or meloxicam (0.2 mg/kg subcutaneous once daily) alone were recently reported in New Zealand White rabbits (*Oryctolagus cuniculus*) undergoing a minor surgical procedure. Postoperative fecal glucocorticoid metabolite concentration, a marker of physiologic stress, in the single-agent groups was significantly higher for the rabbits receiving combination therapy, versus the other groups. Weight gain was also greater in the combination therapy group throughout the 28-day study period.[48] These results support the value of multimodal analgesic therapy in small mammals.

Few studies regarding the use of tramadol in companion small mammal species have been performed. In domestic rabbits, orally administered tramadol (11 mg/kg) failed to reach plasma concentrations deemed analgesic in humans.[49] In a more recent study, subcutaneous administration of 10 and 20 mg/kg tramadol resulted in decreased plasma cortisol levels in rabbits after gastrostomy, compared with controls.[50] A single study in rats demonstrated that intraperitoneal tramadol provided inadequate analgesia for incisional pain.[51] Additional prospective studies are warranted before tramadol can be recommended for use in small mammal species. Additionally, although gabapentin has shown promise in other domestic species, its efficacy as an analgesic in small mammals remains unknown, because PK and PD data are currently lacking.

Although previous research has been performed on a variety of NSAIDs in small mammal species, recent prospective studies have focused on meloxicam. The PK of a single subcutaneous dose of meloxicam (0.2 mg/kg) in ferrets (*Mustela putorius furo*) were recently described and, although achieved plasma concentrations were considered effective compared with other species, significant differences between males and females were reported.[52] The PK of oral meloxicam has been investigated in rabbits following once-daily dosing of 1 mg/kg for 1 day, 5 days,[53] and 29 days.[54] Plasma concentrations were similar following all dosing regimens, and were comparable to concentrations deemed clinically effective in other species. Rabbits in the latter study were euthanized for necropsy on day 31 with no notable abnormal findings. Thus, the investigators concluded that once-daily dosing of meloxicam at 1 mg/kg for up to 29 days may be safe for use in healthy rabbits. Because that dose (1 mg/kg) is higher than that administered to dogs, cats, and other companion exotic animals, further investigation into the analgesic efficacy and adverse effects of this dose in clinically ill rabbits is warranted.

Local anesthetics have traditionally been administered to small mammals via multiple routes, including topically, subcutaneously, and epidurally among others, and their continued use as part of a multimodal analgesic protocol in these species is recommended. There has been recent interest in regional anesthesia for small mammal species, and future prospective studies are indicated. A recent case series and case report described the technique for sciatic-femoral nerve blocks in rabbits[55] and a guinea pig (*Cavia porcellus*),[56] respectively, undergoing hind limb surgery. Although no complications were noted, no assessment of efficacy was made in either species.

Reptiles and Amphibians

A recent study evaluated the antinociceptive efficacy of morphine (2 mg/kg subcutaneously) or butorphanol (20 mg/kg subcutaneously) in red-eared slider turtles (*Trachemys scripta scripta*) undergoing unilateral gonadectomy. Turtles receiving morphine had increased thermal withdrawal latencies for 28 hours postoperatively, compared with those in a sham-saline group, with no significant difference noted for those animals receiving butorphanol. Feeding, breath frequency, and movement scores were similarly reduced in both groups on postoperative day 0; however, breathing frequency remained decreased on days 1 to 2 in those turtles receiving morphine.[57] This study demonstrated that a single subcutaneous injection of morphine can result in prolonged thermal withdrawal latency in this species. Administration of butorphanol 1 mg/kg intramuscularly in juvenile green iguanas (*Iguana iguana*) did not result in thermal antinociception; however, the visible presence of an observer significantly increased the thermal threshold temperature,[58] highlighting the importance of considering the effects of human interactions on companion pet exotic species, especially with regard to pain recognition and assessment. The antinociceptive efficacy of both buprenorphine (0.1, 0.2, 1 mg/kg) and hydromorphone (0.5 mg/kg) were recently evaluated in red-eared slider turtles (*Trachemys scripta elegans*). Following subcutaneous administration, buprenorphine did not significantly increase thermal withdrawal latency at any dosage or time point compared with saline; however, hydromorphone resulted in significantly increased thermal withdrawal latency for up to 24 hours.[59] In a study evaluating the PK of single-dose, subcutaneous buprenorphine at 2 doses (0.02, 0.05 mg/kg) in the forelimb and hindlimb in red-eared slider turtles, it was reported that 11 of 13 turtles maintained minimum effective plasma levels for 24 hours following forelimb administration of the higher dose with only 6 of 13 turtles reaching this benchmark with the lower dose. Lower plasma levels following hindlimb administration were attributable to hepatic first-pass effect.[60]

Several recent studies have been published regarding the PK and PD of tramadol in chelonian species; however, no prospective studies exist regarding tramadol use in other reptiles or amphibians. After oral administration of tramadol to loggerhead sea turtles (Caretta caretta), plasma concentrations of both the parent compound and O-desmethyltramadol (M1) metabolite exceeded concentrations associated with analgesia in humans for 48 and 72 hours following a 5 and 10 mg/kg dose, respectively.[61] Various doses of oral and subcutaneous tramadol were investigated in red-eared slider turtles, and oral administration of 5 and 10 mg/kg increased thermal withdrawal latency for at least 4 days, and resulted in less respiratory depression compared with that reported for morphine. Subcutaneous administration resulted in lower thermal withdrawal latencies, slower onset, and a shorter duration of action compared with the oral route.[62] In yellow-bellied slider turtles, intramuscular administration of 10 mg/kg tramadol in either the forelimb or hindlimb resulted in significantly higher (20%) production of the M1 metabolite in the hindlimb group and significant increases in thermal withdrawal latencies over 8.0 to 48.0 hours and 0.5 to 48.0 hours in the forelimb and hindlimb groups, respectively.[63]

Tapentadol is a newer, centrally acting opioid analgesic similar to tramadol. Because it does not undergo metabolic activation, its use has been investigated in a variety of veterinary species,[64–66] including yellow-bellied slider turtles.[67] Following intramuscular administration, thermal withdrawal latencies were increased for up to 10 hours. Whereas tramadol and tapentadol show promise as long-acting analgesics, in view of the results of these studies, additional research is necessary before their routine, recommended use, especially in nonchelonian species.

As with other species, the bulk of recent evidence-based literature regarding the use of NSAIDs in reptiles and amphibians focuses on the use of meloxicam. In loggerhead sea turtles, bioavailability of meloxicam following intramuscular administration of 0.1 mg/kg was low, and plasma concentrations decreased below the limits of detection by 8 hours.[68] Conversely, in red-eared slider turtles, intramuscular meloxicam at 0.2 mg/kg was demonstrated to have high bioavailability, a long half-life, and no immediate adverse effects.[69] Oral bioavailability after the same dose (0.2 mg/kg) in the same species was found to be low in a separate study.[70] Although none of the studies assessed analgesic efficacy, these results suggest there may be species differences in the PK behavior of meloxicam, especially in response to the route of administration. A study in North American bullfrogs (Rana catesbeiana) evaluated the change in circulating prostaglandin E2 (PGE2), a known downstream effect of NSAIDs in mammalian species, in response to intramuscular meloxicam at 0.1 mg/kg following tissue biopsy. The calculated means of the absolute change in PGE2 between baseline and postbiopsy samples were significantly lower in meloxicam-treated frogs compared with saline control, suggesting anti-inflammatory and analgesic effects in this species.[71] When comparing meloxicam and flunixin meglumine (among other analgesics) in a recent study in African-clawed frogs (Xenopus laevis), no significant difference in analgesic efficacy (as evidenced by response to chemical or thermal noxious stimuli) was noted following surgical intervention; however, in the absence of surgery, flunixin meglumine provided better analgesia.[72] The importance of this disparity is unclear.

No practice-changing research regarding the use of local anesthetics in reptiles and amphibians has been published in the recent past.

SUMMARY

Pain recognition, assessment, treatment, and reassessment are important pillars of pet exotic animal clinical medicine. As the PK and PD responses to an analgesic can vary immensely between species, extrapolation of drugs and doses from similar, yet taxonomically distinct, species should be practiced with discretion. An evidence-based approach to analgesic drug selection should be used whenever possible; however, continual patient reassessment remains essential for appropriate pain management.

REFERENCES

1. IASP Taxonomy - IASP. Available at: http://www.iasp-pain.org/Taxonomy#Pain. Accessed January 4, 2017.
2. Roughan J, Flecknell P. Effects of surgery and analgesic administration on spontaneous behaviour in singly housed rats. Res Vet Sci 2000;69(3):283–8.
3. Roughan J, Flecknell P. Behavioural effects of laparotomy and analgesic effects of ketoprofen and carprofen in rats. Pain 2001;90(1–2):65–74.
4. Shafford HL, Schadt JC. Effect of buprenorphine on the cardiovascular and respiratory response to visceral pain in conscious rabbits. Vet Anaesth Analg 2008; 35(4):333–40.
5. Reichert JA, Daughters RS, Rivard R, et al. Peripheral and preemptive opioid antinociception in a mouse visceral pain model. Pain 2001;89(2–3):221–7.
6. Guzman DS-M, Drazenovich TL, Olsen GH, et al. Evaluation of thermal antinociceptive effects after intramuscular administration of hydromorphone hydrochloride to American kestrels (*Falco sparverius*). Am J Vet Res 2013;74(6):817–22.
7. Guzman DS-M, KuKanich B, Drazenovich TL, et al. Pharmacokinetics of hydromorphone hydrochloride after intravenous and intramuscular administration of a single dose to American kestrels (*Falco sparverius*). Am J Vet Res 2014;75(6): 527–31.
8. Hoppes S, Flammer K, Hoersch K, et al. Disposition and analgesic effects of fentanyl in white cockatoos (*Cacatua alba*). J Avian Med Surg 2003;17(3):124–30.
9. Waugh L, Knych H, Cole G, et al. Pharmacokinetic evaluation of a long-acting fentanyl solution after transdermal administration in helmeted guineafowl (*Numida meleagris*). J Zoo Wildl Med 2016;47(2):468–73.
10. Ceulemans SM, Guzman DS-M, Olsen GH, et al. Evaluation of thermal antinociceptive effects after intramuscular administration of buprenorphine hydrochloride to American kestrels (*Falco sparverius*). Am J Vet Res 2014;75(8):705–10.
11. Gustavsen KA, Guzman DS-M, Knych HK, et al. Pharmacokinetics of buprenorphine hydrochloride following intramuscular and intravenous administration to American kestrels (*Falco sparverius*). Am J Vet Res 2014;75(8):711–5.
12. Paul-Murphy JR, Brunson DB, Miletic V. Analgesic effects of butorphanol and buprenorphine in conscious African grey parrots (*Psittacus erithacus erithacus* and *Psittacus erithacus timneh*). Am J Vet Res 1999;60(10):1218–21.
13. Paul-Murphy J, Hess JC, Fialkowski JP. Pharmacokinetic properties of a single intramuscular dose of buprenorphine in African grey parrots (*Psittacus erithacus erithacus*). J Avian Med Surg 2004;18(4):224–8.
14. Guzman DS-M, Drazenovich TL, KuKanich B, et al. Evaluation of thermal antinociceptive effects and pharmacokinetics after intramuscular administration of butorphanol tartrate to American kestrels (*Falco sparverius*). Am J Vet Res 2014; 75(1):11–8.

15. Riggs SM, Hawkins MG, Craigmill AL, et al. Pharmacokinetics of butorphanol tartrate in red-tailed hawks (*Buteo jamaicensis*) and great horned owls (*Bubo virginianus*). Am J Vet Res 2008;69(5):596–603.
16. Guzman DS-M, Flammer K, Paul-Murphy JR, et al. Pharmacokinetics of butorphanol after intravenous, intramuscular, and oral administration in Hispaniolan Amazon parrots (*Amazona ventralis*). J Avian Med Surg 2011;25(3):185–91.
17. Singh PM, Johnson C, Gartrell B, et al. Pharmacokinetics of butorphanol in broiler chickens. Vet Rec 2011;168:588.
18. Sladky KK, Krugner-Higby L, Meek-Walker E, et al. Serum concentrations and analgesic effects of liposome-encapsulated and standard butorphanol tartrate in parrots. Am J Vet Res 2006;67(5):775–81.
19. Paul-Murphy JR, Krugner-Higby LA, Tourdot RL, et al. Evaluation of liposome-encapsulated butorphanol tartrate for alleviation of experimentally induced arthritic pain in green-cheeked conures (*Pyrrhura molinae*). Am J Vet Res 2009; 70(10):1211–9.
20. Paul-Murphy JR, Sladky KK, Krugner-Higby LA, et al. Analgesic effects of carprofen and liposome-encapsulated butorphanol tartrate in Hispaniolan parrots (*Amazona ventralis*) with experimentally induced arthritis. Am J Vet Res 2009; 70(10):1201–10.
21. Guzman DS-M, KuKanich B, Keuler NS, et al. Antinociceptive effects of nalbuphine hydrochloride in Hispaniolan Amazon parrots (*Amazona ventralis*). Am J Vet Res 2011;72(6):736–40.
22. Keller DL, Guzman DS-M, Klauer JM, et al. Pharmacokinetics of nalbuphine hydrochloride after intravenous and intramuscular administration to Hispaniolan Amazon parrots (*Amazona ventralis*). Am J Vet Res 2011;72(6):741–5.
23. Guzman DS-M, Braun JM, Steagall PVM, et al. Antinociceptive effects of long-acting nalbuphine decanoate after intramuscular administration to Hispaniolan Amazon parrots (*Amazona ventralis*). Am J Vet Res 2013;74(2):196–200.
24. Guzman DS-M, KuKanich B, Heath TD, et al. Pharmacokinetics of long-acting nalbuphine decanoate after intramuscular administration to Hispaniolan Amazon parrots (*Amazona ventralis*). Am J Vet Res 2013;74(2):191–5.
25. Souza MJ, Martin-Jimenez T, Jones MP, et al. Pharmacokinetics of oral tramadol in red-tailed hawks (*Buteo jamaicensis*). J Vet Pharmacol Ther 2011;34(1):86–8.
26. Souza MJ, Guzman DS-M, Paul-Murphy JR, et al. Pharmacokinetics after oral and intravenous administration of a single dose of tramadol hydrochloride to Hispaniolan Amazon parrots (*Amazona ventralis*). Am J Vet Res 2012;73(8):1142–7.
27. Black PA, Cox SK, Macek M, et al. Pharmacokinetics of tramadol hydrochloride and its metabolite O-desmethyltramadol in peafowl (*Pavo cristatus*). J Zoo Wildl Med 2010;41(4):671–6.
28. Souza MJ, Gerhardt L, Cox S. Pharmacokinetics of repeated oral administration of tramadol hydrochloride in Hispaniolan Amazon parrots (*Amazona ventralis*). Am J Vet Res 2013;74(7):957–62.
29. Geelen S, Guzman DS-M, Souza MJ, et al. Antinociceptive effects of tramadol hydrochloride after intravenous administration to Hispaniolan Amazon parrots (*Amazona ventralis*). Am J Vet Res 2013;74(2):201–6.
30. Guzman DS-M, Souza MJ, Braun JM, et al. Antinociceptive effects after oral administration of tramadol hydrochloride in Hispaniolan Amazon parrots (*Amazona ventralis*). Am J Vet Res 2012;73(8):1148–52.
31. Guzman DS-M, Drazenovich TL, Olsen GH, et al. Evaluation of thermal antinociceptive effects after oral administration of tramadol hydrochloride to American kestrels (*Falco sparverius*). Am J Vet Res 2014;75(2):117–23.

32. Desmarchelier M, Troncy E, Fitzgerald G, et al. Analgesic effects of meloxicam administration on postoperative orthopedic pain in domestic pigeons (*Columba livia*). Am J Vet Res 2012;73(3):361–7.

33. Cole GA, Paul-Murphy J, Krugner-Higby L, et al. Analgesic effects of intramuscular administration of meloxicam in Hispaniolan parrots (*Amazona ventralis*) with experimentally induced arthritis. Am J Vet Res 2009;70(12):1471–6.

34. Molter CM, Court MH, Cole GA, et al. Pharmacokinetics of meloxicam after intravenous, intramuscular, and oral administration of a single dose to Hispaniolan Amazon parrots (*Amazona ventralis*). Am J Vet Res 2013;74(3):375–80.

35. Lacasse C, Gamble KC, Boothe DM. Pharmacokinetics of a single dose of intravenous and oral meloxicam in red-tailed hawks (*Buteo jamaicensis*) and great horned owls (*Bubo virginianus*). J Avian Med Surg 2013;27(3):204–10.

36. Montesinos A, Ardiaca M, Gilabert JA, et al. Pharmacokinetics of meloxicam after intravenous, intramuscular and oral administration of a single dose to African grey parrots (*Psittacus erithacus*). J Vet Pharmacol Ther 2016;40(3):279–84.

37. Montesinos A, Ardiaca M, Juan-Sallés C, et al. Effects of meloxicam on hematologic and plasma biochemical analyte values and results of histologic examination of kidney biopsy specimens of African grey parrots (*Psittacus erithacus*). J Avian Med Surg 2015;29(1):1–8.

38. Musser JMB, Heatley JJ, Phalen DN. Pharmacokinetics after intravenous administration of flunixin meglumine in budgerigars (*Melopsittacus undulatus*) and Patagonian conures (*Cyanoliseus patagonus*). J Am Vet Med Assoc 2013; 242(2):205–8.

39. Brandão J, da Cunha AF, Pypendop B, et al. Cardiovascular tolerance of intravenous lidocaine in broiler chickens (*Gallus gallus domesticus*) anesthetized with isoflurane. Vet Anaesth Analg 2015;42(4):442–8.

40. Da Cunha AF, Messenger KM, Stout RW, et al. Pharmacokinetics of lidocaine and its active metabolite monoethylglycinexylidide after a single intravenous administration in chickens (*Gallus domesticus*) anesthetized with isoflurane. J Vet Pharmacol Ther 2012;35(6):604–7.

41. d'Ovidio D, Noviello E, Adami C. Nerve stimulator-guided sciatic-femoral nerve block in raptors undergoing surgical treatment of pododermatitis. Vet Anaesth Analg 2015;42(4):449–53.

42. Brenner DJ, Larsen RS, Dickinson PJ, et al. Development of an avian brachial plexus nerve block technique for perioperative analgesia in mallard ducks (*Anas platyrhynchos*). J Avian Med Surg 2010;24(1):24–34.

43. da Cunha AF, Strain GM, Rademacher N, et al. Palpation- and ultrasound-guided brachial plexus blockade in Hispaniolan Amazon parrots (*Amazona ventralis*). Vet Anaesth Analg 2013;40(1):96–102.

44. Baine K, Jones MP, Cox S, et al. Pharmacokinetics of compounded intravenous and oral gabapentin in Hispaniolan Amazon Parrots (*Amazona ventralis*). J Avian Med Surg 2015;29(3):165–73.

45. Yaw TJ, Zaffarano BA, Gall A, et al. Pharmacokinetic properties of a single administration of oral gabapentin in the great horned owl (*Bubo virginianus*). J Zoo Wildl Med 2015;46(3):547–52.

46. Chum HH, Jampachairsri K, McKeon GP, et al. Antinociceptive effects of sustained-release buprenorphine in a model of incisional pain in rats (*Rattus norvegicus*). J Am Assoc Lab Anim Sci 2014;53(2):193–7.

47. Healy JR, Tonkin JL, Kamarec SR, et al. Evaluation of an improved sustained-release buprenorphine formulation for use in mice. Am J Vet Res 2014;75(7): 619–25.

48. Goldschlager GB, Gillespie VL, Palme R, et al. Effects of multimodal analgesia with low dose buprenorphine and meloxicam on fecal glucocorticoid metabolites after surgery in New Zealand white rabbits (*Oryctolagus cuniculus*). J Am Assoc Lab Anim Sci 2013;52(5):571–6.

49. Souza MJ, Greenacre CB, Cox SK. Pharmacokinetics of orally administered tramadol in domestic rabbits (*Oryctolagus cuniculus*). Am J Vet Res 2008;69(8):979–82.

50. Udegbunam RI, Onuba AC, Okorie-Kanu C, et al. Effects of two doses of tramadol on pain and some biochemical parameters in rabbits post-gastrotomy. Comp Clin Path 2015;24(4):783–90.

51. McKeon GP, Pacharinsak C, Long CT, et al. Analgesic effects of tramadol, tramadol-gabapentin, and buprenorphine in an incisional model of pain in rats (*Rattus norvegicus*). J Am Assoc Lab Anim Sci 2011;50(2):192–7.

52. Chinnadurai SK, Wrenn A, DeVoe RS. Evaluation of noninvasive oscillometric blood pressure monitoring in anesthetized boid snakes. J Am Vet Med Assoc 2009;234(5):625–30.

53. Fredholm DV, Carpenter JW, KuKanich B, et al. Pharmacokinetics of meloxicam in rabbits after oral administration of single and multiple doses. Am J Vet Res 2013;74(4):636–41.

54. Delk KW, Carpenter JW, KuKanich B, et al. Pharmacokinetics of meloxicam administered orally to rabbits (*Oryctolagus cuniculus*) for 29 days. Am J Vet Res 2014;75(2):195–9.

55. d'Ovidio D, Rota S, Noviello E, et al. Nerve stimulator–guided sciatic-femoral block in pet rabbits (*Oryctolagus cuniculus*) undergoing hind limb surgery: a case series. J Exot Pet Med 2014;23(1):91–5.

56. Aguiar J, Mogridge G, Hall J. Femoral fracture repair and sciatic and femoral nerve blocks in a guinea pig. J Small Anim Pract 2014;55(12):635–9.

57. Kinney ME, Johnson SM, Sladky KK. Behavioral evaluation of red-eared slider turtles (*Trachemys scripta elegans*) administered either morphine or butorphanol following unilateral gonadectomy. J Herpetol Med Surg 2011;21(2–3):54–62.

58. Fleming GJ, Robertson SA. Assessments of thermal antinociceptive effects of butorphanol and human observer effect on quantitative evaluation of analgesia in green iguanas (*Iguana iguana*). Am J Vet Res 2012;73(10):1507–11.

59. Mans C, Lahner LL, Baker BB, et al. Antinociceptive efficacy of buprenorphine and hydromorphone in red-eared slider turtles (*Trachemys scripta elegans*). J Zoo Wild Med 2012;43(3):662–5.

60. Kummrow MS, Tseng F, Hesse L, et al. Pharmacokinetics of buprenorphine after single-dose subcutaneous administration in red-eared sliders (*Trachemys scripta elegans*). J Zoo Wildl Med 2008;39(4):590–5.

61. Norton TM, Cox S, Nelson SE, et al. Pharmacokinetics of tramadol and O-desmethyltramadol in loggerhead sea turtles (*Caretta caretta*). J Zoo Wildl Med 2015;46(2):262–5.

62. Baker BB, Sladky KK, Johnson SM. Evaluation of the analgesic effects of oral and subcutaneous tramadol administration in red-eared slider turtles. J Am Vet Med Assoc 2011;238(2):220–7.

63. Giorgi M, Salvadori M, De Vito V, et al. Pharmacokinetic/pharmacodynamic assessments of 10 mg/kg tramadol intramuscular injection in yellow-bellied slider turtles (*Trachemys scripta scripta*). J Vet Pharmacol Ther 2015;38(5):488–96.

64. Lavy E, Lee H-K, Mabjeesh SJ, et al. Use of the novel atypical opioid tapentadol in goats (*Capra hircus*): pharmacokinetics after intravenous, and intramuscular administration. J Vet Pharmacol Ther 2014;37(5):518–21.

65. Lee H-K, Łebkowska-Wieruszewska B, Kim T-W, et al. Pharmacokinetics of the novel atypical opioid tapentadol after intravenous, intramuscular and subcutaneous administration in cats. Vet J 2013;198(3):620–4.

66. Kögel B, Terlinden R, Schneider J. Characterisation of tramadol, morphine and tapentadol in an acute pain model in beagle dogs. Vet Anaesth Analg 2014; 41(3):297–304.

67. Giorgi M, Lee H-K, Rota S, et al. Pharmacokinetic and pharmacodynamic assessments of tapentadol in yellow-bellied slider turtles (*Trachemys Scripta Scripta*) after a single intramuscular injection. J Exot Pet Med 2015;24(3):317–25.

68. Lai OR, Di Bello A, Soloperto S, et al. Pharmacokinetic behavior of meloxicam in loggerhead sea turtles (*Caretta caretta*) after intramuscular and intravenous administration. J Wildl Dis 2015;51(2):509–12.

69. Uney K, Altan F, Aboubakr M, et al. Pharmacokinetics of meloxicam in red-eared slider turtles (*Trachemys scripta elegans*) after single intravenous and intramuscular injections. Am J Vet Res 2016;77(5):439–44.

70. Di Salvo A, Giorgi M, Catanzaro A, et al. Pharmacokinetic profiles of meloxicam in turtles (*Trachemys scripta scripta*) after single oral, intracoelomic and intramuscular administrations. J Vet Pharmacol Ther 2016;39(1):102–5.

71. Minter LJ, Clarke EO, Gjeltema JL, et al. Effects of intramuscular meloxicam administration on prostaglandin E2 synthesis in the North American bullfrog (*Rana catesbeiana*). J Zoo Wildl Med 2011;42(4):680–5.

72. Coble DJ, Taylor DK, Mook DM. Analgesic effects of meloxicam, morphine sulfate, flunixin meglumine, and xylazine hydrochloride in African-clawed frogs (*Xenopus laevis*). J Am Assoc Lab Anim Sci 2011;50(3):355–60.

Advancements in Evidence-Based Anesthesia of Exotic Animals

Julie A. Balko, VMD*,
Sathya K. Chinnadurai, DVM, MS, DACZM, DACVAA

KEYWORDS

• Alfaxalone • Anesthesia • Avian • Reptile • Small mammal

KEY POINTS

- The body of literature regarding anesthesia in companion exotic animal species continues to grow, emphasizing the importance of safe anesthesia and reliable anesthetic monitoring.
- Recent evidence-based advances in anesthetic pharmacology for exotic animal species have allowed for improved multimodal anesthetic management.
- Because very large interspecies variability can exist with regard to the pharmacokinetic and pharmacodynamic responses to anesthetic drugs, extrapolation of drugs and dosages from similar, yet taxonomically distinct species should be practiced with extreme caution.
- Anatomic nuances that make intubation, intravenous access, and monitoring challenging in a certain species are critical factors to understand before attempting to anesthetize a new species.
- Adaptation of anesthetic monitoring devices designed for humans and domestic animals to exotic animals is challenging, and further monitor validation is needed to make informed clinical decisions.

INTRODUCTION

As small exotic animals grow in popularity as companion pets, there is an increased urgency to improve the standard of veterinary care, including with the provision of safe, evidence-based protocols for anesthesia and sedation. Nonetheless, to date much of the current practice of exotic animal anesthesia relies on anecdotal drug dosing recommendations and extrapolation from unrelated species. Anesthesia and sedation of pet nondomestic species is often necessary for both invasive and noninvasive procedures. Even minimally invasive procedures, such as blood collection and

The authors have nothing to disclose.
Brookfield Zoo, Chicago Zoological Society, 3300 Golf Road, Brookfield, IL 60513, USA
* Corresponding author.
E-mail address: jbalkovmd@gmail.com

Vet Clin Exot Anim 20 (2017) 917–928
http://dx.doi.org/10.1016/j.cvex.2017.04.014
1094-9194/17/© 2017 Elsevier Inc. All rights reserved.

vetexotic.theclinics.com

radiographs, can be stressful for small prey species that are not domesticated or acclimated to human contact and restraint.

Extrapolation from domestic dogs and cats to exotics is complicated by differences in physiology, anatomy, and drug metabolism. Those differences affect the pharmacokinetic behavior of anesthetic drugs and can hinder the use of anesthetic monitors designed for domestic mammals or humans. Anatomic and physiologic nuances that make intubation, intravenous (IV) access and monitoring challenging in a certain species are critical factors to understand before attempting to anesthetize a new species.

It is the authors' hope that, with recent advancements in evidence-based practice, the standard of care for exotic pets will continue to improve based on scientifically sound best practices and rely less on anecdotal recommendations. Multiple books and chapters have been published about anesthesia in exotic pets, and this article focus on new scientific literature that has been published in the last 5 years. In many cases, the best evidence may come from studies of related wild or laboratory species; the authors discuss those studies if they clearly affect anesthetic practice in pet exotics. For ease of reading, the authors divide the article to highlight advances in anesthetic pharmacology and discoveries in anesthetic physiology and monitoring. To assist clinicians, **Table 1** summarizes anesthetic protocols for companion exotic animal species, according to currently available published evidence.

ADVANCES IN ANESTHETIC PHARMACOLOGY
Avian

Inhalant anesthetics remain a mainstay of avian anesthesia. The highly efficient respiratory system of birds allows for rapid induction and recovery from inhalants.[1] Volatile (inhalant) anesthetics are considered direct cardiovascular depressants and can cause hypotension due to dose-dependent decreases in myocardial contractility, stroke volume, and systemic vascular resistance.[2,3] Recent studies have examined the potency of certain volatile anesthetics in multiple avian species as well as the cardiopulmonary effects. Potency of inhalant anesthetics is often measured using the minimum alveolar (or anesthetic) concentration (MAC) required to prevent purposeful movement in response to a supramaximal noxious (painful) stimulus in 50% of subjects. Although MAC for individual inhalants is fairly consistent across species, documented variability in isoflurane MAC between avian taxa highlights the difficulty in extrapolating anesthetic drug dosing across multiple species. The mean $\pm$ SD isoflurane MAC in pigeons (*Columba livia*) is $1.8 \pm 0.4\%$,[4] whereas in thick-billed parrots it is reportedly much lower at 1.07% (95% confidence interval [CI] 0.97%–1.16%).[5] If an anesthetist treated the two species in these studies similarly, overdosing of parrots or underdosing of pigeons is possible. Directly comparing MAC studies may be misleading, depending on the type of stimulus used. Mean sevoflurane MAC in thick-billed parrots determined with toe-clamp stimulus was 2.35% (95% CI 2.13%–2.65%), similar to other avian species, whereas the same study found that the mean MAC with electrical stimulation was 4.24% (95% CI 3.61%–8.71%).[6] The MAC for volatile anesthetics can be lowered with the concurrent administration of additional analgesics or sedatives. In chickens, methadone (6 mg/kg intramuscular [IM]) was found to reduce the mean MAC of isoflurane by 30% (range 11%–46%). Butorphanol (4 mg/kg IM) was also evaluated for MAC reduction in guinea fowl but resulted in unacceptable cardiac arrhythmias.[7,8]

When comparing equipotent doses of isoflurane, sevoflurane, and desflurane in red-tailed hawks (*Buteo jamaicensis*), no significant differences were found in

Table 1
Anesthesia protocols commonly used in exotic animals from current published evidence

Drug	Key References	Species	Study Design	No. of Animals	Dose	Route of Administration	Adverse Effects	Comments
Avian								
Diazepam	Prather,[16] 2012	Zebra finch	PD	20	10 mg/kg	IM		Antagonized with 0.3 mg/kg flumazenil
Xylazine	Sadegh,[13] 2013	Budgerigar	Randomized/ crossover	15	25 mg/kg	IN		
Diazepam	Sadegh,[13] 2013	Budgerigar	Randomized/ crossover	15	13 mg/kg	IN		
Midazolam	Sadegh,[13] 2013	Budgerigar	Randomized/ crossover	15	13 mg/kg	IN		
Methadone	Escobar et al,[7] 2016	Chicken	PD	13	6 mg/kg	IM	Rare AV block and VPCs	
Butorphanol	Escobar et al,[8] 2012	Guinea fowl	PD	10	2 mg/kg	IM	Arrhythmias noted at 4 mg/kg	
Midazolam	Mans et al,[15] 2012	Amazon parrots	PD	9	2 mg/kg	IN		Antagonized with 0.05 mg/kg flumazenil
Midazolam/ dexmedetomidine	Hornak et al,[14] 2015	Pigeons	PD	6	5 mg/kg (m) with 80 µg/kg (dm)	IN		Antagonized with 250 µg/kg atipamezole
Reptiles								
Alfaxalone	Knotek et al,[23] 2013	Iguana	PD	13	5 mg/kg	IV		
Alfaxalone	Knotek,[22] 2014	Red-eared slider	PD	10	5 mg/kg	IV		

(continued on next page)

Table 1
(continued)

Drug	Key References	Species	Study Design	No. of Animals	Dose	Route of Administration	Adverse Effects	Comments
Amphibians								
Propofol	Knotek,[22] 2014	Tiger salamanders	Randomized/ crossover	11	25–35 mg/kg	ICe		
Propofol	Wojick et al,[33] 2010	Sonoran Desert toads	Randomized/ crossover	9	35 mg/kg	ICe		Only effective in 1 of 9 animals
Alfaxalone	Posner et al,[34] 2013	American bullfrogs	Randomized/ crossover	8	Up to 17.5 mg/kg	IM		Light sedation
Small mammal								
Detomidine	Phillips et al,[17] 2015	Ferret	PD	8	2–4 mg/m^2	Transmucosal		
Ketamine-medetomidine	Williams & Wyatt,[48] 2007	Rabbit	PD	40	25.0 mg/kg–0.5 mg/kg	IM or SC	Bradycardia, bradypnea, hypoxemia, apnea during recovery	Reversal with 1.0 mg/kg atipamezole
Alfaxalone	Grint et al,[49] 2008	Rabbit	PD	20	2 mg/kg, 3 mg/kg	IV	Apnea	
Fentanyl-fluanisone-midazolam-isoflurane	Benato et al,[50] 2013	Rabbit	PD	32	0.04 mg/kg–2.0 mg/kg–0.2 mg/kg–2.0%	IM, IM, IV, OT	Respiratory acidosis	

Abbreviations: ICe, intracoelomic; IM, intramuscular; IN, intranasal; OT, orotracheal; PD, pharmacodynamic; SC, subcutaneous.

induction time, heart rate, or blood pressure between the 3 drugs, though isoflurane did result in a slightly slower time to full recovery.[9] Although this lack of significant difference between inhalant drugs can justify the choice of isoflurane as a standard inhalant anesthetic for birds, there are other potential adverse effects that should be considered. Isoflurane anesthesia has been associated with second- and third-degree atrioventricular block in pigeons and bald eagles.[4,10] Multiple studies have documented hypotension with isoflurane anesthesia in pigeons, parrots, and vultures.[3,4,11] Isoflurane-associated hypotension can be treated with constant-rate infusions of dopamine or dobutamine. Dopamine produces significantly greater increases in blood pressure than dobutamine and is recommended to be administered at rates of 7 and 10 µg/kg/min to cause the greatest increases in arterial blood pressure.[11] In clinical cases, these treatments should be titrated to effect in conjunction with decreasing anesthetic depth or IV fluid support as appropriate. Later in this article, the authors describe the difficulties in measuring blood pressure under anesthesia in birds. With regard to fluid selection, no significant differences were found in electrolyte or acid base balance when using lactated Ringer solution or 0.9% sodium chloride at 20 mL/kg/h by intraosseous catheter during isoflurane anesthesia in pigeons.[12]

Concerns over pain from IM injection and the technical difficulty of IV injection in many nonmammalian species have prompted investigation of alternative routes of administration, including intranasal. Multiple studies have evaluated both alpha-2 agonists and benzodiazepines administered to small birds by the intranasal route. Reported dose ranges are very wide, and caution is advised when comparing results of different studies. When comparing xylazine (25 mg/kg), diazepam (13 mg/kg), and midazolam (13 mg/kg) administered intranasally to budgerigars, recumbency was achieved with diazepam and midazolam, but only mild sedation resulted from xylazine. However, the duration of sedation with xylazine was markedly longer (mean, 286 ± 28.8 minutes) compared with diazepam (165 ± 19.2 minutes) and midazolam (76 ± 8.9 minutes).[13] In pigeons, intranasal midazolam (5 mg/kg) and dexmedetomidine (80 mcg/kg) produced adequate sedation for positioning a bird in dorsal recumbency but also caused marked decreases in heart rate, respiratory rate, and body temperature.[14] In Amazon parrots, 2 mg/kg of intranasal midazolam provided adequate sedation within 3 minutes and lasted at least 15 minutes. The sedation was easily and rapidly reversible with 0.05 mg/kg of intranasal flumazenil.[15] Similar sedation was induced in zebra finches with 10 mg/kg of diazepam and antagonized with 0.3 mg/kg flumazenil.[16]

Small Mammal

As with birds, many exotic small mammal species require some degree of chemical restraint to avoid injury to the animal and undue stress from handling. Often sedation is useful and preferable to general anesthesia. Oral transmucosal detomidine, formulated and sold for equine use, has been evaluated in domestic ferrets. At a dose of 2 mg/m^2 applied topically to the oral mucosa, animals were sedated within 10 minutes and could be placed in dorsal recumbency for physical examination, nail trimming, and venipuncture. In approximately half of the study animals, venipuncture was successful with no additional anesthetic or sedation required; the remainder did require isoflurane for blood collection. Doubling the dose showed no significant improvement in sedation or success of venipuncture.[17]

As rabbits are commonly used laboratory animals, the effects of numerous anesthetics are well studied, though many of the doses and drugs that have been evaluated for research animals are not practical for clinical use in patients. Reliable, mild sedation was induced with the single agents buprenorphine (0.03 mg/kg), butorphanol

(0.3 mg/kg), and midazolam (2.0 mg/kg), administered IM, whereas deeper sedation was accomplished with combinations of midazolam with either buprenorphine or butorphanol. Full recovery was achieved in less than 3 hours in all cases. At the listed doses, these drug combinations did cause a decrease in respiratory rate but not a significant decrease in oxygenation or ventilation.[18]

The cardiovascular dose effect of isoflurane was determined in New Zealand white rabbits, and it was determined that isoflurane causes dose-dependent compromise of cardiovascular function, mainly by decreasing cardiac contractility and vasodilation. These effects were exacerbated by positive pressure mechanical ventilation.[2] In a separate study, the same group reported that balanced anesthesia with a constant rate infusion of fentanyl (IV) in combination with isoflurane, decreased heart rate but improved blood pressure and cardiac output in New Zealand white rabbits.[19] IV administration of fentanyl or lidocaine also resulted in a significant reduction of mean isoflurane MAC.[20,21] By interpreting these findings in concert, a clinician could use fentanyl or lidocaine (eg, as a continuous rate infusion) to decrease the isoflurane concentration needed for a surgical procedure and, as such, mitigate the negative effects of the inhalant anesthetic on cardiovascular function.

Reptile and Amphibian

Alfaxalone, a neurosteroid with no analgesic properties that was recently approved by the Food and Drug Administration, has been appealing to veterinarians treating reptile and amphibians because of the relative ease of IM administration and short duration of action. Currently, alfaxalone is only labeled for IV administration in the United States; however, it has been administered by the IM route in other countries. Neither propofol nor alfaxalone are appropriate sole agents for painful procedures, and additional analgesic drugs should be used. In green iguanas and red-eared slider turtles, alfaxalone administered IV at 5 mg/kg provided rapid induction (less than 1 minute) and full recovery in 15 minutes for iguanas and 30 minutes for sliders.[22–24]

A continued challenge for anesthetists is controlling the length of anesthetic recovery time for reptile patients. In many cases, reptiles exhibit prolonged recovery from gas anesthesia. Theories explaining this phenomenon include the presence of cardiopulmonary shunting, which can allow the animal to divert blood from the pulmonary circulation into systemic circulation and thereby delay expulsion of the inhalant anesthetic via ventilation. A series of recent articles have examined the effect of adrenergic agonists on the recovery from anesthesia. Epinephrine at 0.1 mg/kg IM was shown to significantly reduce the time from cessation of inhalant anesthesia to spontaneous ventilation and recovery in snapping turtles.[25] These findings may be relevant to other reptilian taxa and are currently being investigated. A second theory that could explain prolonged recovery from inhalation anesthesia relates to the use of oxygen as a carrier gas for the inhalant anesthetic. In most veterinary settings, inhalant gases are delivered in 100% oxygen. The ventilatory drive for many reptile species is thought to be hypoxemia, instead of hypercapnia, as in mammals. The logical conclusion is that when a high concentration of oxygen is administered, a reptile may become hyperoxemic and, thus, lose its drive to breathe. Multiple recent studies have attempted to quantify the effect that varying inspired oxygen fractions (FIO_2) have on the drive to breathe in anesthetized reptiles. In bearded dragons, no significant difference was found in the time to extubation and return to spontaneous respiration in subjects recovered on 21% oxygen (room air) compared with 100% oxygen.[26] These finding could have been affected by small sample size and the fact that the investigators provided intermittent manual ventilation. Similar findings have been documented in Dumeril monitor lizards, in which 100% and 21% FIO_2 did not significantly alter recovery times.[27] To the authors' knowledge, no study has demonstrated consistent improvement in recovery time with room air compared with 100% oxygen; therefore, 21% Fio_2 as a treatment cannot objectively be recommended. Further studies in other taxa, especially aquatic reptiles, are warranted.

Tricaine methanesulfonate (MS-222) as a bath is currently considered the anesthetic of choice for many amphibians, and studies evaluating other anesthetics often compare them with MS-222. Despite the wide use of MS-222 in anurans, objective evaluation of physiologic effects is limited.[28] In African clawed frogs *(Xenopus laevis)*, MS-222 at 1 g/L provided surgical anesthesia for 30 minutes and at 2 g/L for 60 minutes. Both concentrations caused pronounced respiratory depression but no decrease in heart rate or oxygen saturation and no histologic evidence of organ damage.[29]

In leopard frogs *(Rana pipiens)*, MS-222 at 1 g/L provided rapid and reliable surgical anesthesia, whereas clove oil (255 mg/L) and benzocaine cream, applied topically, provided immobilization without sufficient analgesia for surgery.[30] In the same study, a eutectic mixture of lidocaine and prilocaine (EMLA cream) resulted in death of 5 of 12 animals. When comparing the effects of MS-222, clove oil, and ketamine/diazepam on the stress response in cane toads *(Rhinella marina)*,[31] it was noted that clove oil resulted in a significantly greater elevation in serum corticosterone concentration compared with the other two protocols. Clove oil has also been associated with increased mortality in some species and is irritating to many anurans, resulting in gastric eversion or reflux.[32] When comparing clove oil (450 ppm) with injectable propofol (25 or 35 mg/kg intracoelomic) in tiger salamanders *(Ambystoma tigrinum)*, both drugs provided surgical anesthesia; however, clove oil had a faster onset of action and longer duration. When propofol (35 mg/kg intracoelomic) was compared with MS-222 (1 g/L as a bath) in Sonoran Desert toads *(Bufo alvarius)*, MS-222 produced surgical anesthesia in 9 of 9 toads, whereas propofol produced surgical anesthesia in only 1 of 9.[33] In a study of American bullfrogs, IM alfaxalone at 10.0, 12.0, 15.0, or 17.5 mg/kg produced immobilization in frogs but did not provide sufficient anesthesia to prevent response to noxious stimuli. In the same study, bath immersion of 2 g/L of alfaxalone for up to 30 minutes did not result in anesthesia.[34]

Inhalant anesthetics administered by chamber can also induce anesthesia in anurans. Isoflurane, sevoflurane, and desflurane all caused loss of righting reflex within 15 minutes in cane toads at (median and range) 1.4% (0.9–1.4), 1.75% (1.1–1.9), and 4.4% (4.3–5.5), respectively. Although induction times were similar, recovery time was almost twice as long with isoflurane or sevoflurane compared with desflurane.[35] Volatile anesthetics have also been evaluated in amphibians by other routes. A jelly formulation of sevoflurane was evaluated for use in cane toads. A solution made up of 3.5 mL sevoflurane with 3.0 mL aqueous lubricant jelly and 1.5 mL distilled water and 37.5 µL of the combination per gram body weight applied topically to the dorsum resulted in loss of righting reflex. Formulations using higher concentrations of sevoflurane failed to achieve a homogenous mixture, and the anesthetic separated from the gel.[36]

RECENT ADVANCES IN ANESTHETIC PHYSIOLOGY AND MONITORING
Temperature Monitoring

Traditional understanding indicates that most, if not all, reptiles and amphibians are ectothermic; their basic physiologic functions strictly depend on ambient temperature. These species have numerous physiologic and behavioral adaptations to allow changes in body temperature in relation to ambient temperature.[37] Recent studies have indicated that several reptilian species can maintain their core body temperature greater than the ambient temperature even in the absence of an external heat source. Some clinicians may forgo monitoring core body temperature under the erroneous assumption that the core temperature under anesthesia is simply the ambient temperature. However, although only a limited number of species were studied, results of a recent study suggest that assumptions of complete ectothermy in both anesthetized and awake animals is likely unfounded.[38]

Lung Volume and Body Position

In most nonmammalian species, the lack of a true diaphragm and pleural space limits the ability to generate negative intracavitary pressure to facilitate pulmonary expansion. Many species require active involvement of skeletal muscles during ventilation for pulmonary expansion. Body position can also play a major role in lung expansion, which can also affect ventilation and oxygenation and potentially affect interpretation of the lung fields on imaging studies. Three recent studies have examined the effect of body position in two species of birds and one species of chelonian.

In penguins (Spheniscus humboldti), body position had minimal effect on lung volume but had a large effect on air sac volume. This finding could be expected as most avian species have very little physiologic expansion of the lungs and the bellows action of the air sacs is what allows for bulk air movement during breathing. Awake penguins in sternal recumbency had the largest expansion of the air sacs. Anesthetized, dorsally recumbent penguins had the smallest air sac expansion and the highest lung density on computed tomography, indicating compression of pulmonary tissue and accumulation of blood or fluid in the dorsal part of the lungs. The authors, therefore, suggest that dorsal recumbency is not a physiologically appropriate positon and may result in poor pulmonary function and gas exchange under anesthesia.[39]

These findings are similar to a previous study in red-tailed hawks, which determined that sternal recumbency was also the preferred position for highest air sac expansion and lowest lung density.[1] But a follow-up study in the same species revealed that respiratory rate was greater in right lateral recumbency and tidal volume was greater in dorsal recumbency.[40] The net result was no difference in minute ventilation between the two positions. This finding suggests that there is minimal true physiologic difference between right lateral and dorsal recumbency under anesthesia, but that study did not compare either of these positions with sternal recumbency. Although neither species is a companion pet, these findings are important to note as they may have implications for companion birds.

In red-eared slider turtles (Trachemys scripta elegans), gravity-dependent changes in lung volume were documented when animals were placed vertically, in right and left lateral recumbencies, as well as a head-up-tail-down vertical position. Additional differences were found between a sternal recumbent position with and without limbs and head extended. This information indicates that the optimal position for lung expansion in this species is sternal recumbency with the limbs extended. Although this study was not examining the effects of general anesthesia or positive pressure ventilation on lung volume, it is critical to note that large changes in lung volume are documented with different body positions. For this reason, care should be made when positioning an anesthetized chelonian, which will not have control over its limbs and, thus, cannot contribute to active ventilation, compounding the detrimental effects of poor positioning.[41]

Tracheal Intubation in Birds

Tracheal strictures after intubation have been anecdotally reported in avian species. The prevailing thought is that an inflated endotracheal tube cuff or a large tube diameter may place excessive pressure on the tracheal mucosa. This pressure may result in mucosal necrosis due to the complete tracheal rings and the noncompliant trachea of birds. Tracheal strictures can necessitate resection and anastomosis and can result in death. Sykes and colleagues[42] investigated risk factors for tracheal stricture in two zoo collections. Tracheal obstruction was noted in 1.8% of intubated birds in the study and carried a 70% mortality rate. Interestingly, a wide range of species was affected but no raptors or parrots, despite their relatively high numbers in the study population.

Blood Pressure

In domestic animals and human patients, noninvasively measured arterial blood pressure is the standard practice for indirect assessment of adequacy of cardiac output and tissue perfusion. The gold standard for measuring blood pressure, via direct arterial catheterization, is less commonly used. There are intrinsic limitations when devices designed and validated for humans or domestic mammals are applied to nonmammalian species. Two studies in avian species showed poor correlation between direct systolic arterial blood pressure measurements and indirect measurements with either Doppler or oscillometric devices. In red-tailed hawks, oscillometric measurements were unreliable and Doppler measurements were closer approximations of mean arterial blood pressure measurements versus systolic blood pressure.[43] In a similar study with Hispaniolan Amazon parrots, there was significant disagreement between direct systolic arterial blood pressure and Doppler measurements; attempts to obtain oscillometric blood pressure measurements were unsuccessful.[44] In fact, an additional study in multiple parrot species brings into questions whether it is possible to obtain repeated indirect measurements of blood pressure with Doppler in the same animal. In that study, blood pressure measurements varied significantly between cuff placements on the same limb from the same bird. The overall precision of Doppler blood pressure measurements was poor. Therefore, the use of Doppler measurements to monitor trends in blood pressure in an individual bird is likely dubious clinical practice.[45]

Similar findings have also been reported in boid snakes[46] and green iguanas.[47] In iguanas, an oscillometric device failed to provide a blood pressure reading for most attempts and correlated poorly with directly measured values. When used on the tail of anesthetized boid snakes, the same device more frequently provided a reading but consistently overestimated systolic blood pressure while underestimating diastolic and mean.

SUMMARY

Clinical anesthesia of nondomestic companion animals continues to develop as a field with increasing research activity to improve the evidence base. Many comprehensive sources provide anecdotal dosages and techniques from years of clinical experience and serve as a valuable starting point for future study. Continued pharmacokinetic and pharmacodynamic evaluation of anesthetic protocols will bring the standard of practice in exotic companion animal anesthesia to the level of domestic animals. Integral to advancing anesthetic care in these species is the objective evaluation and refinement of monitoring techniques.

REFERENCES

1. Malka S, Hawkins MG, Jones JH, et al. Effect of body position on respiratory system volumes in anesthetized red-tailed hawks (*Buteo jamaicensis*) as measured via computed tomography. Am J Vet Res 2009;70(9):1155–60.

2. Barter LS, Epstein SE. Cardiopulmonary effects of three concentrations of isoflurane with or without mechanical ventilation and supramaximal noxious stimulation in New Zealand white rabbits. Am J Vet Res 2013;74(10):1274–80.

3. Seok SH, Jeong DH, Hong IH, et al. Cardiorespiratory dose-response relationship of isoflurane in cinereous vulture (*Aegypius monachus*) during spontaneous ventilation. J Vet Med Sci 2016;79(1):160–5.

4. Botman J, Dugdale A, Gabriel F, et al. Cardiorespiratory parameters in the awake pigeon and during anaesthesia with isoflurane. Vet Anaesth Analg 2016;43(1): 63–71.

5. Mercado JA, Larsen RS, Wack RF, et al. Minimum anesthetic concentration of isoflurane in captive thick-billed parrots (*Rhynchopsitta pachyrhyncha*). Am J Vet Res 2008;69(2):189–94.

6. Phair KA, Larsen RS, Wack RF, et al. Determination of the minimum anesthetic concentration of sevoflurane in thick-billed parrots (*Rhynchopsitta pachyrhyncha*). Am J Vet Res 2012;73(9):1350–5.

7. Escobar A, da Rocha RW, Pypendop BH, et al. Effects of methadone on the minimum anesthetic concentration of isoflurane, and its effects on heart rate, blood pressure and ventilation during isoflurane anesthesia in hens (*Gallus gallus domesticus*). PLoS One 2016;11(3):e0152546.

8. Escobar A, Valadão CAA, Brosnan RJ, et al. Effects of butorphanol on the minimum anesthetic concentration for sevoflurane in guineafowl (*Numida meleagris*). Am J Vet Res 2012;73(2):183–8.

9. Granone TD, de Francisco ON, Killos MB, et al. Comparison of three different inhalant anesthetic agents (isoflurane, sevoflurane, desflurane) in red-tailed hawks (*Buteo jamaicensis*). Vet Anaesth Analg 2012;39(1):29–37.

10. Joyner PH, Jones MP, Ward D, et al. Induction and recovery characteristics and cardiopulmonary effects of sevoflurane and isoflurane in bald eagles. Am J Vet Res 2008;69(1):13–22.

11. Schnellbacher RW, da Cunha AF, Beaufrère H, et al. Effects of dopamine and dobutamine on isoflurane-induced hypotension in Hispaniolan Amazon parrots (*Amazona ventralis*). Am J Vet Res 2012;73(7):952–8.

12. Carregaro AB, Gehrcke MI, Marques JS, et al. Lactated Ringer's solution or 0.9% sodium chloride as fluid therapy in pigeons (*Columba livia*) submitted to humerus osteosynthesis. Pesqui Veterinária Bras 2015;35(1):95–8.

13. Sadegh AB. Comparison of intranasal administration of xylazine, diazepam, and midazolam in budgerigars (*Melopsittacus undulatus*): clinical evaluation. J Zoo Wildl Med 2013;44(2):241–4.

14. Hornak S, Liptak T, Ledecky V, et al. A preliminary trial of the sedation induced by intranasal administration of midazolam alone or in combination with dexmedetomidine and reversal by atipamezole for a short-term immobilization in pigeons. Vet Anaesth Analg 2015;42(2):192–6.

15. Mans C, Guzman DS-M, Lahner LL, et al. Sedation and physiologic response to manual restraint after intranasal administration of midazolam in Hispaniolan Amazon parrots (*Amazona ventralis*). J Avian Med Surg 2012;26(3):130–9.

16. Prather JF. Rapid and reliable sedation induced by diazepam and antagonized by flumazenil in zebra finches (*Taeniopygia guttata*). J Avian Med Surg 2012; 26(2):76–84.

17. Phillips BE, Harms CA, Messenger KM. Oral transmucosal detomidine gel for the sedation of the domestic ferret (*Mustela putorius furo*). J Exot Pet Med 2015; 24(4):446–54.

18. Schroeder CA, Smith LJ. Respiratory rates and arterial blood-gas tensions in healthy rabbits given buprenorphine, butorphanol, midazolam, or their combinations. J Am Assoc Lab Anim Sci 2011;50(2):205–11.
19. Tearney CC, Barter LS, Pypendop BH. Cardiovascular effects of equipotent doses of isoflurane alone and isoflurane plus fentanyl in New Zealand white rabbits (*Oryctolagus cuniculus*). Am J Vet Res 2015;76(7):591–8.
20. Schnellbacher RW, Carpenter JW, Mason DE, et al. Effects of lidocaine administration via continuous rate infusion on the minimum alveolar concentration of isoflurane in New Zealand white rabbits (*Oryctolagus cuniculus*). Am J Vet Res 2013;74(11):1377–84.
21. Barter LS, Hawkins MG, Pypendop BH. Effects of fentanyl on isoflurane minimum alveolar concentration in New Zealand white rabbits (*Oryctolagus cuniculus*). Am J Vet Res 2015;76(2):111–5.
22. Knotek Z. Alfaxalone as an induction agent for anaesthesia in terrapins and tortoises. Vet Rec 2014;175(13):327.
23. Knotek Z, Hrdá A, Knotková Z, et al. Alfaxalone anaesthesia in the green iguana (*Iguana iguana*). Acta Vet Brno 2013;82(1):109–14.
24. Shepard MK, Divers S, Braun C, et al. Pharmacodynamics of alfaxalone after single-dose intramuscular administration in red-eared sliders (*Trachemys scripta elegans*): a comparison of two different doses at two different ambient temperatures. Vet Anaesth Analg 2013;40(6):590–8.
25. Goe A, Shmalberg J, Gatson B, et al. Epinephrine or GV-26 electrical stimulation reduces inhalant anesthestic recovery time in common snapping turtles (*Chelydra serpentina*). J Zoo Wildl Med 2016;47(2):501–7.
26. O O, Churgin SM, Sladky KK, et al. Anesthetic induction and recovery parameters in bearded dragons (*Pogona vitticeps*): comparison of isoflurane delivered in 100% oxygen versus 21% oxygen. J Zoo Wildl Med 2015;46(3):534–9.
27. Bertelsen MF, Mosley C, Crawshaw GJ, et al. Inhalation anesthesia in Dumeril's monitor (*Varanus dumerili*) with isoflurane, sevoflurane, and nitrous oxide: effects of inspired gases on induction and recovery. J Zoo Wildl Med 2005;36(1):62–8.
28. Chinnadurai SK, Kane LP. Advances in amphibian clinical therapeutics. J Exot Pet Med 2014;23(1):50–5.
29. Lalonde-Robert V, Beaudry F, Vachon P. Pharmacologic parameters of MS-222 and physiologic changes in frogs (*Xenopus laevis*) after immersion at anesthetic doses. J Am Assoc Lab Anim Sci 2012;51(4):464–8.
30. Guenette SA, Lair S. Anesthesia of the leopard frog, *Rana pipiens*: a comparative study between four different agents. J Herp Med Surg 2006;16:38–44.
31. Hernández SE, Sernia C, Bradley AJ. The effect of three anaesthetic protocols on the stress response in cane toads (*Rhinella marina*). Vet Anaesth Analg 2012;39(6):584–90.
32. Mitchell MA, Riggs SM, Singleton CB, et al. Evaluating the clinical and cardiopulmonary effects of clove oil and propofol in tiger salamanders (*Ambystoma tigrinum*). J Exot Pet Med 2009;18(1):50–6.
33. Wojick KB, Langan JN, Mitchell MA. Evaluation of MS-222 (tricaine methanesulfonate) and propofol as anesthetic agents in Sonoran desert toads (*Bufo alvarius*). J Herpetol Med Surg 2010;20(2–3):79–83.
34. Posner LP, Bailey KM, Richardson EY, et al. Alfaxalone anesthesia in bullfrogs (*Lithobates catesbeiana*) by injection or immersion. J Zoo Wildl Med 2013;44(4):965–71.
35. Morrison KE, Strahl-Heldreth D, Clark-Price SC. Isoflurane, sevoflurane and desflurane use in cane toads (*Rhinella marina*). Vet Rec Open 2016;3(1):e00018.

36. Stone SM, Clark-Price SC, Boesch JM, et al. Evaluation of righting reflex in cane toads (Bufo marinus) after topical application of sevoflurane jelly. Am J Vet Res 2013;74(6):823-7.
37. Seebacher F, Franklin CE. Physiological mechanisms of thermoregulation in reptiles: a review. J Comp Physiol B 2005;175(8):533-41.
38. Raske M, Lewbart GA, Dombrowski D, et al. Body temperatures of selected amphibian and reptile species. J Zoo Wildl Med 2012;43(3):517-21.
39. Nevitt BN, Langan JN, Adkesson MJ, et al. Comparison of air sac volume, lung volume, and lung densities determined by use of computed tomography in conscious and anesthetized Humboldt penguins (Spheniscus humboldti) positioned in ventral, dorsal, and right lateral recumbency. Am J Vet Res 2014; 75(8):739-45.
40. Hawkins MG, Malka S, Pascoe PJ, et al. Evaluation of the effects of dorsal versus lateral recumbency on the cardiopulmonary system during anesthesia with isoflurane in red-tailed hawks (Buteo jamaicensis). Am J Vet Res 2013;74(1):136-43.
41. Mans C, Drees R, Sladky KK, et al. Effects of body position and extension of the neck and extremities on lung volume measured via computed tomography in red-eared slider turtles (Trachemys scripta elegans). J Am Vet Med Assoc 2013; 243(8):1190-6.
42. Sykes JM IV, Neiffer D, Terrell S, et al. Review of 23 cases of postintubation tracheal obstructions in birds. J Zoo Wildl Med 2013;44(3):700-13.
43. Zehnder AM, Hawkins MG, Pascoe PJ, et al. Evaluation of indirect blood pressure monitoring in awake and anesthetized red-tailed hawks (Buteo jamaicensis): effects of cuff size, cuff placement, and monitoring equipment. Vet Anaesth Analg 2009;36(5):464-79.
44. Acierno MJ, da Cunha A, Smith J, et al. Agreement between direct and indirect blood pressure measurements obtained from anesthetized Hispaniolan Amazon parrots. J Am Vet Med Assoc 2008;233(10):1587-90.
45. Johnston MS, Davidowski LA, Rao S, et al. Precision of repeated, Doppler-derived indirect blood pressure measurements in conscious psittacine birds. J Avian Med Surg 2011;25(2):83-90.
46. Chinnadurai SK, Wrenn A, DeVoe RS. Evaluation of noninvasive oscillometric blood pressure monitoring in anesthetized boid snakes. J Am Vet Med Assoc 2009;234(5):625-30.
47. Chinnadurai SK, DeVoe R, Koenig A, et al. Comparison of an implantable telemetry device and an oscillometric monitor for measurement of blood pressure in anaesthetized and unrestrained green iguanas (Iguana iguana). Vet Anaesth Analg 2010;37(5):434-9.
48. Williams AM, Wyatt JD. Comparison of subcutaneous and intramuscular ketamine – medetomidine with and without reversal by atipamezole in Dutch belted rabbits (Oryctolagus cuniculus). J Am Assoc Lab Anim Sci 2007;46(6):16-20.
49. Grint NJ, Smith HE, Senior JM. Clinical evaluation of alfaxalone in cyclodextrin for the induction of anesthesia in rabbits. Vet Rec 2008;163(13):395-6.
50. Benato L, Chesnerl M, Eatwell K, et al. Arterial blood gas parameters in pet rabbits anaesthetized using a combination of fentanyl–fluanisone–midazolam–isoflurane. J Small Anim Pract 2013;54(7):343-6.

Information Resources for the Exotic Animal Practitioner

Laura L. Pavlech, DVM, MSLS

KEYWORDS

- Animals • Databases as topic • Databases, bibliographic
- Evidence-based medicine • Information storage and retrieval/methods • Research
- Veterinarians • Veterinary medicine

KEY POINTS

- When deciding where to search, consider what resources are accessible and where, or by whom, information about the topic and species of interest is likely to be published.
- The evidence pyramid provides a framework for selecting evidence-based information resources. If available, consult resources at the top of the pyramid first.
- Information relevant to exotic animals is published in a variety of veterinary medical, human medical, zoologic, and wildlife journals, which may not be indexed by easily accessible databases.
- A structured approach to searching a database enhances the efficiency and effectiveness of the search.
- All studies should be evaluated for validity and applicability of the results to patient care.

INTRODUCTION
What Sources Do Veterinarians Use to Find Information?

The increasing number of electronic resources available to veterinarians, along with widespread Internet access, means that, theoretically, answers to clinical questions are no more than a few clicks away. Surveys have shown that veterinarians use a variety of resources to find answers to the questions that arise in the course of daily practice. A survey conducted in 2000 found that veterinarians in the United Kingdom (UK) preferred to obtain diagnostic, therapeutic, and drug information from journal articles, textbooks, and conferences.[1] Databases and web sites ranked low on the list of preferred information sources. A decade later, when UK veterinarians were asked to choose which electronic resources they accessed for information from a predefined

Disclosure: The author has nothing to disclose.
Department of Research and Instruction, Hirsh Health Sciences Library, Tufts University, 145 Harrison Avenue, Boston, MA 02111, USA
E-mail address: laura.pavlech@tufts.edu

Vet Clin Exot Anim 20 (2017) 929–946
http://dx.doi.org/10.1016/j.cvex.2017.05.001
1094-9194/17/© 2017 Elsevier Inc. All rights reserved.

list, Google was the most accessed resource, with 71% of respondents reporting that they used this search engine.[2] Google was also considered the most useful electronic resource, followed by PubMed and Veterinary Information Network (VIN). Nonclinical veterinarians considered PubMed more useful than clinical veterinarians did. In survey of veterinarians practicing outside of the UK, VIN, International Veterinary Information Source, and PubMed were the most accessed and most useful electronic resources.[3] Similar to the survey of UK veterinarians, nonclinical veterinarians accessed PubMed more frequently than clinical veterinarians. In a 2014 roundtable discussion, 8 exotic animal veterinarians in academic and private practice reported using electronic databases (BIOSIS Previews, CAB Abstracts, Scopus and Web of Science), search engines (Google Scholar), VIN, and the web sites of professional organizations when investigating a topic.[4]

The survey of UK veterinarians reported that, when confronted with a difficult case, clinicians preferred to ask a colleague, consult a textbook, or contact a specialist. Less than 5% selected 'general Internet search' as their first source for information on a difficult case. In a survey of Belgian veterinarians, 64% of respondents contacted a colleague when confronted with an unusual case, 85% contacted a specialist, 86% consulted a laboratory, and 68% used the Internet.[5] Only 2.5% reported using PubMed, perhaps due to a language barrier. Collectively, these surveys suggest that clinicians prefer to receive information passively, in a summarized form, from a colleague, specialist, or textbook.[2]

Do Veterinarians Feel There Is Information Available on Exotic Animals?

Although there are no formal surveys that focus exclusively on the information sources of exotic animal practitioners, the study of UK veterinarians did include clinicians who had exotic animal patients. The survey asked clinicians to list the 4 species they saw most frequently, the 3 most common presenting conditions for each of those species, and the amount of information they perceived to be available for each condition (none, a little, some, a lot, don't know).[6] Among veterinarians who performed clinical work, rabbits were the third most commonly seen species, after dogs and cats, and guinea pigs were the sixth most commonly seen species. Although clinicians felt there was a lot of information available on the most common presenting complaints in dogs, cats, horses, and cattle, they indicated that a lot of information was available for only 18% of common conditions in rabbits and 5% of common conditions in guinea pigs. The authors of this study hypothesized that the perceived low amount of information available on rabbits and guinea pigs was due to an actual dearth of published information about these species, difficulty finding or accessing information, or a combination of these factors.

EVIDENCE-BASED INFORMATION RESOURCES
What Are Evidence-Based Information Resources?

Evidence-based information resources provide "processed information on [the] best available research evidence which are critically appraised, integrated, concisely summarized, and regularly updated as new research evidence becomes available."[7] In human medicine, evidence-based information resources have proliferated, facilitating evidence-based practice (EBP) for doctors, nurses, and other human health care professionals. Veterinary medicine lags behind human medicine in the availability of evidence-based resources.

The evidence pyramid provides a model for evaluating information resources (**Fig. 1**).[8,9] Although there are many variations of this model, the relative rank of the major study designs within the pyramid remains reasonably consistent.[8] As one moves

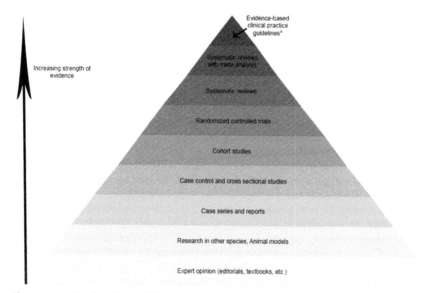

Increasing strength of evidence

Evidence-based clinical practice guidelines[a]

Systematic reviews with meta-analysis

Systematic reviews

Randomized controlled trials

Cohort studies

Case control and cross sectional studies

Case series and reports

Research in other species, Animal models

Expert opinion (editorials, textbooks, etc.)

Fig. 1. Pyramid of evidence. [a] See text for definition of clinical practice guidelines. (*Adapted from* Sargeant JM, Kelton DF, O'Connor AM. Study designs and systematic reviews of interventions: building evidence across study designs. Zoonoses Public Health 2014;61 Suppl 1:14; and Vandeweerd JM, Clegg P, Buczinski S. How can veterinarians base their medical decisions on the best available scientific evidence? Vet Clin North Am Food Anim Pract 2012;28(1):4; with permission.)

from the bottom of the pyramid to the top, the level of evidence that a study provides increases. If properly designed and executed, studies at the top of the pyramid have less risk of bias and greater relevance to clinical practice.[10] The resources that veterinarians report using to answer clinical questions, namely, colleagues and textbooks, provide lower levels of evidence because they rely on personal experience and/or are not designed to answer specific clinical questions. Personal experience is inherently subjective; Holmes and Ramey[11] noted that "good clinicians routinely overestimate the value of their experience" and have a tendency to recall cases that went either extraordinarily well or poorly. A recent viewpoint in *Veterinary Record*, proclaimed, "Undocumented anecdote derived from the fallible recollections of great men is no longer considered a sufficient basis for valid clinical opinion."[12] Experience is an essential component of EBP,[13] but relying solely on experience can perpetuate incorrect practices, leading to dogma.[14] In addition to the risk of personal bias, textbooks (and review articles) may be out of date by the time they are published.[15] Therefore, a search for an answer to a clinical question should begin at the top of the evidence pyramid, and progress down if no resources are available in a higher category.

What Are the Barriers to Finding and Using Evidence-Based Information Resources?

The principal barrier to finding and using evidence-based information resources in veterinary medicine in general, and exotic animal medicine in particular, is the paucity of studies that provide high levels of evidence, and preappraised resources that synthesize those studies. The deficiency of systematic reviews, meta-analyses, and randomized controlled trials in veterinary medicine can be attributed to difficulty enrolling high numbers of patients, lack of validated outcome measures, insufficient funding, and few veterinarians trained as clinical researchers.[12,16–18] These problems are even more pronounced in exotic animal medicine. The second, often insurmountable, barrier that veterinarians encounter in their quest for evidence-based information is access to electronic resources. The database that provides the best coverage of the veterinary literature, CAB Abstracts,[19] is only accessible through an institutional subscription. If a veterinarian does find a relevant article, then the electronic full text is often either not freely available or not available at all, because the archives of many veterinary journals have not been digitized. For example, electronic issues of the *Journal of the American Veterinary Medical Association* are available only back to 2000. A 2013 survey of UK veterinarians found that although a majority of respondents had access to the Internet both at home and at work (89% and 83%, respectively), far fewer had regular access to either electronic journals (32%) or a professional library (19%).[20] Access to the Internet, personal and professional libraries, and electronic journals was significantly higher for veterinarians who worked in zoos/wildlife/exotics, universities, or industry than for those who worked in first-opinion practice, referral/consultancy, or for the government. Presumably, veterinarians who practice in the United States experience the same problems with access to electronic resources as their British colleagues, with those in private practice faring the worse. As of 2015, approximately 60% of the veterinary positions held in the United States were in private clinical practice.[21] In recent years, the increasing number of veterinary open access journals and journals that publish open access articles has alleviated, but certainly not eliminated, the problem of access to electronic full text. The authors of a 2011 editorial in the *Journal of Veterinary Medical Education* stated, "In the face of the enormous volume of digital information and its prolific growth, access still remains the largest problem."[22] Insufficient high-quality studies, lack of evidence-based resources that provide preappraised information, and limited access to electronic resources have hindered veterinarians' ability to fully engage in EBP.

CHOOSING AN EVIDENCE-BASED INFORMATION RESOURCE

Given these barriers, it can seem impossible to find evidence-based information on exotic animal species. The remainder of this article is devoted to strategies for overcoming those barriers. When selecting a resource to answer a clinical question, consider the following questions: What resources do you have access to? Where, or by whom, is information about your question likely to be published?

What Resources Do You Have Access to?

Your search will obviously be restricted to those resources to which you have access. Unless you are associated with an academic institution or have a personal or practice subscription to a resource, then you are limited to those that are available at no cost. This limitation may be particularly frustrating for exotic animal practitioners because information about the species you treat is unlikely to be available only in free resources. Some veterinary medical libraries offer services, such as searching and electronic delivery of articles, for alumni and/or local practitioners. However, the time delay for such services makes them impractical in emergent situations.

Where, or by Whom, Is Information About Your Question Likely to Be Published?

Consider the species that you are treating and the condition in which you are interested. A question about parasites in koi may prompt a search of both the veterinary and fisheries literature. A question about mice may necessitate a search of both human and veterinary medical literature. For questions about zoonotic disease, look at animal and human health organizations and regulatory agencies, such as the World

Organisation for Animal Health, Centers for Disease Control and Prevention, or World Health Organization.

With the answers to these questions in mind, try to find a resource at the top of the evidence pyramid, such as a clinical practice guideline, systematic review or meta-analysis (**Table 1**). These resources synthesize and summarize studies from the lower levels of the pyramid, and may provide recommendations on the management of a specific clinical condition.[23,24] Clinical practice guidelines, according to the Institute of Medicine, are "statements that include recommendations intended to optimize patient care that are informed by a systematic review of evidence and an assessment of the benefits and harms of alternative care options."[25] Several professional veterinary organizations generate guidelines on the care of animals. Although these guidelines do not always meet the rigorous definition of clinical practice guidelines set forth by the Institute of Medicine, they do provide standards of care. Critically appraised topics are brief summaries of the best available evidence on a particular clinical topic. Critically appraised topics have been used in veterinary education to teach students

Table 1
Summary and synthesis resources in veterinary medicine

Resource	Description	Access
Clinical practice guidelines	Evidence-based recommendations on patient care	Published in journals and/or available on web sites of professional organizations (may require membership)
Vetlexicon	Online, peer-reviewed, point-of-care resource Evidence-based summaries of diseases, diagnostic and surgical techniques, and drugs, with links to primary literature in PubMed and VetMed Resource Separate 'services' for dogs (Canis), cats (Felis), rabbits (Lapis), horses (Equis) and cattle (Bovis, forthcoming)	Individual, practice, association, or institutional subscriptions https://www.vetstream.com/
VetCompanion	Evidence-based, point-of-care resource for canine and feline conditions Exotic animal species may be added in the future	Individual or practice subscriptions http://vetcompanion.com/
BestBETs for Vets	Collection of critically appraised topics (Best Evidence Topics, or BETs) Exotic animals do not have their own category, but there is a BET for rabbits	Free https://bestbetsforvets.org/
Veterinary Evidence	Open access journal that publishes knowledge summaries, systematic reviews, commentaries and research articles	Free https://www.veterinaryevidence.org
VetsRev	Citation and abstract database of systematic reviews, meta-analyses and critically appraised topics relevant to veterinary medicine, veterinary science, animal health, animal reproduction and animal nutrition	Free Links out to full text, which may require subscription or purchase of single article http://webapps.nottingham.ac.uk/refbase/

the principles of EBP.[26–28] There are a few online resources that aggregate critically appraised topics and systematic reviews, eliminating the need to search multiple databases. Unfortunately, these resources do not typically cover exotic animals because there are no existing studies to synthesize and summarize. Nevertheless, practitioners should be aware of these resources, because the information they offer about common domestic animals may be relevant to exotic animals and they may (eventually) include information about exotic animals.

BIBLIOGRAPHIC DATABASES

If a clinical summary, systematic review or meta-analysis cannot be found in one of the resources listed in **Table 1**, then searching a bibliographic database is the most efficient way to find published research articles. Bibliographic databases (henceforth, databases) are organized collections of references to published literature, typically journals articles, conference proceedings, books, and book chapters. Databases differ from one another in the subjects, dates, and types of material they cover. Veterinary literature, and exotic animal literature in particular, can be difficult to find because relevant articles may be published in journals from a variety of disciplines, including human and veterinary medicine, zoology and wildlife management, which are indexed by different databases (**Table 2**). A 2012 study of 9 databases found that none of the databases indexed all of the titles on core and extended lists of veterinary journals.[19] CAB Abstracts, a database from the Centre for Agriculture and Biosciences International, provided the best overall coverage of the veterinary literature, indexing 95% of the journals on the core list and 90.2% of the journals on the extended list. MEDLINE, the database that provides the content in PubMed, indexed 82.6% of the core journals and 36.5% of the journals on the extended list. The authors of this study concluded, "MEDLINE, PubMed, or Embase . . . cannot be relied upon to give comprehensive coverage of the veterinary literature on their own."[19] Another investigation found that CAB Abstracts provided the best coverage of a selected set of avian journals, indexing all journals in the set.[29] Even when 2 databases include the same journals, they may cover different years of those journals, have different ways of indexing, and distinct search options. Paul-Murphy[29] showed that when different databases indexed the same journals, the number of avian articles retrieved from each journal differed depending on which database was searched. The multidisciplinary nature of veterinary medicine, and variability in what and how journals are indexed by each database, means that a search for evidence, and certainly for any type of thorough review (narrative review, scoping review, systematic review), should include more than 1 database.[19,30] **Tables 3** and **4** list core and other bibliographic databases for exotic animal literature.

The approach to searching a database for evidence is the same, regardless of which database you choose to search. The structured approach described herein may seem laborious, and it need not be executed in full for every question that arises in the course of daily practice. However, once it becomes routine, this approach will hopefully make searching more effective and efficient. The structured approach can be distilled into 5 steps (**Box 1**).

Step 1: Develop a Focused Clinical Question

This is the first step (Ask) in EBP. Incorporate the 4 PICO elements, where P stands for patient, population or problem, I for intervention, C for comparison, and O for outcome. Once you have the 4 elements, generate a question that starts with 'In patients with…'. The clinical question will help you formulate a search strategy and determine the relevance of search results.

Table 2
Inclusion of select journals relevant to exotic animal medicine in 7 bibliographic databases

Journal	BIOSIS Previews	CAB Abstracts	PubMed	Scopus	VetMed Resource	Web of Science Core Collection	Zoologic Record
American Journal of Veterinary Research	X	X	X	X	X	X	—
Avian Diseases	X	X	X	X	X	X	X
Avian Pathology	X	X	X	X	X	X	X
Comparative Medicine	X	X	X	X	X	X	—
Journal of the American Association for Laboratory Animal Science	X	X	X	X	X	X	X
Journal of the American Veterinary Medical Association	X	X	X	X	X	X	X
Journal of Aquatic Animal Health	X	X	X	X	X	X	X
Journal of Avian Medicine and Surgery	—	X	X	X	X	X	X
Journal of Comparative Pathology	X	X	X	X	X	X	—
Journal of Exotic Pet Medicine	—	X	—	—	X	X	X
Journal of Fish Diseases	X	X	X	X	X	X	X
Journal of Herpetological Medicine and Surgery	—	X	—	—	X	—	X
Journal of Herpetology	X	X	—	X	X	X	X
Journal of Small Animal Practice	X	X	X	X	—	X	—
Journal of Wildlife Diseases	X	X	X	X	X	X	X
Journal of Zoo and Aquarium Research	—	X	—	—	X	—	—
Journal of Zoo and Wildlife Medicine	X	X	X	X	X	X	X
Veterinary Clinics of North America - Exotic Animal Practice	—	X	X	X	X	—	X
Veterinary Record	—	X	X	X	X	X	—
Veterinary Record Open	—	X	—	—	X	—	—
BMC Veterinary Research	—	X	X	X	X	X	X
Zoo Biology	X	X	X	X	X	X	X

Table 3
Core bibliographic databases for veterinary medicine

Database	Subjects/Dates Covered	Type of Material	Controlled Vocabulary	Features	Access
BIOSIS Previews	Life sciences from agriculture to zoology, including animal studies 1926–present	Journal articles Meeting abstracts Book chapters	No	Taxa Notes Veterinary medicine filter Citing and cited articles View related records	Institutional subscription only
CAB Abstracts	Applied life sciences, including veterinary and animal science Best coverage of the veterinary literature 1973–present	Journal articles Conference proceedings Book chapters Reports	CAB Thesaurus		Institutional subscription only
PrimateLit	Nonhuman primates 1940–present	Journal articles Conference proceedings Book chapters Technical reports Theses	No	Taxonomic search genus, species or subspecies	Free
PubMed	Biomedical literature 1946–present	Journal articles	Medical Subject Headings (MeSH)	Veterinary science filter Find similar articles	Free

	Description	Content types	Thesaurus	Features	Access
Scopus	Sciences, social sciences, and arts and humanities Good international coverage 1970–present (some to 1823)	Journal articles Conference proceedings Book chapters Trade publications	No	Citing and cited articles Related documents	Institutional subscription only
VetMed Resource	Veterinary medicine references from CAB abstracts Commissioned reviews, news, and datasheets 1972–present	Journal articles Conference proceedings Book chapters CAB reviews Datasheets	CAB Thesaurus	Preformulated searches for exotic animal topics, for example, 'Koi herpesvirus' Topic page for 'Exotics, zoo and wild animal' Some full text	Individual, practice and institutional subscriptions
Web of Science Core Collection	Sciences, social sciences, arts and humanities Good historical coverage 1900–present	Journal articles Conference proceedings Book chapters	No	Veterinary sciences filter Citing and cited articles View related records	Institutional subscription only
Zoologic Record	Animal biology, including veterinary science Taxonomic reference 1864–present	Journal articles Conference proceedings Book chapters Reports	Zoologic Record Thesaurus	Organism and taxa notes filters Citing and cited articles View related records	Institutional subscription only

Table 4
Other bibliographic databases for veterinary medicine

Database	Subjects/Dates Covered	Type of Material	Controlled Vocabulary	Features	Access
Aquatic Sciences and Fisheries Abstracts	Marine and freshwater environments, including fisheries and aquatic organisms 1971–present	Journal articles Conference proceedings Book chapters Reports	Aquatic Sciences and Fisheries Abstracts Thesaurus Taxonomic terms	Some full text	Institutional subscription only
Biological and Agricultural Index Plus	Biological and agricultural studies, including veterinary medicine 1982–present	Journal articles Conference proceedings Trade publications Magazine articles	Biological and Agricultural Index Plus Thesaurus	Some full text	Institutional subscription only
Embase	Biomedical literature Includes MEDLINE content Good coverage of pharmaceutical, medical device and international literature 1988–present (Embase Classic, back to 1947)	Journal articles Conference proceedings	Emtree		Individual and institutional subscriptions
Fish, Fisheries and Aquatic Biodiversity Worldwide	All aspects of fish and aquatic biology, including marine mammals Good international coverage 1970s–present	Journal articles Conference proceedings Book chapters Reports Theses	No	Links to FishBase, a global biodiversity information system that provides species profiles (FishBase is freely available)	Institutional subscription only
PubAg	Agricultural research 1990s–present	Journal articles Reports	National Agricultural Library Thesaurus Medical Subject Headings (MeSH)	Some full text	Free
Wildlife and Ecology Studies Worldwide	Wild mammals, birds, reptiles and amphibians 1935–present	Journal articles Conference proceedings Trade publications Magazine articles	No		Institutional subscription only

---

Box 1
Structured approach to searching a bibliographic database

- Step 1: Develop a focused clinical question.
- Step 2: Identify key concepts of question.
- Step 3: Generate a list of keywords and standardized terms to describe each concept.
- Step 4: Search each concept separately, then combine, using AND, OR, and NOT.
- Step 5: Apply filters to limit results.

Example:
    Patient/problem: ferrets with adrenal disease
    Intervention: gonadotropin-releasing hormone agonists
    Comparison: adrenalectomy
    Outcome: resolution of clinical signs
    Question: In ferrets with adrenal disease, do gonadotropin-releasing hormone agonists reduce clinical signs as effectively as adrenalectomy?

Step 2: Identify the Key Concepts of Your Question

If you have used the PICO framework to formulate your question, then you already have your key concepts. If not, then dissect your question into its essential parts. Each question should have at least 2 distinct concepts. These concepts will be used to create a structured search.

Step 3: Generate a List of Keywords and Standardized Terms to Describe Each Concept

Keywords are the natural language you would use to discuss your question with a colleague or client. When generating a list of keywords, include synonyms, abbreviations, acronyms, and alternate spellings (eg, hematuria and haematuria). Standardized terms are a set of predefined words and definitions used to describe the references in a database. These sets of terms are also called controlled vocabularies. Medical subject headings (MeSH), the controlled vocabulary for PubMed/MEDLINE, is perhaps the best-known biomedical vocabulary. Indexers at the National Library of Medicine read each article that is included in PubMed/MEDLINE and apply MeSH terms that describe the content of the article and the type of study or publication (eg, randomized controlled trial; editorial). Standardized terms help you find articles about a topic regardless of how an author has referred to that topic. For example, one author may use 'chronic kidney disease,' whereas another may use 'end-stage renal disease.' If you only include 'chronic kidney disease' in a search, then you will miss relevant articles with the phrase 'end-stage renal disease.' Using the MeSH term for this topic, namely 'Kidney failure, chronic,' eliminates this problem because, regardless of which term the author used, this is the MeSH term that would be applied to articles about chronic kidney disease. Standardized terms are typically arranged in a hierarchy of progressively more specific terms (**Boxes 2** and **3**). This structure can be helpful for finding articles on a broad topic, such as cancer, or a narrow topic, such as insulinoma. A search that includes the MeSH term for cancer, 'Neoplasms,' will retrieve all references indexed with this term as well as any of the terms nested below, such as leukemia or carcinoma. The hierarchical structure of controlled vocabularies allows you to include all species within a taxonomic category or identify related species, which can be helpful when searching for articles about exotic animals.[29,31] Some databases, such as BIOSIS Previews and Zoologic Record, allow you to choose which

Box 2

Hierarchical structure for term 'leukemia' in the Medical Subject Heading (MeSH) controlled vocabulary for PubMed/MEDLINE

All MeSH categories
  Diseases category
    Neoplasms
      Neoplasms by histologic type
        Leukemia
          Enzootic bovine leukosis
          Leukemia, experimental

            Avian leukosis

            Leukemia L1210

            Leukemia L5178

            Leukemia P388
          Leukemia, feline
          Leukemia, hairy cell
          Leukemia, lymphoid

            Leukemia, B-cell +

            Leukemia, biphenotypic, acute

            Leukemia, prolymphocytic +

            Leukemia, T-cell +

            Precursor cell lymphoblastic leukemia-lymphoma +
          Leukemia, mast cell
          Leukemia, myeloid

            Leukemia, myelogenous, chronic, BCR-ABL positive +

            Leukemia, myeloid, acute +

            Leukemia, myeloid, chronic, atypical, BCR-ABL negative

            Leukemia, myelomonocytic, acute

            Leukemia, myelomonocytic, chronic

            Leukemia, myelomonocytic, juvenile

            Sarcoma, myeloid
          Leukemia, plasma cell
          Leukemia, radiation-induced

level of a taxonomic hierarchy to include in your search. The use of standardized terms in a search strategy should improve the sensitivity and specificity of the search. The use of keywords ensures that the search does not miss articles that have not yet been indexed, been indexed improperly, or address a concept not captured in the controlled vocabulary. Some databases do not have a controlled vocabulary. **Table 5** provides an example of keywords and standardized terms for a clinical question.

Step 4: Search Each Concept Separately, Then Combine Using AND, OR, and NOT

Once you have a list of keywords and standardized terms for each concept, then you are (finally) ready to start searching. The words AND, OR, and NOT, known as Boolean operators, tell the database how to interpret a string of words (**Table 6**). The word 'OR'

Box 3
Hierarchical structure for term 'carcinoma' in the Medical Subject Heading (MeSH) controlled vocabulary for PubMed/MEDLINE

All MeSH categories
  Diseases category
    Neoplasms
      Neoplasms by histologic type
        Neoplasms, glandular and epithelial
          Carcinoma
            Adenocarcinoma
              Adenocarcinoma in situ
              Adenocarcinoma, bronchioloalveolar
              Adenocarcinoma, clear cell
              Adenocarcinoma, follicular +
              Adenocarcinoma, mucinous
              Adenocarcinoma, papillary +
              Adenocarcinoma, scirrhous +
              Adenocarcinoma, sebaceous
              Adrenocortical carcinoma
              Carcinoid tumor +
              Carcinoma, acinar cell
              Carcinoma, adenoid cystic
              Carcinoma, ductal +
              Carcinoma, endometrioid
              Carcinoma, hepatocellular
              Carcinoma, intraductal, noninfiltrating +
              Carcinoma, islet cell +
              Carcinoma, lobular
              Carcinoma, mucoepidermoid
              Carcinoma, neuroendocrine +
              Carcinoma, renal cell +
              Carcinoma, signet ring cell +
              Carcinoma, skin appendage
              Cholangiocarcinoma +
              Choriocarcinoma +
              Cystadenocarcinoma +
              Eccrine porocarcinoma
              Paget disease, extramammary
              Pulmonary adenomatosis, ovine

will always broaden a search and is used to separate similar terms for one concept. The word 'AND' will always narrow a search, and is used to combine 2 or more concepts to retrieve articles with at least 1 term from each concept. The word 'NOT' can be used to exclude terms that you do not want in your search results. For example,

Table 5
Keywords and standardized terms (MeSH) for clinical question: "In ferrets with adrenal disease, do GnRH agonists reduce clinical signs as effectively as adrenalectomy?" (Step 3 in structured approach to searching)

	Concept 1 (Patient): Ferrets	Concept 2 (Problem): Adrenal Disease	Concept 3 (Intervention): GnRH Agonist
Standardized Terms (MeSH)	Ferrets	Adrenocortical hyperfunction Cushing syndrome Hyperandrogenism	Gonadotropin-releasing hormone Leuprolide
Keywords	Ferrets Mustela putorius furo	Adrenal disease Adrenocortical disease Hyperadrenocorticism Hyperandrogenism	Gonadotropin-releasing hormone agonist GnRH agonist Leuprolide Leuprorelin Lupron Deslorelin Suprelorin

Abbreviations: GnRH, gonadotropin-releasing hormone; MeSH, Medical Subject Heading.

'NOT' could be used to eliminate articles about poultry from a search for avian information: "Avian NOT poultry."[29] Enter all the terms that describe one concept in the database search box, separating these terms with OR. Run the search; repeat for each concept. After you search each concept separately, then combine the concepts using 'AND' (**Tables 7** and **8**). Searching each concept separately allows you to detect problems with a term before creating a complicated search, and gives you flexibility when combining concepts. You may not need to include all the concepts in your search. When using the PICO format, the outcome concept is often excluded because specific outcomes are often not indexed and/or mentioned in an abstract.

Table 6
Boolean operators (AND, OR, NOT) used to combine words and concepts when searching bibliographic databases

Operator	Example	Search Results	Venn Diagram
AND	Fracture AND hyperparathyroidism	Articles containing BOTH fracture and hyperparathyroidism	
OR	Fracture OR hyperparathyroidism	Articles containing EITHER fracture, hyperparathyroidism, or both	
NOT	Fracture NOT hyperparathyroidism	Articles containing ONLY fracture, not hyperparathyroidism	

Table 7
Combine keywords and standardized terms for each concept using 'OR'; combine separate concepts using 'AND' (step 4 in structured approach to searching)

Concept 1 (Patient): Ferrets	AND	Concept 2 (Problem): Adrenal Disease[a]	AND	Concept 3 (Intervention): GnRH Agonist[a]
"Ferrets"[MeSH] OR Ferrets OR "Mustela putorius furo"		"Adrenocortical hyperfunction"[MeSH] OR "Adrenal disease" OR "Adrenocortical disease" OR Hyperadrenocorticism		"Leuprolide"[MeSH] OR "Gonadotropin-releasing hormone agonist" OR "GnRH agonist" OR Leuprorelin

Abbreviations: GnRH, gonadotropin-releasing hormone; MeSH, Medical Subject Headings.
   [a] Owing to space constraints, all keywords and standardized terms generated for this concept are not displayed.

Step 5: Apply Filters to Limit Results

Once you have run your search, then you can apply filters to limit your results, if necessary. Although each database has different filters, most allow you to limit results by date, language, and publication or article type. It is tempting when confronted with a large number of results to apply several filters to reduce the number of references you have to review. If you are confronted with an overwhelming number of results, then modify your search strategy by adding another concept or removing terms that are retrieving irrelevant results. Be judicious when applying filters to a search for exotic animal literature. Resist the urge to limit results to articles published in the past 5 years, or similarly arbitrary date restrictions, because the only report of a particular condition in an exotic species may have been published 20 years ago.[31] Some databases provide an option to filter results to a veterinary science (PubMed) or veterinary medicine (BIOSIS Previews) subset. If your species and/or topic are likely to be addressed in the human medical, zoologic, or other literature, then do not limit your results to veterinary medicine.

Tips for Finding Exotic Animal Literature in a Bibliographic Database

More often than not, you will have too few results when searching for evidence to answer a clinical question in exotic animal medicine. Here are a few strategies to deploy when confronted with this problem: include terms for related species, check

Table 8
Complete search strategy for clinical question: 'In ferrets with adrenal disease, do GnRH agonists reduce clinical signs as effectively as adrenalectomy?'

Database	Search Strategy
PubMed	("Ferrets"[MeSH] OR "Ferrets"[All Fields] OR "Mustela putorius furo"[All Fields]) AND ("Adrenocortical hyperfunction"[MeSH] OR "Cushing syndrome"[MeSH] OR "Hyperadrogenism"[MeSH] OR "Adrenal disease"[All Fields] OR "Adrenocortical disease"[All Fields] OR "Hyperadrenocorticism"[All Fields] OR "Hyperandrogenism"[All Fields]) AND ("Gonadotropin-releasing hormone"[MeSH] OR "Leuprolide"[MeSH] OR "Gonadotropin-releasing hormone agonist"[All Fields] OR "GnRH agonist"[All Fields] OR "Leuprolide"[All Fields] OR "Leuprorelin"[All Fields] OR "Lupron"[All Fields] OR "Deslorelin"[All Fields] OR "Suprelorin"[All Fields])

Abbreviations: GnRH, gonadotropin-releasing hormone; MeSH, Medical Subject Headings.

the controlled vocabulary terms applied to an article, view similar or related articles, view citing and cited articles, and restrict your search to a specific journal.

Include terms for related species
Just as you do when faced with a novel species in practice, think of related or physiologically equivalent species, and include terms for those species, families, classes, and so on in your search.

Check the controlled vocabulary terms applied to an article
If you find 1 good article in PubMed, or another database that uses a controlled vocabulary, then look at the controlled vocabulary terms (MeSH in PubMed) applied to that article and include those terms to your search.

View similar or related articles
If you have that 1 good article, then look for an option to view similar or related articles. Many databases provide this option, which uses an algorithm to find articles related to the one of interest.

View citing and cited articles
Another technique if you have a useful article is to review the articles that have cited it (citing articles) and its references (cited articles). The databases on the Web of Science platform (BIOSIS Previews, Web of Science Core Collection, Zoological Record) and the Scopus database allow you to easily view citing and cited articles for each article.

Restrict your search to a specific journal
Use AND to combine a broad topic search with the tile of a journal. For example, "guinea pigs"[MeSH] AND "dystocia"[MeSH] AND "The Veterinary Clinics of North America. Exotic Animal Practice"[Journal]. This strategy is particularly useful for finding information quickly in the clinic.

OTHER RESOURCES
Google Scholar

Google Scholar uses a distinct algorithm to find scholarly material, such as journal articles, books, reports, and theses, on the web. Google Scholar is not considered a bibliographic database because it is a search engine, not a predefined collection of material. Google Scholar can be useful for finding evidence in exotic animal practice because it searches across all disciplines and types of material. Google Scholar also provides links to full text and citing articles. However, it is important to recognize the limitations of Google Scholar. Like in Google, there are few options to create a structured search and an overwhelming number of results, which cannot be filtered, are often returned. The content that Google Scholar searches is not controlled, as it is in a database. Therefore, information resources retrieved in a Google Scholar search must be evaluated carefully. Finally, Google Scholar does not search all web content, so important literature may be missed.

Veterinary Information Network

VIN was one of the earliest online resources exclusively for veterinarians and remains popular. Indeed, in the survey of UK veterinarians, VIN was considered the third most useful electronic resource among all respondents, and the second most useful among those who practiced small animal (including exotic) medicine.[2] VIN was the most accessed electronic resource in the survey of non-UK veterinarians.[3] VIN is a professional networking and continuing education site that offers message boards, rounds with specialists, a collection of veterinary journals, and the full text of conference proceedings and select drug formularies. Recent improvements to the search feature of VIN allow users to search by year, species, or folder (eg, Aquatic Animal Medicine) and filter by source (eg, conference proceeding, guidelines, notes, lecture, or journals). VIN is a unique and valuable resource, particularly for exotic animal practitioners, because it provides knowledge and material, such as conference proceedings from the American Association of Zoo Veterinarians and the Association of Avian Veterinarians, to which clinicians may not otherwise have access. However, the features for which VIN is typically used, namely, its message boards and rounds, are expert opinion, and therefore provide lower levels of evidence.

SUMMARY

The barriers to finding and using the best available evidence in exotic animal practice can seem insurmountable. In the editorial that codified the definition of evidence-based medicine, Sackett and colleagues[13] acknowledged that "if no randomised trial has been carried out for our patient's predicament, we must follow the trail to the next best external evidence and work from there." With an awareness of the resources that do exist and a structured approach to selecting, searching and evaluating the evidence from those resources, clinicians can follow the trail of evidence and integrate EBP into patient care.

REFERENCES

1. Wales T. Practice makes perfect? Vets' information seeking behaviour and information use explored. Aslib Proc 2000;52(7):235–46.
2. Nielsen TD, Dean RS, Massey A, et al. Survey of the UK veterinary profession 2: sources of information used by veterinarians. Vet Rec 2015;177(7):172.
3. Huntley SJ, Dean RS, Massey A, et al. International evidence-based medicine survey of the veterinary profession: information sources used by veterinarians. PLoS One 2016;11(7):e0159732.
4. Powers LV, Benson KC, Brandao J, et al. Avian health information management in the digital age. J Avian Med Surg 2014;28(3):251–6.
5. Vandeweerd JM, Vandeweerd S, Gustin C, et al. Understanding veterinary practitioners' decision-making process: implications for veterinary medical education. J Vet Med Educ 2012;39(2):142–51.
6. Nielsen TD, Dean RS, Robinson NJ, et al. Survey of the UK veterinary profession: common species and conditions nominated by veterinarians in practice. Vet Rec 2014;174(13):324.
7. Asokan GV, Kasimanickam RK, Asokan V. Surveillance, response systems, and evidence updates on emerging zoonoses: the role of one health. Infect Ecol Epidemiol 2013;3(1).
8. Sargeant JM, Kelton DF, O'Connor AM. Study designs and systematic reviews of interventions: building evidence across study designs. Zoonoses Public Health 2014;61(Suppl 1):10–7.
9. Vandeweerd JM, Clegg P, Buczinski S. How can veterinarians base their medical decisions on the best available scientific evidence? Vet Clin North Am Food Anim Pract 2012;28(1):1–11.
10. Roudebush P, Allen TA, Dodd CE, et al. Application of evidence-based medicine to veterinary clinical nutrition. J Am Vet Med Assoc 2004;224(11):1765–71.
11. Holmes MA, Ramey DW. An introduction to evidence-based veterinary medicine. Vet Clin North Am Equine Pract 2007;23(2):191–200.

12. Lanyon L. Collecting the evidence for EBVM: who pays? Vet Rec 2016;178(5): 120–1.

13. Sackett DL, Rosenberg WMC, Gray JAM, et al. Evidence based medicine: what it is and what it isn't. BMJ 1996;312(7023):71–2.

14. Adamantos S. In search of evidence in small animal emergency medicine - a speciality of its own. J Small Anim Pract 2010;51(5):240–1.

15. Cockcroft P, Holmes M. Evidence-based veterinary medicine 2. Identifying information needs and finding the evidence. In Pract 2004;26(2):96–102.

16. Lanyon LE. A scientifically based profession? Vet Rec 2012;171(5):128–9.

17. Schulz KS, Cook JL, Kapatkin AS, et al. Evidence-based surgery: time for change. Vet Surg 2006;35(8):697–9.

18. Toews L. The information infrastructure that supports evidence-based veterinary medicine: a comparison with human medicine. J Vet Med Educ 2011;38(2): 123–34.

19. Grindlay DJ, Brennan ML, Dean RS. Searching the veterinary literature: a comparison of the coverage of veterinary journals by nine bibliographic databases. J Vet Med Educ 2012;39(4):404–12.

20. Dale VHM, Pierce SE, May SA. Motivating factors and perceived barriers to participating in continuing professional development: a national survey of veterinary surgeons. Vet Rec 2013;173(10):247.

21. American Veterinary Medical Association. Market research statistics: U.S. veterinarians 2015. 2016. Available at: https://www.avma.org/KB/Resources/Statistics/Pages/Market-research-statistics-US-veterinarians.aspx. Accessed November 25, 2016.

22. Nault AJ, Baker HJ. The power of information. J Vet Med Educ 2011;38(1):3–4.

23. Dicenso A, Bayley L, Haynes RB. Accessing pre-appraised evidence: fine-tuning the 5S model into a 6S model. Evid Based Nurs 2009;12(4):99–101.

24. Haynes RB. Of studies, syntheses, synopses, summaries, and systems: the "5S" evolution of information services for evidence-based healthcare decisions. Evid Based Med 2006;11(6):162–4.

25. Clinical practice guidelines we can trust. Washington, DC: The National Academies Press; 2011. Available at: https://www.nationalacademies.org/hmd/Reports/2011/Clinical-Practice-Guidelines-We-Can-Trust.aspx.

26. Arlt SP, Haimerl P, Heuwieser W. Training evidence-based veterinary medicine by collaborative development of critically appraised topics. J Vet Med Educ 2012; 39(2):111–8.

27. Hardin LE, Robertson S. Learning evidence-based veterinary medicine through development of a critically appraised topic. J Vet Med Educ 2006;33(3):474–8.

28. Steele M, Crabb NP, Moore LJ, et al. Online tools for teaching evidence-based veterinary medicine. J Vet Med Educ 2013;40(3):272–7.

29. Paul-Murphy J. Finding avian health information. J Exot Pet Med 2010;19(2): 151–9.

30. O'Connor AM, Anderson KM, Goodell CK, et al. Conducting systematic reviews of intervention questions I: writing the review protocol, formulating the question and searching the literature. Zoonoses Public Health 2014;61:28–38.

31. Alpi KM, Stringer E, Devoe RS, et al. Clinical and research searching on the wild side: exploring the veterinary literature. J Med Libr Assoc 2009;97(3):169–77.

Basic Statistics for the Exotic Animal Practitioner

 CrossMark

Michelle A. Giuffrida, VMD, MSCE, DACVS

KEYWORDS

- Evidence-based practice • Evidence-based medicine • Clinical epidemiology
- Biostatistics

KEY POINTS

- Descriptive statistics are used to organize and summarize data obtained from study samples, whereas inferential statistics are used to generalize sample data to larger populations.
- The main framework for inferential statistics in medicine is hypothesis testing, which uses *P* values to judge whether observed results are likely to occur due to chance alone.
- The specific statistical methods depend on the distribution of data, but the general principles, interpretation, and limitations are consistent across hypothesis testing methods.
- Confidence intervals provide estimates of population parameters and associations along with a measure of how precise the estimate is likely to be.

Evidence-based practice (EBP) depends on clinicians' access to best research evidence, as determined through the process of critical appraisal. In veterinary medicine, the work of critical appraisal is still largely the responsibility of clinicians themselves. Clinical epidemiology guidelines such as those outlined earlier in this issue can help practitioners identify the strengths and weaknesses of different research methods. However, many studies' conclusions are based on statistical inference, so a working knowledge of basic biomedical statistics is also extremely helpful to the EBP practitioner.

The purpose of most clinical research is to explore whether causal associations exist between exposures (such as treatments, environment factors, or patient characteristic) and outcomes (such as the development, progression, or resolution of disease). Because it would be impractical to try achieve this by studying every single animal with a given exposure or outcome, most clinical research relies on data obtained from samples of subjects drawn from and presumed to represent the larger populations of similar animals. This setup means that a research study needs to do

Disclosure Statement: The author has nothing to disclose.
Small Animal Surgery, Department of Surgical and Radiological Sciences, University of California, Davis School of Veterinary Medicine, One Shields Avenue, Davis, CA 95616, USA
E-mail address: magiuffrida@ucdavis.edu

Vet Clin Exot Anim 20 (2017) 947–959
http://dx.doi.org/10.1016/j.cvex.2017.04.007
1094-9194/17/Published by Elsevier Inc.
vetexotic.theclinics.com

2 different things: (1) describe the data obtained from the immediate sample of animals in a useful and organized way, and (2) draw inferences from the data about cause-effect associations in the overall population. Descriptive and inferential statistics are used to accomplish these respective aims.

DESCRIPTIVE STATISTICS

Descriptive statistics refer to methods of organizing, summarizing, and displaying data. It would be hard for readers to understand what the data are showing if articles presented raw research data, especially if there are many animals, data points, or measurements. Descriptive statistics are thus very important for communicating the results of most clinical research studies, with the exception of case reports. In addition to reporting results, descriptive statistics are also used by researchers to identify data errors and to determine which inferential statistical methods are appropriate.

Exposures, outcomes, and other measured data points are referred to as variables. Variables are broadly categorized for biostatistics as being categorical or continuous (**Table 1**); these labels refer to characteristics of the data itself and help determine the appropriate type of descriptive and inferential statistics for each variable.

The distribution of a variable refers to what the data look like if a graph were made showing all the possible measurement values and how many times each value occurred in the data set. Data that have a bell-shaped curve follows the normal (Gaussian) distribution; data that take a non-bell-shaped form have a nonnormal distribution, of which there are many types[1] (**Fig. 1**). Continuous data can have either a normal or nonnormal distribution; categorical data alway take a nonnormal distribution. Although graphs are very helpful ways to summarize data, it would not be practical for journal articles to include graphs of every single variable. Instead, the distributions are summarized using measures of central tendency and variability, which are called summary statistics.

Central Tendency: Numbers that Describe the Middle of the Data Set

- Mean: the arithmetical average of the data values
  - Distorted by outliers (extreme data points)
  - Commonly used to describe continuous and ordinal data
- Median: the value above and below which half the data points lies
  - The data value at the 50th percentile
  - Not distorted by outliers
  - Commonly used to describe continuous and ordinal data
- Mode: the most frequently obtained values
  - Not distorted by outliers
  - Used to describe categorical data, or nonnormal continuous data cluster that are around 2 different points (bimodal)

Variability: Spread of the Data Around the Central Value

- Range: interval between the lowest and highest values obtained
  - Simple, only considers extreme values
  - Typically used to describe variability around the median or mode
- Interquartile range (IQR): interval between 25th and 75th percentile values
  - An estimate of spread around the median; the middle 50% of data points relative to the median
  - Recommended to describe variability of nonnormal data[2]

Table 1
Basic descriptive and inferential statistics for continuous and categorical variables

	Continuous Variables	Categorical Variables
Description	Characteristics that are measured along a continuous numerical scale, sometimes within a fixed interval of possibilities	Characteristics that are measured on discrete or qualitative scales; 2 main types *Nominal* ≥2 groups with no inherent order *Ordinal* ≥2 groups that can be ordered or ranked
Example variables	Age, body weight, systolic blood pressure, packed cell volume, survival time	Sex Neuter status Treatment type *Variables categorized as:* Yes/no Present/absent	Disease stage Body condition score Preanesthetic status *Grouped continuous variables such as:* Age groups Drug dose ranges
Distribution	Normal (bell curve) Not normal	Not normal	Not normal
Descriptive statistics	Mean, SD Median, IQR	Frequency and % proportions	Frequency and % proportions Mean and SD Median and range
Inferential statistics	*Parametric* t tests ANOVA *Non-parametric* Wilcoxon rank sum Wilcoxon signed rank Sign test Kruskal-Wallis	Fisher's exact χ^2 McNemar's test Binomial probability	Fisher's exact χ^2 McNemar's test Nonparametric tests

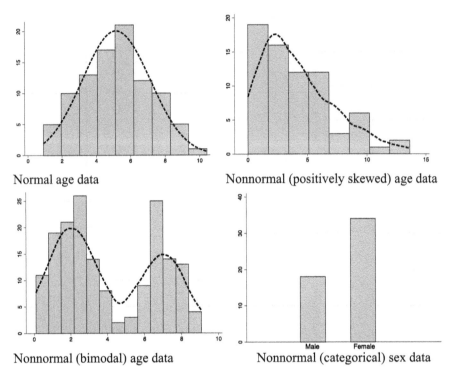

Normal age data

Nonnormal (positively skewed) age data

Nonnormal (bimodal) age data

Nonnormal (categorical) sex data

Fig. 1. Normal and nonnormal data distributions. In all graphs, frequency (number of subjects) is on the y-axis and variable data are on the x-axis.

- Standard deviation (SD): calculated value that estimates data spread around the mean in normally distributed data
  - About 68% of data points will fall within ±1 SD of the mean
  - Recommended to describe variability of normal data[2]

Descriptive Statistics in Study Results

Descriptive statistics are reported in study results in either tables, graphs, or charts, or in the text. Most clinical study results sections will begin with descriptive statistics of the study population so that the reader has an understanding of the basic characteristics of the animals that were studied. If the study intends to compare 2 or more different groups of animals, the descriptive statistics for each group should be presented separately, often in tabular form. In addition to describing features of the study sample, descriptive statistics are also used to summarize exposures and outcomes before any attempts to evaluate associations between them.

Limitations of Descriptive Statistics

Descriptive statistics can only summarize data in the subjects that were actually studied; they cannot be used to generalize results to other animals or clinical situations.[2] For example, if a study of tibiotarsal fractures in 10 Amazon parrots reports that 5 birds had short oblique mid-diaphyseal fractures, it would be incorrect to claim that this type of fracture accounts for 50% of tibiotarsal fractures in Amazons in general. Alternatively, imagine a study that tested 2 antibiotic regimens in Guinea pigs with pododermatitis and found that regimens X and Y resulted in 50% and 20% cure rates, respectively; even though the cure rate for X was higher in the study sample, it would be incorrect to claim that these proportions are the treatment responses in the general population of guinea pigs with this condition, or even that treatment X is more effective than Y in the general population. In fact, inferential statistics are needed to support such claims.

Descriptive study results alone should not automatically be generalized to nonstudy animals (ie, your patients). There is a very real chance that these numbers do not reflect what is truly expected in the larger population. In the absence of any inferential statistics, you can assess the study methods for obvious threats to internal validity (such as very small sample size, selection bias, imbalanced study groups), and how similar your patient is to the study sample. If the study appears to be at risk of these threats, or the study animals are unlike your patient, the rationale for expecting similar results in your patient is weak.

INFERENTIAL STATISTICS

Inferential statistics are used to estimate population parameters and associations based on data obtained from just a sample of the population. Samples of animals are unlikely to perfectly represent the larger populations from which they are drawn, so ways are needed quantify potential errors in the immediate data set relative to what would be obtained if the whole population were studied. Focused on here are the basic inferential concepts that exotic animal practitioners are likely to encounter during the course of EBP.

Classical Hypothesis Testing

Hypothesis testing, the main paradigm for inferential statistics in medicine,[3] is based on the idea that for any clinical question we might have, there is a true effect that a single research study can only estimate. In hypothesis testing, the researchers create a null hypothesis that they wish to test and possibly disprove.[3] Typically, the null hypothesis is that there is no difference in the variable of interest between groups of animals. However, what does "no difference" actually mean? Even if the null hypothesis is true, chance alone will ensure some differences are observed, particularly if the study samples are small.[4] Therefore, we need parameters for what differences to attribute to chance and what differences to consider significant (ie, not due to chance). If the study data show a difference between groups that is more extreme than the preset parameters, it is concluded that the difference is significant and the null hypothesis can be rejected because it is sufficiently unlikely. One of the mistakes that could be made with this method is to conclude there is a non-chance difference between groups, when in fact no difference exists in the population. This mistake is called a false positive or type I error. For example, imagine flipping a coin 10 times in order to determine if the coin is fair. The null hypothesis is that if the coin is fair, you will observe no difference in the number of head and tail results. You set the parameter that if you get a result of more than 8 heads or tails, you will reject the null hypothesis of a fair coin. Obviously, it is possible that a fair coin could fall the same way 9 or 10 times out of 10, but it is pretty unlikely, so most of the time our parameter would lead us to a correct estimate of the coin's fairness. The probability of making a type I error (designated α) is the parameter used in hypothesis testing to separate out significant and chance results and is commonly referred to as the significance level of a test.[5] By convention, α is usually set at less than .05, meaning a 1 in 20 probability of making a false positive conclusion.

P Values

Probability functions, called P values, are used to evaluate where the study data fall with respect to the chosen significance level, and thus whether we will reject or not reject the null hypothesis. A P value refers to the probability of observing a given difference between groups, or an even more extreme difference, due to chance alone.[4] For example, a P value of .01 means that if the null hypothesis were in fact true and we repeated the study 100 times, only once (1% of the time) would we expect to find a difference in groups as large or larger than what was observed.[3] When the exact P value for a comparison is less than the preset α level (usually <.05), the result is considered "statistically significant"; that is to say, the result is unlikely enough that we are willing to reject the null hypothesis and consider that something other than chance is responsible for the result. Note, we never "accept" the null hypothesis with this method; we simply examine the strength of evidence against it (**Box 1**).[4]

Test Procedures

Classical tests of hypotheses involve first generating at test statistic that represents how well the distribution of the study data compares to a theoretic distribution that would be expected if the null hypothesis were true.[5] Different data distributions require different comparison procedures and test statistics. Next, the P value is calculated, which is the probability of obtaining an equally or more extreme test statistical if the null hypothesis is true. Finally, we examine where the P value falls with respect to the preset significance level and decide whether to reject or not reject the null hypothesis.

Tests can be 1- or 2-sided (also referred to as 1-tailed or 2-tailed). When we specify a null hypothesis of no difference, we are in effect contrasting it to an alternative hypothesis that states: the difference between the 2 groups is *not* zero. This hypothesis makes sense, because even if there is truly a difference between groups, we generally have no idea ahead of time what size or direction that difference could be.[5] For example, if researchers are comparing surgical site infection rates with 2 different

---

Box 1
Additional guidelines for understanding and interpreting P values

- When the P value is significant, we reject the null hypothesis. This means one of the following is true, but we cannot know for sure which one:
  - There is a real (non-chance) difference between the groups.
  - There is no difference and in rejecting the null we make a false positive or type I error.

- When the P value is not significant, we do not reject the null hypothesis. This means one of the following is true, but we cannot know for sure which one:
  - There is truly no difference between the groups.
  - There is a real (non-chance) difference, but we failed to identify it. If we fail to reject the null hypothesis when a difference actually exists, we make a false negative or type II error.

- The P value depends on the sample size. This is because the chance effect diminishes as more subjects are studied. For a given significance parameter, a larger study can identify smaller differences as significant and is less likely to result in type II error.

- A P value is NOT the probability that the null hypothesis is true,[4] and it cannot prove or disprove the null hypothesis.

- A P value is NOT equivalent to the actual type I error rate.[14]

skin antiseptics, they do not know ahead of time which preparation technique is more effective; the infection rate with antiseptic A could be higher or lower than the rate for B. Two-sided tests set significance parameters at both the high and the low ends of any potential difference between groups. One-sided tests only set a significance parameter at one end (either high or low) and therefore will only identify significant differences in a certain direction. In the skin preparation example, a 1-sided test could be set up so that a difference in infection would only be considered significant if it favors antiseptic A. Obviously, the potential problem with this approach is that very large differences in infection rate that favor antiseptic B would not be considered significant. Compared with 2-sided tests, 1-sided tests will give a lower *P* value for differences in the direction of interest, so researchers could be tempted to use 1-sided tests to improve the chance of "significant" results if they think they can anticipate the direction of results. In most cases, 2-sided tests should be used in order not to miss important but unanticipated differences. Using a 1-sided test is generally only appropriate when the consequences of missing an effect in the untested direction are negligible and ethical.[6]

Common Parametric Tests of Hypotheses

Parametric statistical methods are used to compare the distribution of a normally distributed continuous variable in 2 or more groups of subjects.

- T tests are a method used to compare 2 different mean values. There are different types of *t* tests:
  - One-sample *t* test: compares the sample mean to a hypothesized mean
    - Example usage: to compare whether the mean body temperature measured in a group of chinchillas differs from 101°F
  - Two-sample *t* test: compares the mean in 2 independent samples
    - Example usage: to compare body weights of 1-year-old budgies obtained from 2 different breeders
  - Paired-sample *t* test: compares the mean in 2 related samples
    - Used to compare measurements in 2 groups of subjects that have been matched on key characteristics, or to compare 2 measurements taken in succession in the same group of subjects
    - Example usage: to compare systolic blood pressure measurements obtained in the fore paws versus hind paws in a group of ferrets
    - Example usage: to compare heart rate in a group of ferrets before and after a dose of acepromazine
  - Null hypothesis: the difference between the 2 sample means is zero
  - Interpretation: if *P* is statistically significant, reject the hypothesis of no difference in mean between the groups
- Analysis of variance (ANOVA) is a test method used to compare multiple mean values. Two common types are as follows:
  - One-way ANOVA: compares the mean in 3 or more independent samples
    - An extension of the 2-sample *t* test that examines whether there is a difference between *any 2* of the samples
    - Example: to compare body weights of 1-year-old budgies obtained from 4 different breeders
  - Repeated-measures ANOVA: compares the mean in 3 or more related samples
    - An extension of the paired-sample *t* test that examines whether there is a difference between *any 2* of the samples

- Example: to compare heart rate measured at 5, 30, and 60 minutes after induction of general anesthesia in a group of ferrets
- Example: to compare blood uric acid levels in a group of African gray parrots after being fed each of 4 different diets
  - Null hypothesis: the difference between *any 2* sample means is zero
  - Interpretation: if *P* is statistically significant, reject the hypothesis of no difference in mean between *any 2* samples
    - The ANOVA *P* value should NOT be interpreted that the means in all samples are different from one another. It only tells you that at least 2 of the samples are "significantly" different, but importantly, *it does not tell you which samples.*
    - Example: if the *P* value for the 1-way ANOVA comparing mean body weight in budgies from 4 breeders is significant, it means that the body weights of birds from at least 2 breeders differed, but we do not know if the differences was in breeder groups 1 versus 2, or 2 versus 4, and so forth.
    - If the ANOVA *P* value is significant, the statistician should perform and report additional tests that examine each possible pairwise comparison (1 vs 2, 1 vs 3, 1 vs 4, 2 vs 3, and so forth). Most methods used to do this are based on 2-sample *t* tests and involve an additional procedure that adjusts the significance parameters in order to limit false positive results that can occur when a large number of tests are performed.[7] Examples of this are Tukey and Bonferroni tests.

Common Nonparametric Tests of Hypotheses

Nonparametric statistical methods are based on the assumption that the variable being analyzed is continuous or ordinal and does not necessarily follow the normal (bell-shaped) distribution.[5] Ordinal data are categorical variables (see **Table 1**) that can be put in a specific rank or order, but the different levels do not have an inherent numerical value. For example, cancer is often categorized according to degree of disease progression, a property called "stage," which can be given a numeric value. We know that low stage is less advanced that high stage, but the difference between stages 1, 2, and 3 do not have mathematical value, nor are they necessarily equivalent differences. These tests are used to compare the distribution of continuous or ordinal variables in 2 or more groups of subjects.

- Wilcoxon rank sum test is a nonparametric analogue of the 2-sample *t* test. This test compares data points based on their relative ranks rather than actual numeric values, so is slightly less intuitive.
  - Equivalent to the Mann-Whitney *U* test, which compares ranks in a different way but arrives at the same *P* value.[5]
  - Null hypothesis: the difference between the 2 rank distributions is zero.
  - Interpretation: if *P* is statistically significant, reject the hypothesis of no difference in distribution between the 2 samples.
- Wilcoxon signed rank sum test is a nonparametric alternative to the paired-sample *t* test. Like the rank sum test above, it also compares data based on their relative ranks rather than actual numeric values.
  - Null hypothesis: the difference between the 2 rank distributions is zero.
  - Interpretation: if *P* is statistically significant, reject the hypothesis of no difference in distribution between the 2 samples.

- Sign test is another nonparametric alternative to paired-sample t test. Rather than use ranks like the Wilcoxon sign rank test, it compares the *median* values in 2 related groups.
  - Null hypothesis: the difference between the 2 medians is zero.
  - Interpretation: if P is statistically significant, reject the hypothesis of no difference in median between the two samples.
- Kruskal-Wallis test is a nonparametric alternative to the 1-way ANOVA and is used to compare rank distributions across 3 or more independent samples.
  - Null hypothesis: the difference between *any* 2 samples' rank distributions is zero.
  - Interpretation: if P is statistically significant, reject the hypothesis of no difference in distribution between *any* 2 samples.
    - Like in ANOVA, the Kruskal-Wallace P value should NOT be interpreted that distributions of all samples are different from one another. It only tells you that at least 2 of the samples are significantly different, but importantly, *it does not tell you which samples.*
    - Like in ANOVA, if the Kruskal-Wallace P value is significant, the statistician should perform and report additional tests to examine each pairwise comparison. A common nonparametric test for this is called Dunn's procedure, which performs pairwise comparisons that are analogous to individual Wilcoxon rank sum tests.

Common Hypothesis Tests for Categorical Data

Categorical data take different distributions from continuous variables and are therefore analyzed across groups using a different set of tests. Categorical data are summarized as sample frequencies or proportions and can be arranged in contingency tables showing the frequency of one variable in rows and another in columns, as seen in this 2×2 table of 80 animals:

| | Variable 1: Sex | | |
Variable 2: Weight group	Male	Female	Total
<100 g	10	30	40
≥100 g	20	20	40
Total	30	50	80

To compare whether the distribution of sex is different across weight categories, the observed contingency table is compared with a theoretic table that of values that would be expected if no relationship existed between sex and weight group. The null hypothesis is that there is no difference in sex distribution between the weight categories. If the null hypothesis is true, we expect that the proportions of males and females in each weight category should not differ significantly.

Common statistical methods that can be used to test contingency table data are the χ^2 test, Fisher's exact test, and McNemar's test. These tests are used to compare the distribution of a categorical variable across 2 or more groups of subjects. The χ^2 test and Fisher's exact test are both used for independent (unpaired) samples. Between the 2 tests, Fisher's is recommended when the total number of subjects being compared is 20 or fewer; for larger samples, either test can be used.[8] McNemar's test is used for matched pairs or related data. All of these tests share the following characteristics:

- Compare the observed frequencies of a variable to a theoretic distribution in which the variable is equally distributed across groups.
- Null hypothesis: the proportions of the variable are not different between the groups.
- Interpretation: if P is statistically significant, reject the hypothesis of no difference in the proportions between the groups.

The distribution of a categorical variable in a single group can also be used to estimate the distribution in the entire population. The binomial probability test compares an observed proportion to a hypothesized proportion under the null hypothesis of no difference between the proportions. A significant P value is interpreted to mean that study results were not consistent with the hypothesized proportion.

Inferential Statistics in Study Results

In order for readers to interpret the results of inferential statistics, articles must provide basic information about the methodology and sample (**Box 2**). In the author's experience, detailed information about statistical procedures and results is not always

---

Box 2
Basic information that should be reported in a paper using hypothesis testing for statistical inference, with examples

Methods

- Name of test performed and any test variations or options
- Whether the test is 1 -or 2-sided (1- or 2-tailed)
- Preset significance level of the test

Results

- Sample size and summary statistics of group or groups being tested
- The exact P value for the test (eg, $P = .25$, rather than just "not significant")
- A measure of the difference between groups and surrounding CI

Example A:

We compared the length (cm) of 6-month-old captive bearded dragons obtained from 2 different states using a 2-sample t test. The test was 2-sided and $P<.05$ was considered significant.

58 lizards were studied: 23 from California and 35 from Florida. Mean ± SD body length was length 32 ± 12 cm for California lizards and 37 ± 5 cm for Florida lizards. Lizards from Florida were on average 5 cm longer (mean difference 5 cm, 95%CI 0.4–9.6) than lizards from California, and the difference was statistically significant ($P = .04$).

Example B:

We compared the hospital discharge rate of rabbits treated surgically for acute and chronic liver lobe torsions using a 2-tailed Fisher exact test. $P<.05$ was considered statistically significant.

8/11 (72.7%) rabbits with chronic liver lobe torsions and 4/8 (50.0%) rabbits with acute liver lobe torsions were discharged alive following surgery. The difference in discharge rate for acute torsions was −22.7% (95%CI −66.2% to 20.8%) relative to chronic torsions, but the difference was not statistically significant ($P = .38$).

reported in veterinary clinical studies. Study results should be interpreted with caution if the article does not report the results of all tests performed or does not include all the information necessary for you to interpret the results. Inferential statistics should also be interpreted in light of the study's overall design and its potential for bias or confounding, which might be reflected in the results.

Limitations of Hypothesis Testing

Despite commonplace use in veterinary medical research, hypothesis testing has major drawbacks. Overemphasis on P values has led to a clinical research culture that focuses on dichotomizing results as significant or not significant, rather than estimating the size and direction of outcome differences between groups of patients.[9] This practice is problematic because the yes-no result obtained is often incorrect or misinterpreted, for example,

- Studies with nonsignificant results are often incorrectly interpreted as "negative" when in fact they are inconclusive.[10,11] This is of particular concern in veterinary medicine because these errors are much more likely to occur when sample sizes are small.
- False positive results are very likely to occur when researchers comb the data for statistically significant findings,[12,13] as often occurs in retrospective and other observational study designs that compose much of the veterinary literature. This is called the multiple comparisons problem and means that the risk of type I errors increases as more tests are performed. Problematic approaches include the following[13]:
  - Excessive numbers and permutations of variables tested
  - Repeated tests across different subgroups of subjects
  - Repeated comparisons at different time points
  - Addition or removal subjects until significance is met
- Statistically significant differences are not necessarily medically important or biologically relevant.[9]

Part of the problem is that P values convey no information about the size or precision of any estimated difference in outcome between groups of patients, but in fact this is the information clinicians most need to know.[9] Many experts recommend that studies limit excessive reliance P values and focus instead on reporting the actual estimate of the association (difference) between groups and a surrounding measure of precision.[9,10] When comparing the mean or proportion of a variable between 2 groups, the estimate of association is the difference in mean or proportion between groups, and a confidence interval (CI) (see later discussion).

It is essential to remember that statistical inference will not overcome bias in the study design or execution. Furthermore, none of the statistical techniques presented here will control for confounding. If there is bias or confounding, the results of statistical inference are likely to be incorrect, which in turn can result in incorrectly finding or not finding significant differences, or making mistaken estimates of the magnitude or direction of associations. Such errors are major problems that could have real implications for patient care when they occur in clinical studies and point to why EBP practitioners must examine a study's methods before making judgments about the validity or applicability of its results.

CONFIDENCE INTERVALS

CI are calculated values that provide estimates of precision around observed study parameters or differences between groups. A 95% CI is most common and can be interpreted as a range of values that would include the true population parameter 95% of the time, if the study were repeated over and over again.[4] There is a close link between hypothesis testing and CIs, such that by calculating the 95%CI, one can infer the result of a 2-sided hypothesis test with a significance level of $\alpha < .05$.[9] If the 95%CI includes the value that represents no difference (eg, zero, for comparisons of means or proportions), the result is not statistically significant at the .05 level. Compared with hypothesis testing methods, which give yes/no answers, CIs also show a range of actual values within which the true population parameter or difference is expected to lie.

CIs can be used to estimate population parameters from a single group of data or provide an estimate of precision around an association.[4] They can be used in addition to classical hypothesis tests or other statistical inference techniques to aid interpretation of the results, as illustrated in the examples in **Box 2**. In example A, a significant difference in length between the 2 groups of bearded dragons has been identified using a t test. However, that test alone gives no information about the magnitude or direction of the difference. Is it a huge difference or negligible one? Remember, statistical significance does not equate to clinical significance. The report of a 4-cm difference and accompanying 95%CI of 0.2 to 7.8 shows us that the estimated true difference is likely to fall within a range that includes both clinically relevant and clinically insignificant values. Therefore, although the study identified a difference between groups, the estimate is not very precise, so we should leave open the possibility that the true difference between these groups could either be negligible or of larger magnitude that was observed. In example B, a null hypothesis of no difference in hospital discharge rate between 2 groups of rabbits was not rejected using a Fisher's exact test. Does this mean there is truly no difference in outcome between rabbits with acute and chronic torsions? The CI shows that the true difference in discharge rates could range anywhere from 66% worse in the acute group to 20% better in the acute group. Clearly a clinically relevant difference in outcome between groups has not been excluded, so we would interpret that the study results are inconclusive rather than negative.

An unfortunate reality of veterinary clinical research is that sample sizes are often quite small, which means that samples often do not accurately represent the larger populations, and that estimates are likely to be imprecise. CIs are often encouraged because they can help readers interpret the meaning of a negative statistical test and thus avoid dismissing potentially valuable treatments or accepting harmful ones.[9,11]

SUMMARY

Clinical research studies often contain descriptive statistics and make conclusions based on the results of statistical inference. EBP practitioners should have a basic understanding of how to interpret summary statistics, P values, and CIs in order to understand the conclusions derived in clinical studies.

REFERENCES

1. Gaddis ML, Gaddis GM. Introduction to biostatistics: part 1, basic concepts. Ann Emerg Med 1990;19(1):86–9.
2. Gaddis ML, Gaddis GM. Introduction to biostatistics: part 2, descriptive statistics. Ann Emerg Med 1990;19(3):309–15.
3. Guyatt G, Jaeschke R, Heddle N, et al. Basic statistics for clinicians: 1. hypothesis testing. CMAJ 1995;152(1):27–32.

4. Campbell MJ, Swinscow TDV. Statistics at square one. 11th edition. Chichester (United Kingdom): Wiley-Blackwell/BMJ Books; 2009.
5. Rosner B. Fundamentals of biostatistics. 7th edition. Boston: Brooks/Cole; 2011.
6. What are differences between one-tailed and two-tailed tests?. UCLA: Statistical Consulting Group. Available at: http://www.ats.ucla.edu/stat/mult_pkg/faq/general/tail_tests.htm. Accessed November 30, 2016.
7. Cabral HJ. Multiple comparisons procedures. Circulation 2008;117(5):698–701.
8. Campbell I. Chi-squared and Fisher-Irwin tests of two-by-two tables with small sample recommendations. Stat Med 2007;26:3661–75.
9. Gardner MJ, Altman DG. Confidence intervals rather than P values: estimation rather than hypothesis testing. Br Med J (Clin Res Ed) 1986;292:746–50.
10. Lang TA, Altman DG. Basic statistical reporting for articles published in biomedical journals: the "Statistical Analysis and Methods in the Published Literature" or SAMPL Guidelines. Int J Nurs Stud 2015;52:5–9.
11. Wagg CR, Kwong GPS, Pang DSJ. Application of confidence intervals to data interpretation. Can Vet J 2016;57:547.
12. Austin PC, Mamdani MM, Juurlink DN, et al. Testing multiple statistical hypotheses resulted in spurious associations: a study of astrological signs and health. J Clin Epidemiol 2006;59(9):964–9.
13. Proschan MA, Waclawiw MA. Practical guidelines for multiplicity adjustment in clinical trials. Control Clin Trials 2000;21(6):527–39.
14. Goodman SN. Toward evidence-based medical statistics. 1: the P value fallacy. Ann Intern Med 1999;130(12):995–1004.

Advanced Statistics for Exotic Animal Practitioners

John Hodsoll, PhD*, Jennifer M. Hellier, BSc (Hons), Elizabeth G. Ryan, PhD

KEYWORDS

- Statistics • Exotic animals • Correlation • Regression

KEY POINTS

- Correlation estimates the strength and direction of an association between 2 random variables.
- Linear regression aims to quantify and predict the values of a continuous random variable based on the values of an explanatory variable or variables.
- Logistic regression extends linear models to binary outcomes.
- Statistical models rely on assumptions which should be critically evaluated.

VISUALISING THE RELATIONSHIP BETWEEN 2 VARIABLES

Scatter plots are an important graphical method to understand the nature of the association between 2 random variables. In a scatter plot, x and y coordinate points on a graph are determined by the numerical value of the variables. If there is no correlation between the variables, the points of the variables are scattered randomly across the plane. In contrast, if there is a linear correlation, the distribution of points will follow a straight line and be scattered randomly above and below the line, with most data close to the line. The strength of the association depends on the spread of the data around the line. An apparently strong linear association is shown in **Fig. 1**, which shows a scatter plot for the heart weight of 143 cats weighing more than 2 kg against their body weight. The line here represents the best-fit line through the data, which approximates the overall trend of the data most completely. There are various distance measures used to calculate this line. Most typically the least squares approach is used, as in linear regression (discussed later).

Disclosure: Dr J. Hodsoll receives salary support from the National Institute for Health Research (NIHR) Mental Health Biomedical Research Center at South London and Maudsley NHS Foundation Trust and King's College London. This article is independent research part funded by the National Institute for Health Research (NIHR) Biomedical Research Centre at South London and Maudsley NHS Foundation Trust and King's College London. The views expressed are those of the author(s) and not necessarily those of the NHS, the NIHR or the Department of Health. Department of Biostatistics, Institute of Psychiatry, Psychology & Neuroscience, King's College London, 16 De Crespigny Park, London SE5 8AF, UK
* Corresponding author.
E-mail address: john.hodsoll@kcl.ac.uk

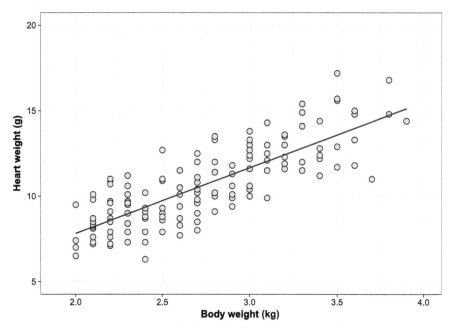

Fig. 1. Linear association between body and heart weight in a sample of adult cats weighing more than 2 kg.

The value of graphical analysis can be shown in **Fig. 2**, which shows 4 data sets created by the statistician Anscombe, each with 2 random variables X and Y.[1] Each of the variables in the 4 data sets have very similar descriptive statistics; the mean and standard deviation are the same, as is (of particular relevance) the linear line of best fit. However, the relationship between the 2 variables in the 4 data sets is very different and this becomes clear when the associations are inspected visually. Only example 2A is a good candidate for linear correlation or regression. For 2B, the relationship between X and Y is curvilinear or quadratic, set 2C has a large outlier, and for 2D there is no variability in X apart from 1 large observation.

CORRELATION

Correlation assesses the strength of an association between 2 random variables. For linear associations between 2 continuous variables, the appropriate statistic is the Pearson product moment correlation coefficient (commonly referred to as r). The value for r estimates how 2 random normally distributed variables X and Y covary with one another or how variations in one variable are related to variations in the other. For example, for a particular animal, whether a value exceeding the mean for one variable suggests a value higher than the mean for another variable. Alternatively, it may imply a value less than the mean or no systematic relationship. The correlation coefficient is calculated as the covariance divided by the standard deviations for the two variables, and ranges from -1 to 1. Variables are positively correlated if, when x increases, y also increases, or if, when x decreases, y also decreases. A negative correlation between 2 variables is identified when, as X increases, Y decreases, or as X decreases, Y increases. As such, calculation of r allows measurement of the extent to which knowing the value of X helps to predict the value of Y. It is scaled according to standard deviation, and the value is independent of the units of measurement for X and Y.

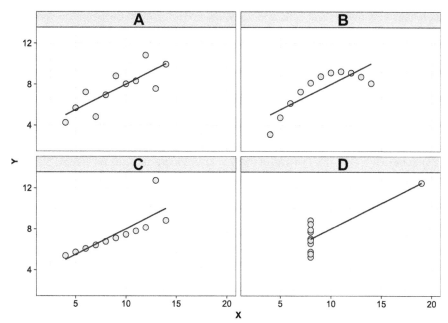

Fig. 2. Scatter plots of the Anscombe quartet. The data sets are difficult to tell apart with simple descriptive statistics but differences are seen clearly on plots. (*A*) Linear relationship, appropriate for linear regression. (*B*) Curvilinear relationship. (*C*) Large outlier in Y. (*D*) No variability in X apart from 1 observation.

Fig. 3 shows scatter plots and best-fit lines for various correlation coefficients. In 3A, there is a perfect negative correlation. Increases in Y are matched by decreases in X or decreases in Y are matched by increases in X. 3B shows a perfect positive correlation of 1, in which increases or decreases in Y are matched by increases or

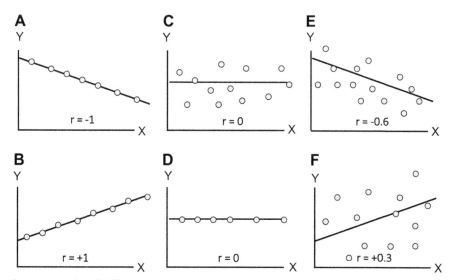

Fig. 3. Examples of different types of correlation between variables in terms of strength and direction. (*A*) r = -1; (*B*) r = 1; (*C*) r = 0; (*D*) r = 0; (*E*) r = -0.6; (*F*) r = 0.3.

decreases in X respectively. 3C and 3D show no association between the variables ($r = 0$). In the first there is no consistent change in Y across the values of X. In the second there is no change in y for the different values of x. The final 2 plots (3E and 3F) show intermediate negative and positive correlations and show the amount of variation around the line. Strong associations show little spread around the line, whereas weak associations show a wide spread. As a general rule, r values of 0.5, 0.3, and 0.1 indicate strong, moderate, and weak associations.[2]

To generalize from sample to population it is possible to set up a hypothesis test to determine whether the correlation coefficient is different from 0. A P-value can be determined from the t-distribution with degrees of freedom determined by the number of observations minus 2 (n – 2). The size of the p-value strongly depends on sample size. For example, to be significant at the 0.05 level with a 2-tailed test, a sample size of 50 would mean that a moderate correlation coefficient of 0.28 would be significant. A sample size of 16 would be needed to conclude that a strong correlation of 0.5 is different from chance. Alternatively, a large sample of 1000 could detect a correlation as small as 0.062. Although it can be important to determine whether the correlation is different from chance, it is important to know whether the size of the correlation is meaningful. One way to interpret correlation coefficients is using the coefficient of variation, which is r^2. This value can be interpreted as the amount of variance that 2 variables share. A moderate correlation of 0.3 translates to a coefficient of variation of $0.3^2 = 0.09$. Each variable explains 9% of the variance in the other; they have a shared variance of 9%. A further aid to interpretation is calculating confidence intervals to give the range of possible values of r. However, generic confidence intervals are based on the assumption that the parameter to be estimated is normally distributed, but correlation coefficients have a skewed distribution with the degree of skew dependent on the size of r. Confidence intervals must thus be calculated using the Fisher Z-transformation.[3]

The assumptions of the Pearson correlation coefficient are that both variables are continuous and normally distributed and that the relationship between them is linear. In **Fig. 2**, plots B to D show scenarios in which these assumptions do not hold. If the data do not conform to the assumptions of linear correlation, one option is to use alternative forms of correlation coefficient that are more appropriate to the data. **Table 1** shows different types of correlation coefficient matched to different types of data. In addition, the polychoric and tetrachoric correlation coefficients are appropriate if categorical variables reflect discretization of an underlying continuous latent variable.[4]

SIMPLE LINEAR REGRESSION

Correlation gives an estimate of the strength of association between 2 variables. Linear regression allows investigators to find the best-fit straight line describing the association between 2 numerical variables. The variable to be predicted is generally

Table 1 Correlation coefficients according to type of data	
Coefficient	Types of Variable
Pearson r	Both continuous
Spearman rank	Both ordinal
Phi	Both dichotomous
Biserial	1 continuous, 1 ordinal
Point biserial	1 continuous, 1 dichotomous
Rank biserial	1 ordinal, 1 dichotomous

called the dependent or outcome variable, with the predicting variable known as the predictor, independent, or explanatory variable. As for correlation, before formal analysis it is good practice to plot the data. By convention, the dependent variable is shown graphically on the y axis and the independent variable on the x axis. **Fig. 4** shows the hypothetical data set with the best-fit line superimposed.

The line of best fit is defined by the straight line equation seen in **Fig. 4**: expected value of $Y = \alpha + \beta X$.

However, the variability in the outcome is typically not just to do with the predictor or independent variable. Other variables affect Y and so the best-fit line describes the average or expected value of several values of Y. Individual observations differ from Y and the error term or residuals (ε, compare with **Fig. 4**) is the difference between the observed and predicted values. The best-fit line can be estimated in 2 ways. The first approach is called ordinary least squares and minimizes the squared deviation or distance between the data points and the fitted line. A more general method is called maximum likelihood estimation (MLE), which determines the line for which the data would most likely have occurred. For maximum likelihood, the distribution of the errors is needed. If the errors are normally distributed, MLE is equivalent to ordinary least squares and the estimated model parameters are the same.

The parameter of interest in the regression line is most commonly β, the slope of the line. The key statistical hypothesis of regression is whether the change estimate β is different from 0. No association usually follows from a horizontal straight line (see **Fig. 3**C and D). The intercept is interpreted as the mean value of Y at the minimum value of X (often 0). The regression intercept and coefficient for the cat heart weight versus body weight example are shown in **Table 2**. Here, there is strong evidence of an association between body and heart weight for cats. Each change of 1 kg in body

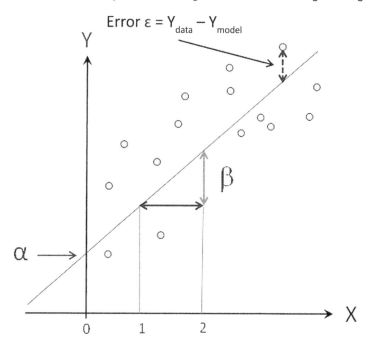

Fig. 4. Understanding the regression line and how it relates to the observed data. Y, scalar outcome variable; α, intercept or value of Y when X = 0; β, slope of line or how Y changes with unit changes in X; X, explanatory variable.

Table 2
Regression table for heart weight versus body weight for cats weighing more than 2 kg

	Coefficient	SE	t	P	95% CI
Body Weight (kg)	3.85	0.24	15.7	<0.001	3.36, 4.33
Intercept	0.12	0.67	−0.18	0.861	−1.21, 1.45

Abbreviations: CI, confidence interval; SE, standard error.

weight is associated with a change of 3.85 g in heart weight. The 95% confidence interval differs by 0.5 g in each direction, indicating a low degree of uncertainty in the estimate.

The regression line can be used to predict the expected values of Y based on X. In the example here, the regression equation would be Y = 0.12 + 3.85 X. Thus a cat of 3 kg would have an expected heart weight of 0.12 + 11.55 = 11.7g.

In correlation analysis, the larger the values of r the less variability of the data around the line. In regression, the spread of the data around the line of best fit is indicated by the coefficient of determination, R^2 (the square root of R-squared is equivalent to the correlation coefficient). As for correlation, it is the variability of the regression line around the mean of Y as a proportion of the total variance around the mean. Hypothesis tests for R^2 derive p-values obtained from the F-distribution. Used as such, the F-test can compare regression models and here is equivalent to comparison with a model with just an intercept in which there is no relation between Y and X. The R^2 statistic has an additional functional role in multiple regression (detailed later).

Binary and Categorical Variables

It is possible to use binary and categorical variables as predictors. The simplest case is for binary variables in which there are 2 groups. One group is assigned to the value 1 and the other 0; for example, gender could be coded as 1 for female and 0 for male. The regression line now connects the mean of the 2 groups and the beta coefficient in the regression model represents the group difference between the two. The intercept now represents the mean value of Y for the group coded 0.

Variables with multiple categories can be represented by dummy coding the categories with multiple binary variables. Each binary variable represents a level of the categorical variable. With k categories, k − 1 binary variables will be needed with the noncoded category being the reference level. Note that the regression coefficients in this case represent the mean difference between each category and the chosen reference level. **Table 3** shows an example for rectal temperature categories for

Table 3
Dummy coding of categorical body temperature of rabbits

Rabbit	Temperature Category	Hypothermic (<38°C)	Normothermic (≥38°C and ≤40°C)	Hyperthermic (>40°C)
1	Hypothermic	1	0	0
2	Hypothermic	1	0	0
3	Normothermic	0	1	0
4	Normothermic	0	1	0
5	Hyperthermic	0	0	1
6	Hyperthermic	0	0	1

rabbits (hypothermic, normothermic, and hyperthermic),[5] derived from the continuous temperature variable.

Assumptions of Linear Regression

The assumptions of linear regression are not about the dependent variable alone but about the distribution of Y given the values of the independent variable X. The upshot of this is that the investigator needs to take out the effects of X on Y and then look at the distribution of the remainder, otherwise known as the residuals or error terms. The 4 basic assumptions of linear regression are:

1. The relationship between the independent variable and dependent variable is linear.
2. The variance of residuals are constant across values of X (homoscedasticity).
3. Observations are independent.
4. Residuals are normally distributed.

The graphical analysis in **Fig. 5** shows how violations of these assumptions might look. **Fig. 5B** shows a typical example with nonconstant variance, with the variability of the errors increasing with the fitted values. 5C shows an example of residuals that are not independent and 5D shows how residuals might look if the relationship between Y an X is nonlinear. Returning to **Fig. 2C**, this shows a clear outlier and an important consideration is how influential these points can be on model parameters.

If the data do not meet the assumptions, various options are possible before the analysis is discounted. For nonconstant variance, a transformation of the dependent variable or predictor may help. Note that, if the sample size is large, then the model may not be sensitive to violations of the assumptions. More complex models may be required to explore nonlinearity and nonindependence. For example, repeated measures on the

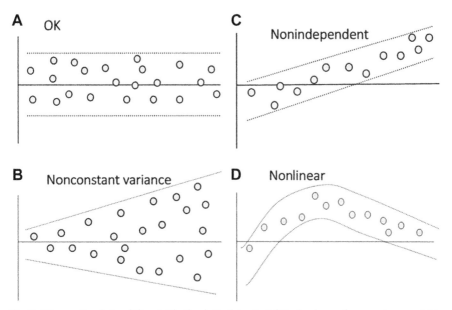

Fig. 5. Diagnostic plots of the residuals plotted against fitted values of regression model to check regression assumptions. Only panel (A) suggests the data fit with assumptions. (A) Residuals which are independent and of constant variance across X. (B) Residuals with nonconstant variance. (C) Residuals related to X. (D) Residuals non-linearly related to X.

same individual can be investigated using linear mixed effects models.[6] For outliers, there may be mistakes in the data set that can be corrected and a sensitivity analysis with outliers excluded can be performed to see whether the results change.

MULTIPLE REGRESSION

In simple linear regression, the association between an outcome and 1 independent variable (or exposure) is evaluated. However, in some cases it may be desirable to model the association between several independent variables and the outcome rather than just 1. Multiple linear regression extends the simple model by allowing 2 or more independent variables to be included in the model. In general, there are 2 reasons for wanting to do this. First, to control confounding of associations between variables of interest, to ensure that the association between variable and outcome is solely identified with that variable. For example, in comparing the weight outcome of groups on some exposure variable (eg, diet), there may be other variables that may relate to the outcome, such as gender, age, or area of living quarters, which need to be taken into account. If groups differ in age as well as diet, it becomes unclear which of the 2 variables is determining differences in weight between the groups. Including age in the regression model allows the effects of diet to be estimated controlling or adjusting for differences in weight between the groups. The second reason is that the uncertainties for parameter estimates in a regression model depend on the variability of the residuals or error terms. For larger residual error, the parameter estimates are more uncertain. Including more explanatory variables in the model can reduce the residual error, increasing the precision of estimates and the statistical power. Reducing error means that any true differences associated with hypothesis tests will be more likely to be found if true. However, there is no such thing as a free lunch: inclusion of too many variables leads to overfitting (discussed later) and difficulties in interpretation.

The basic form of the regression model is similar between simple and multiple regression. In both cases there is only 1 intercept with the addition of extra variables (each requiring an additional coefficient) for multiple regression. The following analysis is based on data from Di Girolamo and colleagues[5] on the prognostic value of temperature on outcomes for hospitalized rabbits. The analysis here is of the association of age, weight, and disease status with body temperature on admission to hospital. **Table 4** shows the

Table 4
Multiple regression for temperature of rabbits against age, weight, and disease status

	B (95% CI)	P	B (95% CI)	P	B (95% CI)	P
Intercept	38.2 (38.0–38.5)	<0.001	37.3 (36.7, 37.8)	<0.001	37.7 (37.1, 38.2)	<0.001
Age (y)	−0.08 (−0.13, −0.02)	0.011	−0.09 (−0.15, −0.04)	0.001	−0.07 (−0.13, −0.01)	0.016
Weight (kg)	—	—	0.62 (0.33, 0.91)	<0.001	0.57 (0.29, 0.86)	<0.001
Disease Status (Yes/No)	—	—	—	—	−0.64 (−0.98, −0.29)	<0.001
Observations	274	—	274	—	274	—
R^2/adjusted R^2	0.024/0.020	—	0.084/0.077	—	0.126/0.116	—
F-statistics	6.6[a]	—	12.5[b]	—	13.0[b]	—

[a] $P<0.05$.
[b] $P<0.001$.

coefficients resulting from fitting 3 models (as might be found in a journal article). The interpretation of the coefficients now being the association between the predictor variable and outcome, adjusted for the effects of the other variable in the model. The effect of disease status in **Table 4** shows the difference in temperature for diseased versus nondiseased rabbits, controlling for any differences in age and weight. Again, overall model fit can be calculated using coefficient of variation R^2, giving the percentage of variation in the Y variable explained by the predictor variables. In addition, the change in R^2 can be calculated, which gives the additional variance explained for each variable.

Multicollinearity

Multiple regression has the same assumptions as simple linear regression, but multicollinearity between predictor variables may also be an issue. Predictors in multiple regression should be strongly correlated with the outcome variable but weakly correlated with each other. Strongly correlated ($r>0.75$) variables are often measuring the same thing and are associated with the same variance in the dependent variable. Computing the model estimates using the least square fit algorithm becomes imprecise, greatly increasing the standard errors and confidence intervals for the individual parameter estimates. Inflated standard errors and variable coefficients changing substantially when another variable is added to the regression model are signs of multicollinearity. A more formal way to assess multicollinearity is to calculate the variance inflation factor (VIF), which estimates how much a coefficient is inflated because of linear correlation with other variables. A VIF of 2 indicates that the variance of a coefficient is twice as large as it would be if it was uncorrelated with the other variables. As a general rule, VIF greater than 10 suggests high multicollinearity.[7] Options to deal with high multicollinearity are (1) to remove redundant variables from the model (as providing the same information), and (2) leave variables in and highlight the presence of multicollinearity. Only individual parameter estimates are affected by multicollinearity; it has no effect on overall model fit or R^2.

Overfitting

Another important issue in multiple regression is overfitting. The key point is that independent variables in the regression model are explaining random error rather than systematic variance. When this happens, associations are not true associations and cannot be generalized or replicated in other data sets. This situation can happen when the model is excessively complex; for example, if there are a small number of observations relative to the number of variables. In general, having 10 observations for each variable is considered reasonable as a general rule, and ensuring that this is the case may be the simplest way to avoid overfitting. Another solution is to use metrics for evaluating how well the regression models fit the data, which are penalized according to the number of variables in the model, with the more variables the greater the penalty. For example, the adjusted R^2 in **Table 4**. Aggregating variables and other data reduction procedures can alleviate the problem, as can having a defined list of candidate variables a priori.[8]

LOGISTIC REGRESSION

Frequently in the clinical literature, the outcome is a binary variable such as mortality or diagnosis, with the event typically coded as 1 and the nonoccurrence of the event by 0. In modeling such an outcome, investigators are interested in the probability of an event occurring. Although in some scenarios it is appropriate to use linear regression, in general the assumptions of the normality of the residuals and homoscedasticity of variance are not met. Furthermore, predicted values of probabilities may be outside the bounds of 0 and 1. Logistic regression relaxes these assumptions by modeling the outcome using the binomial distribution and linking the outcome to the linear predictor by the logit function or the logarithm of the odds. Key to understanding logistic regression is the concept of odds ratios.

Odds Ratios

Odds ratios are very closely related to the relative risk ratios, which give the risk (or probability of an event) in one condition relative to the risk in another. The preference for odds ratios rather than risk ratios is based on their better mathematical properties. The odds of an event are the probability of an event occurring over the probability of the event not occurring. For example, in the rabbit prognostic data set used earlier, the probability or risk of death during hospitalization is 0.3 and the risk of not dying is 0.7. Thus, the odds of death are 0.3 / 0.7 = 0.43. In more concrete terms, for every 43 rabbits that die in hospital, 100 survive. Odds ratios show the odds of an event in one condition relative to the other; that is, the odds of 1 event in a certain condition divided by the other (condition). So if the odds of death for diseased rabbits is 0.73 and for nondiseased rabbits is 0.08, the odds of death are 0.73 / 0.08 = 9.1 times higher for diseased than nondiseased rabbits. For rare events, odds and relative risk ratios are numerically about the same.

Logistic Regression in Practice: Interpreting Model Parameters

Using odds ratios, logistic regression allows the association between the probability of an outcome or event and candidate variables of interest to be understood. Conceptually the idea is similar to multiple regression, with the difference that the model coefficients are log odds ratios rather than unit change on the outcome scale. Log odds ratios can be transformed to odds ratios by exponentiation, which makes them easier to interpret. This example starts with the 2-parameter case from the rabbit mortality data set and interprets the coefficients in concrete terms, as described earlier. **Table 5** shows the outcome of the regression of disease state and temperature with mortality as the dependent variable with both the log odds ratios, as in a fitted model output, and the exponentiated odds ratios.

The easiest to interpret are categorical predictors. In the example here, disease state has a strong association with mortality. The odds of dying for a rabbit admitted to hospital with a positive disease diagnosis are almost 6 times the odds of dying for a nondiseased rabbit. In more concrete terms, for every nondiseased rabbit that dies, 6 diseased rabbits die. Note that, as in multiple regression, the interpretation of disease is the effect of disease state, controlling for rectal temperature. For continuous variables, the interpretation is the change in odds ratio for each unit increase in the measure. Here, in terms of temperature, each 1°C increase in rectal temperature decreased the odds of death by 0.55, or alternatively a 45% decrease. To facilitate interpretation, it can be useful to calculate the odds over a meaningful interval, with odds ratios raised to the power of the interval size. For example, for an increase of 2°C, the odds ratio would be $(0.55)^2 = 0.30$. To interpret this in more concrete terms,

Table 5
Logistic regression model for death (yes or no) versus disease state and temperature. Parameter estimates and 95% confidence intervals are log odds ratios

Variable	Log Odds	95% CI	z	P	Odds Ratio	95% CI
Intercept	−2.3	−3.17, −1.59	−5.79	<0.001	0.10	0.04, 0.20
Disease Status (Yes/No)	1.78	0.99, 2.71	4.11	<0.001	5.94	2.69, 15.1
Temperature (°C)	−0.59	−0.83, −0.37	−4.95	<0.001	0.55	0.43, 0.69

for every 30 rabbits admitted with a temperature of 39°C that die, 100 rabbits admitted with a temperature of 37°C die. Alternatively, continuous measures can be dichotomized in a meaningful way. Di Girolamo and colleagues[5] dichotomotized the temperature scale for hypothermic (<38°C) versus greater than or equal to normothermic and (≥38°C), giving an odds ratio of 5.4 hypothermic rabbits versus normothermic. However, this involves refitting the model with temperature as a binary categorical variable.

Estimating a Logistic Regression Model

The coefficients in a logistic regression are estimated using MLE, with the errors or residuals assumed to follow the binomial distribution. As stated earlier, the likelihood is the probability of observing a set of data given the model parameters. Changes in the value of the likelihood can be used to statistically assess whether adding variables to a model improves model fit, and the likelihood can also be used to test overall model fit.

Overall Model Fit and Model Assumptions

As for linear regression, it is important to understand how the logistic regression model is performing; that is, how well the predicted and observed values match. The log likelihood χ^2 test test is constructed from the difference between the log likelihood of an intercept-only model (with no explanatory variables) and the model of interest. This test can be used as an omnibus test of model fit with a large p-value indicating no difference between the models. Further, it is possible to calculate a pseudo-R^2, which is based on the proportion of the likelihood rather than variance explained; for example, the Cox and Snell or Nagelkerke R^2 statistics. One caveat is that different versions of pseudo-R^2 can produce different values for the same data set and model. The Hosmer-Lemeshow test takes a different approach by calculating the Pearson χ^2 test from the (model) predicted and observed frequency table. A good fit is determined by large p-values.

Although the assumptions of constant variance and normality of residuals are relaxed in logistic regression, the assumptions of (1) linear association between the log odds of the dependent variable and the explanatory variables, and (2) independence of observations are still necessary. Evaluation of residuals focusses on identifying influential observations using deviance or Pearson residuals. These residuals are transformed residuals because the raw data residuals do not have particularly good properties. As for multiple linear regression, multicollinearity can be a problem in logistic regression. However, the approach to dealing with this issue is largely the same as for multiple regression (calculate VIF and deal with any redundant information).

SUMMARY

The association between 2 or more variables can be assessed with correlation or, more generally, regression models. The choice of which to use depends on the objectives of the research, with correlation allowing investigators to describe the strength of the association and regression, allowing more complex modeling of the relationship as well as generating predictions of outcomes depending on predictors. In all cases, the assumptions underlying the application of the techniques to the data should be critically assessed.

REFERENCES

1. Anscombe FJ. Graphs in statistical analysis. Am Stat 1973;27(1):17–21.
2. Cohen J. Statistical power analysis for the behavioral sciences. 2nd edition. Hillsdale (NJ): Erlbaum; 1988.

3. Mudholkar GS. Fisher's Z-transformation. Encyclopedia of statistical sciences. 4. Hoboken (NJ): Wiley; 2006.
4. Hershberger SL. Polychoric correlation, tetrachoric correlation. Encyclopedia of statistics in behavioral science. Hoboken (NJ): Wiley-Blackwell; 2005.
5. Di Girolamo N, Toth G, Selleri P. Prognostic value of rectal temperature at hospital admission in client-owned rabbits. J Am Vet Med Assoc 2016;248(3):288–97.
6. Leyland AH, Goldstein H. Multilevel modelling of health statistics. Chichester (UK): Wiley; 2001.
7. Allison PD. Multiple regression: a primer. Thousand Oaks (CA): Pine Forge Press; 1999.
8. Babyak MA. What you see may not be what you get: a brief, nontechnical introduction to overfitting in regression-type models. Psychosom Med 2004;66(3):411–21.

An Introduction to Systematic Reviews and Meta-Analyses for Exotic Animal Practitioners

Reint Meursinge Reynders, DDS, MS (Oral Biology),
MSc (Evidence-Based Health Care), PhD[a,b,*]

KEYWORDS

- Systematic review • Meta-analysis • Risk of bias • Applicability
- Veterinary medicine • Limitations • Guidelines

KEY POINTS

- Developing and conducting systematic reviews and meta-analyses is a complex process.
- How to develop, conduct, and report these research studies is discussed.
- Veterinary clinicians should seek systematic reviews to address their research questions.
- Criteria for including meta-analyses in a systematic review are also presented.
- Before applying the findings of systematic reviews and meta-analyses to a particular patient, clinicians should weigh a variety of issues. Consulting high-quality systematic reviews is particularly important in this context.

CHARACTERISTICS OF SYSTEMATIC REVIEWS AND META-ANALYSES
Introduction

Systematic reviews synthesize the current best evidence on a particular research question and are considered to provide the highest level of medical evidence.[1,2] This top validity ranking depends on the quality of conducting and reporting of these reviews. Cochrane systematic reviews of interventions are regarded as the reference standard for performing and reporting such reviews.[3]

Conducting systematic reviews of clinical studies has become common practice in medicine since the early 1990s and forms the foundation of evidence-based medicine.

Disclosure Statement: The author has nothing to disclose.
[a] Department of Oral and Maxillofacial Surgery, Academic Medical Center, University of Amsterdam, Meibergdreef 9, Amsterdam 1105 AZ, The Netherlands; [b] Private Practice of Orthodontics, Via Matteo Bandello 15, Milan 20123, Italy
* Department of Oral and Maxillofacial Surgery, Academic Medical Center, University of Amsterdam, Meibergdreef 9, Amsterdam 1105 AZ, The Netherlands.
E-mail address: reyndersmail@gmail.com

Vet Clin Exot Anim 20 (2017) 973–995
http://dx.doi.org/10.1016/j.cvex.2017.04.005
1094-9194/17/© 2017 Elsevier Inc. All rights reserved.

The number of PubMed-indexed articles labeled "Systematic Review" or "Meta-analysis" has been growing exponentially since 1986 to more than 28,000 new articles published in 2014 alone.[4] Veterinary medicine has been slower at adopting these reviews than human health care,[5] but a database of veterinary systematic reviews is now available.[6]

This article (1) explains what systematic reviews and meta-analyses do and how they differ from narrative reviews, (2) assesses their strengths and limitations, and (3) gives an overview of how to conduct and report them and how to implement their findings in clinical practice. This article provides an introduction to these research procedures.

Systematic Reviews Versus Narrative Reviews

Before the 1990s data from multiple studies were synthesized in narrative reviews, which were usually conducted by a single topic expert.[7] These traditional reviews have several limitations,[7,8] such as (1) personal bias of the reviewer; (2) bias in the selection of studies and the extraction and analysis of data; (3) difficulty in reproducing these reviews, because methods are often not systematic and transparent; (4) becoming less useful when large numbers of studies are available, because in those circumstances it becomes difficult to assess the appropriate weight of individual studies and how different covariates influence outcomes.[7]

To avoid these limitations, researchers from the 1990s onward have moved away from narrative reviews and have started to implement systematic reviews. The differences between narrative and a high-quality systematic review are presented in **Table 1**.[5,9–11] The parameter of high quality is a crucial characteristic of a systematic review, as explained later. The 4 key principles on which systematic reviews are based are (1) systematic use of tested research methods, (2) methodologic rigor, (3) transparency, and (4) reproducibility.[8,9,12] Systematic reviews have been adopted by various sciences,[2] but this article focusses exclusively on such reviews in health care.

Why Systematic Reviews Are Important and for Whom

Systematic reviews are important for a variety of reasons: (1) unlike single studies, systematic reviews are representative of the total body of evidence on a research question and provide the highest level of evidence[1,2]; (2) systematic reviews assign a quality score to the total body of evidence, which is essential for the confidence in their outcomes; (3) a systematic review accompanied by a meta-analysis facilitates decision making, because it provides the best estimate of the effect and its precision; (4) systematic reviews include a broader range of patients than individual studies, and their outcomes therefore generally have a wider external validity; (5) they save considerable time, energy, and resources for a wide variety of stakeholders (this issue should be considered in the context of the unmanageable amounts of health care research that are published every year and that searching of the literature and critically appraising research evidence requires specific knowledge and skills[2,12]); and (6) systematic reviews identify the current knowledge status on a specific health issue. This information helps to plan future research agendas. For example, when the quality of evidence is high, no further research is probably necessary on this topic, which avoids wasting additional resources. In contrast, when the quality of evidence is low, researchers can learn from the deficiencies of the eligible studies by improving research methods and possibly fine-tuning or even formulating new research questions.

These 6 reasons explain why systematic reviews are so important for medical decision making and for developing clinical guidelines.[13] Health care providers,

Table 1
High-quality systematic reviews versus narrative reviews[a,b]

Item	High-Quality Systematic Reviews	Narrative Reviews
Operators	At least 2 topic experts, a methodologist, and an information specialist	1 or more topic experts
Research question	Focused and explicit questions according to the PICO acronym[b]	Often broad-scope question and not explicit
Protocol of the research methods	Always present and registered or published	Seldom present
Eligibility criteria	Defined in great detail	Usually not defined
Information sources and study selection	Systematic search of all eligible studies (if possible) in a wide variety of information sources according to a predefined search strategy by at least 2 topic experts	A usually nonextensive and potentially biased selection of studies
Data extraction	Systematic data extraction by at least 2 topic experts	Potentially biased
Risk of bias assessment	Assessment of bias with a tested risk of bias tool by at least 2 topic experts	Risk of personal bias of the reviewer
Study results	Full and transparent reporting of all predefined outcomes and other relevant results	Often selective reporting of outcomes according to the interpretation of the reviewer
Synthesis of findings	Always a narrative synthesis that considers variables such as heterogeneity and risk of bias. A quantitative synthesis (meta-analysis) is conducted when specific criteria are met	Often only a narrative synthesis without statistical analyses. The weight that is given to a given study could easily be misinterpreted because of personal bias
Quality rating	Always a rating of the quality of the total body of evidence	Often no rating of the quality
Conclusions	Based on the totality of evidence and considering the risk of bias and other study limitations	Often not based on the totality of evidence and often without considering bias and other study limitations
Research methods overall	Use of tested, systematic, and transparent research methods that are reproducible	Not systematic and not transparent research methods and therefore difficult to reproduce
Reporting overall	Transparent, systematic, and full reporting of research methods and outcomes, thereby facilitating its reproducibility	Often poor reporting of research methods and outcomes and therefore difficult to reproduce

[a] High quality is an important parameter, because low-quality systematic reviews can be damaging.[4]
[b] The acronym PICO stands for participants, interventions, comparisons, and outcomes.
Data from Refs.[5,9–11]

consumers, researchers, guideline developers, policy makers, and research sponsors all benefit from the findings of systematic reviews[12] and this applies to both human and veterinary medicine.

Types of Systematic Reviews in the Health Care Sciences

Systematic reviews in the health care sciences are evolving fast. Initially these reviews were mostly limited to studies that measure the effects of interventions, but now systematic reviews are also used to assess outcomes of clinical tests, public health and health promotion interventions, research on adverse effects, economic evaluations, diagnostic accuracy tests, individual patients, incidence and prevalence studies, prognostic studies, qualitative research, and so forth.[14–18] Special types of reviews, such as overviews of systematic reviews and rapid reviews, have also been developed to address specific demands. Overviews of systematic reviews have been developed by the Cochrane Collaboration to compile evidence from multiple systematic reviews of interventions.[19] Rapid reviews are important when decisions on health care issues cannot be delayed; for example, on the Ebola epidemic.[20]

What Are Meta-Analyses, Why They Are Important, and for Whom

A meta-analysis uses specific statistical techniques to combine and summarize outcomes of multiple studies.[13] Combining the results of these studies increases the overall sample size and therefore the power of the outcome of interest. To perform such an analysis, the following steps are made: (1) compute the pertinent outcome and variance for each eligible study, then (2) compute a weighted mean of these outcomes.[21] More weight is assigned to the more precise studies (ie, the larger studies).

When used appropriately, meta-analyses can be powerful tools because they can (1) improve statistical power by summarizing results from multiple studies (this is particularly useful when the sample sizes of the included studies are small); (2) improve precision of the effect size (summary effect); (3) answer questions that are not posed or evident in the single eligible studies; (4) show the possibility of conducting subgroup analyses; and (5) determine whether additional studies are indicated and help develop new research questions.[7,22,23] Meta-analyses can provide valuable information for clinicians, patients, researchers, policy makers, guideline developers, and research sponsors.[23]

Fig. 1 presents a hypothetical example of a forest plot with a meta-analysis on the risk of death among ferrets as a result of administering the hypothetical drug X versus a placebo drug. The effect size (risk ratio) is calculated for each individual study (A–E) and is represented by the blue square boxes. The black diamond at the bottom of the forest plot represents the meta-analysis. In **Fig. 2**, the number of events and the number of total events in study B (and not in the other studies) were increased by 6 times to show their effects on several statistics. Various features of forest plots with and without meta-analyses are explained in **Table 2** using **Figs. 1** and **2** as examples.[24–28]

Criteria for Conducting Meta-Analyses

Not all systematic reviews include meta-analyses. Reviewers should consider a series of criteria for whether to conduct a meta-analysis or not. Well-documented criteria for undertaking meta-analyses include (1) summarizing the same outcome measures for individual studies (if this is not possible, outcome measures should be standardized to a uniform scale,[22] and if this is also not possible a meta-analysis should not be conducted, because summarizing different outcomes is like mixing a banana with 10 different fruits and calling it a banana shake); (2) low heterogeneity between studies

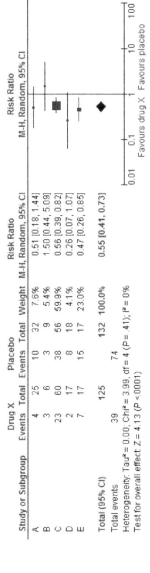

Fig. 1. Impact of drug X on death rates in ferrets. CI, confidence interval. M-H, Mantel-Haenszel.

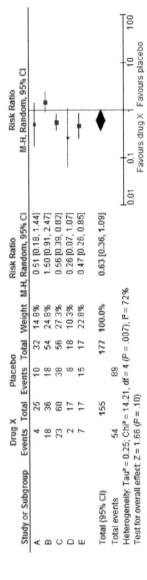

Fig. 2. Impact of drug X on death rates in ferrets (event rates and sample sizes in study B were increased by a factor of 6).

Table 2
Features of forest plots with or without meta-analyses

Item	Description
Drug X and the placebo	For drug X, the number of events (deaths) is presented among the total number of events (death and alive) for all eligible studies A–E. The same events are also listed for the placebo group
Effect size	The effect sizes in **Figs. 1** and **2** are the risk ratio, which reflects the magnitude of the treatment effect in each study. A risk ratio of 1.0 means that the risk of death is the same for both treatment groups (drug X and placebo). A risk ratio <1 indicates fewer events (death) among the patients who received drug X compared with those in the placebo group
Weight and precision	The percentage of the study weight among the eligible studies is assigned to each individual study and adds up to 100%. The higher the precision (the narrower the CIs), the larger the weight. Because precision is primarily driven by sample size, more weight is assigned to the larger studies. Precision is also affected by the design of the study and other unique factors[24]
Fixed-effect vs random-effects models	Two models are used to assign weight to individual studies, which are based on specific assumptions about the distribution of the effect sizes of the individual studies. For the fixed-effect model, it is assumed that all eligible studies share the same common true effect size, whereas the random-effects model assumes that the true effect sizes differ from study to study. Additional explanation of these models goes beyond the objectives of this article
Interpreting effect sizes in forest plots and meta-analyses	• The forest plots of **Figs. 1** and **2** consist of blue square boxes (the effect sizes [ie, the risk ratios] of each individual study) and the black diamond (the meta-analysis; ie, the weighted summary effect size). The larger the weight of the individual study, the larger the blue square boxes • Researchers have to decide whether the criteria for conducting a meta-analysis are met. If not, they should opt to present just the forest plot without the meta-analysis (without the summary diamond) • An effect size to the left of the vertical line (ie, risk ratio <1) favors drug X, meaning a lower risk of death when using drug X compared with placebo • The horizontal lines that cross these blue square boxes are the CIs, which represent the precision of the effect size (risk ratio). The wider the CIs, the less precise is the effect size. When the CIs cross the vertical line (risk ratio = 1), this indicates that there is no significant difference (CI 95%) in the risk of death between drug X and placebo (eg, studies A, B, and D) • The summary diamond at the bottom of the forest plot represents the meta-analysis; ie, the weighted effect size of the 5 studies combined. When the diamond crosses the vertical line (risk ratio = 1), this indicates that there is no significant difference in the overall risk (for all 5 studies combined) of death between drug X and placebo treatment. In **Fig. 2** this diamond crosses the vertical line • In **Figs. 1** and **2**, a meta-analysis is shown for the summary risk ratio. In **Fig. 1**, a risk ratio of 0.55 (95% CI = 0.41–0.73) was calculated; ie, 45% less risk of death when drug X is administered. The test for the overall effect had a Z = 4.13 and a $P<.0001$, indicating a significant difference in risk of death between drug X and placebo; ie, the likelihood of obtaining such a difference is <1 in 10,000. This outcome is visualized by the diamond that does not cross the vertical line (risk ratio = 1)

(continued on next page)

Table 2
(continued)

Item	Description
Interpreting heterogeneity in forest plots	Forest plots are also used to visualize inconsistency (heterogeneity) between studies. The forest plot in **Fig. 1** shows that the effect sizes are reasonably consistent (range, 0.26–0.56) between studies except for study B. This visualization was shown by the overlapping CIs and confirmed by the statistical assessment of heterogeneity. A χ^2 test was conducted for this purpose (null hypothesis: there is no heterogeneity). The calculated $P = .41$ showed that the null hypothesis could not be rejected. However, this test should be considered in the context that a nonsignificant P value ($P = .41$) does not provide sufficient evidence that effect sizes are consistent (no heterogeneity), because this statistic is strongly influenced by a lack of power; ie, small number of studies and small studies (small n) with large within-study variance[25] The I^2 statistic is a useful measure for inconsistency and depends on the extent of the overlap of the CIs of the eligible studies.[26–28] It represents the ratio of true heterogeneity to the total heterogeneity.[26,27] Approximate rules are presented to assign a rough quality to I^2.[22,27] For example, an $I^2 = 72\%$ (see **Fig. 2**) may represent substantial heterogeneity
Fig. 1 vs **Fig. 2**	The sample sizes and the number of events in **Figs. 1** and **2** are identical except for study B. In **Fig. 2**, all events and total events in study B were multiplied by a factor of 6. This increase in sample size had important effects on a variety of statistics: • The 95% CIs of study B were reduced from 0.44–5.09 (see **Fig. 1**) to 0.91–2.47 (see **Fig. 2**) indicating greater precision. Note that the effect size (1.50) of study B did not change • The weight of all eligible studies (A–E) changed • The summary effect size and the width of the CIs changed from RR 0.55 (95% CI = 0.41–0.73) to RR 0.63 (95% CI = 0.36–1.09). The summary diamond in **Fig. 2** crossed the vertical line and the test of the overall effect changed to Z = 1.66 ($P = .10$) indicating that there is no significant difference in the risk of death between drug X and placebo • The null hypothesis of no heterogeneity was rejected in **Fig. 2** (P went from .41 to .007) and I^2 went from 0% (see **Fig. 1**) to 72% (see **Fig. 2**) indicating that it may represent substantial heterogeneity[22,27]

Abbreviation: CI, confidence interval.

(eg, eligible studies should use the same treatments and comparators); (3) outcomes of the included studies should not be too diverse, and synthesizing outcomes with inconsistent directions should be avoided; (4) low risk of bias in the eligible studies; (5) low risk of publication and/or reporting biases; and (6) a high number of eligible studies, preferably with large sample sizes.[22,23,29] However, even applying these 6 criteria correctly is not enough, because the validity of a meta-analysis depends on the quality of the conduct of the systematic review. For example, poor defining of outcomes, searching and selecting of eligible studies, data extraction, data analyses, assessments of risk of bias, and so forth can jeopardize the validity of a review, especially when the outcomes of the eligible studies are synthesized in a meta-analysis. In this context it should be considered that the outcomes of 1 large, well-conducted randomized controlled trial on a specific population is more reliable for that population than a meta-analysis of numerous small studies with heterogeneous populations.[23]

Limitations of Systematic Reviews and Meta-Analyses

Suboptimal systematic reviews and meta-analyses are generally more harmful than poorly conducted single studies because of (1) their high-quality evidence rating and the associated trust in these publications,[4] and (2) their wide external validity. Ioannidis[4] reported that production of systematic reviews and meta-analyses has reached epidemic proportions[4,30]; he suggests that most of these studies are probably unnecessary, and/or are not carefully done, and/or are conducted with conflicts of interest. He summarized this disturbing picture as follows: "Few systematic reviews and meta-analyses are both non-misleading and useful."[4] Before implementing the findings of systematic reviews, clinicians should therefore critically appraise the validity of these articles using 1 or more of the following tools: Critical Appraisal Skills Programme (CASP), A Measurement Tool to Assess Systematic Reviews (AMSTAR), tool to assess Risk Of Bias In Systematic Reviews (ROBIS), Scottish Intercollegiate Guidelines Network (SIGN), and Graphic Approach To Epidemiology-Critical Appraised Topics (GATE-CAT).[31–36]

DEVELOPING, CONDUCTING, AND REPORTING OF SYSTEMATIC REVIEWS AND META-ANALYSES

The process of developing, conducting, and reporting of systematic reviews and meta-analyses consists of 4 action phases, which are outlined here (**Fig. 3**).[37–39]

Phase 1. Preparing of the Review

Phase 1 consists of 6 steps (see **Fig. 3**). These steps should be conducted iteratively with most steps providing feedback from a previous step or for a next step. This iterative process moves slowly forward until the eventual desired research questions and eligibility criteria are fine-tuned. These procedures should be conducted with great attention for detail, because the consequences of a revocation or modification of a research question or eligibility criteria or other items in the protocol could be costly and could downgrade the validity of the systematic review.

The review team

The review team preferably consist of at least 2 topic experts, an information specialist, a methodologist, and a statistician. Conflicts of interest of team members should be assessed and could be important exclusion criteria for certain stakeholders.[16]

Prioritizing research questions

Before developing review questions researchers should assess which questions are important for patients, because often there is a mismatch between questions that are relevant for patients and those asked by researchers.[40] Researchers should therefore consult with patients, caregivers, and clinicians and should subsequently prioritize the treatment uncertainties with these stakeholders.[41]

Formulating research questions and defining eligibility criteria

Research questions on interventions are generally formulated according to the PICO acronym, indicating the types of participants, interventions, comparisons, and outcomes (see J Hodsoll and colleagues' article, "Advanced Statistics for the Exotic Animal Practitioner," in this issue).[42] Other types of acronyms are also used and depend on the research topic and the type of question. For example, the acronym PIRT (patient, index test, reference standard, and target condition) is used for diagnostic accuracy questions.[43] *The Cochrane Handbook for Systematic Reviews of Interventions* recommends to limit the number of primary outcomes and to include both a beneficial and at least 1 adverse outcome into the primary research question.[42]

Phase 1. Preparing the review

- Creating a review team
- Prioritizing research questions for a systematic review
- Formulating initial research questions and eligibility criteria
- Assessing the need for undertaking a systematic review on the research question(s)
- Fine-tuning the research question(s) and eligibility criteria
- Finding research sponsors

Phase 2. Developing, registering, and publishing of the review protocol

- Consulting the PRISMA-P statement[37,38]
- Developing the review protocol
- Registering and/or publishing the review protocol

Phase 3. Conducting the systematic review

- Conducting the methods described in the protocol
- Possibly conducting methods that were not described in the protocol

Phase 4. Reporting of the systematic review

- Consulting the PRISMA statement[13,39]
- Reporting the introduction, methods, results, discussion and conclusions
- Reporting where (with rationale) methods differ from the protocol

Fig. 3. The 4 action phases of systematic reviews and meta-analyses. PRISMA-P, preferred reporting items for systematic review and meta-analysis protocols.

Inclusion and exclusion criteria of studies need to be carefully defined at the time of fine-tuning of the research questions.

Assessing the need for undertaking a systematic review
Before developing the review questions, researchers should conduct scoping searches to investigate whether systematic reviews on a particular health issue are

already available or are ongoing.[16,41] This step is particularly important, because systematic reviews typically take years to complete.[20] When such reviews exist, researchers should evaluate whether these reviews are up to date. If so, they should assess the quality and the risk of bias in these reviews using, respectively, the AMSTAR[34,35] and ROBIS tools.[44] In addition, researchers should assess what uncertainties still exist after these assessments and fine-tune research questions accordingly.[41] If a systematic review is of suboptimal quality, reproducing such a research study could also be a valid option.

Sponsors of systematic reviews
After having completed these 4 research steps, the research questions and eligibility criteria have to be fine-tuned. Subsequently, research sponsors can be searched. Conducting systematic reviews (depending on the research topic) is generally a time-consuming process and therefore costly.[20] Research sponsors should pay at least 2 investigators for the predicted time period for completing the review. Ideally, these sponsors should not have a conflict of interest but, if they do, these stakeholders should be strictly excluded from all research phases of the review as well as the publication phase.

Phase 2: Developing, Registering, and Publishing the Systematic Review Protocol
Rationale for developing a review protocol
Conducting a systematic review is complex, requires input from many different stakeholders, and involves many judgements.[45] Preparation in advance of a thorough review protocol is therefore indicated. A protocol is also developed to minimize the potential bias in the review process.[45] For example, prior knowledge of existing research studies and their outcomes could influence review investigators when formulating their research questions; defining study eligibility criteria; and selecting specific participants, interventions, comparisons, outcomes, and time points for measuring outcomes.

Rationale for registering and publishing a review protocol
Registering and publishing of the review protocol before conducting the systematic review is important, because it (1) reduces the risk of reviewer biases associated with prior knowledge of available studies, (2) improves the transparency of research methods, (3) reduces the risk of duplication, (4) allows peer reviewing of the research questions and methods, and (5) enables comparison of what is reported in the review and what was planned in the protocol.[45–47] Registering and publishing of the review protocol increases the reliability of the published review.[37] Review protocols in the health sciences should first be registered in the PROSPERO database[47] or in institutional repositories.[48–50] The Cochrane Library[51] and the journal *Systematic Reviews* publish entire protocols for the health sciences.[52]

Developing and reporting of a review protocol
Review investigators should first explore whether a specific guideline exists for conducting a systematic review on their type of research design. Such guidelines are available for systematic reviews of interventions, diagnostic accuracy tests, qualitative research, incidence and prevalence data, and so forth.[14–18] Besides these guidelines, reviewers should also carefully scrutinize *The Cochrane Handbook for Systematic Reviews of Interventions*, the guidance provided by the Centre for Reviews and Dissemination (CRD), and the PRISMA-P 2015 statement.[16,17,37,38] The PRISMA-P 2015 statement presents a detailed reporting guideline and a preferred reporting (17-item) checklist for protocols of systematic reviews and meta-analyses.

A systematic review protocol consists of 3 sections: (1) administrative information; (2) the introduction, which presents background information, the rationale, and the objectives of the review with an explicit statement of the review questions; and (3) the planned methodology.[38] In this article all 10 key items of the planned methodology are described: (1) eligibility criteria, (2) information sources, (3) search strategy, (4) study records, (5) data items, (6) outcomes and prioritization, (7) risk of bias in individual studies, (8) data synthesis, (9) meta-biases, and (10) confidence in the cumulative estimate.

The review questions and the eligibility criteria The prespecification of eligibility criteria for including and excluding studies is one of the key features that distinguishes a systematic review from the traditional narrative review. These criteria should be defined early in the review process; that is, during the development of the review questions (see phase 1). Transparent and careful defining of eligibility criteria is important for understanding what was done and is essential for reproducing and updating of systematic reviews. The type and number of eligibility criteria depend on the research topic and the type of question. Eligibility criteria are generally selected for (1) study designs, (2) participants, (3) interventions, (4) comparators, (5) outcomes, (6) timing, (7) setting, and (8) language.[38]

Information sources Searches in the information sources are responsible for identifying the relevant references to address the review questions (see J Hodsoll and colleagues' article, "Advanced Statistics for the Exotic Animal Practitioner," in this issue). Searching for eligibility studies in just 1 electronic database (eg, Pubmed [Medline]) is therefore not considered adequate because this can introduce publication bias and language bias. Reviewers should generally consult a wide variety of information sources, such as (1) electronic databases (eg, Veterinary Science Database,[53] Pubmed [Medline], VetSRev - database of veterinary systematic reviews[6]); (2) trial registers (3) gray literature databases, such as Google Scholar; (4) manual screening of references of review articles and eligible studies; and (5) correspondence with study investigators or researchers to identify unpublished or ongoing studies.[38] Selecting appropriate information sources is very question and topic sensitive. When choosing information sources, reviewers are advised to consult information specialists or health sciences librarians with experience in searches for systematic reviews.[54]

Search strategy Information specialists or health sciences librarians should also be consulted for developing search strategies. The Medline search strategy is generally developed first and is subsequently adapted to the other pertinent databases. Search strategies should aim for high sensitivity (high comprehensiveness), which may imply low precision. Pilot testing and subsequent fine-tuning of search strategies is necessary. To improve transparency, review investigators should include the complete search strategy of at least 1 of the major databases (eg, Medline) in their protocol.[38] Search terms should also be listed, as well as the limits (language or search dates) that will be applied.[38]

Study records and data items Investigators should indicate whether they are planning to use data management software (eg, Distiller Systematic Review software). These instruments are useful during the various phases of conducting a systematic review.

The study selection and data collection processes should be reported in full either in the main text or in appendices to the protocol. These procedures need to be conducted by 2 topic experts independently. A methodologist should be consulted when questions arise or when disagreements between operators need to be resolved. Uncertainties in research studies or persisting disagreements between reviewers can be addressed by contacting the investigators of the eligible studies. Before implementing the study selection and data collection methods, all procedures (including the validity of the data extraction forms) have to be pilot-tested and fine-tuned. Data extraction forms need to be developed with a precise description of all pertinent data items and require input from all team members. These forms have to be listed as an appendix to the protocol.

Outcomes and prioritization Careful prioritization and defining of outcomes in a registered or published protocol (1) allows the verification of selective outcome reporting, (2) facilitates updating or reproducing the review, and (3) saves considerable amounts of time when all eligible articles have to be revisited to verify an important outcome that was not included or not carefully defined a priori.[38] Whenever possible, investigators should define both primary (with at least 1 adverse effect) and secondary outcomes, including the end points of interest, and if possible the measure or scale used to quantify these outcomes. Systematic reviews with multiple outcomes are often difficult to handle and it is therefore recommended to limit the number of outcomes. Preferably, the primary outcomes focus on a patient-important outcome; however, it is not always possible to foresee which outcomes are used in the literature and at times it is difficult to give a precise definition of outcomes a priori, because outcome measures (eg, scales or time points for recording them) vary between studies. Investigators should therefore state in their protocols how they are going to deal with such uncertainties in their reviews.

Risk of bias individual studies The Grading of Recommendations Assessment, Development and Evaluation (GRADE) working group defines bias as "A systematic error or deviation in results or inferences from the truth."[55] Limitations in the study design, conduct, and reporting can bias the effect size, which could decrease confidence in the validity of such an outcome. The assessment of risk of bias therefore plays a critical role in the conduct of a systematic review. Numerous tools have been developed to assess risk of bias for both randomized and nonrandomized studies and other research designs. Like most research procedures in a systematic review, bias assessments also need to be conducted by at least 2 operators independently and disagreements should be resolved through discussions or consulting a third author for arbitration. These procedures should first be pilot-tested by these operators on a series of articles that are comparable with the eligible studies. **Fig. 4**[55–57] presents the types of bias that can occur during the various phases of a randomized controlled trial and **Table 3**[55–57] presents the definitions of these biases.

Data synthesis Data can be synthesized either quantitatively (through a meta-analysis) or qualitatively, or both. As explained previously, meta-analyses are only indicated when specific criteria for conducting such quantitative syntheses are met. For a quantitative synthesis investigators should describe items such as (1) the summary measures that they plan to synthesize in the meta-analysis (eg, dichotomous or continuous outcomes), (2) the methods that will be used to handle data (eg, unit of analysis or missing data issues), (3) methods for combining data (ie, fixed-effect or random-effects model), (4) methods for exploring heterogeneity (see **Table 1**), and (5) planned sensitivity and subgroup analyses and meta-regressions.[38]

Qualitative or narrative syntheses are always indicated independent of whether a meta-analysis will be undertaken or not. The CRD and PRISMA-P present guidance on how to conduct and report such syntheses.[16,38] For both quantitative and qualitative data syntheses it is important to consult all members of the review team.

Meta-biases Meta-biases refer to the biased selection of research outcomes. This bias can occur before (selective outcome reporting) or after (publication bias) the

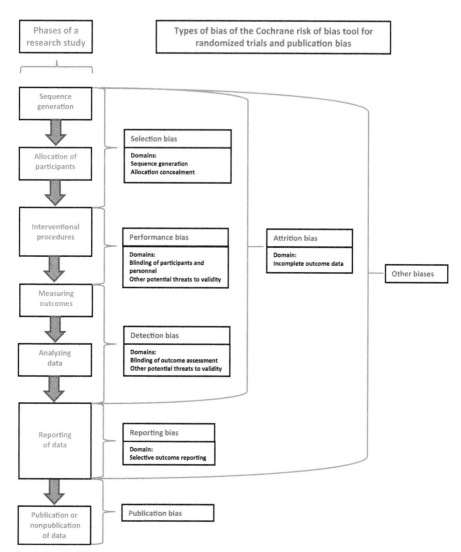

Fig. 4. Types of bias of the Cochrane risk of bias tool for randomized trials and publication bias. (*From* Higgins JPT, Altman DG, Sterne JAC. Chapter 8: assessing risk of bias in included studies. In: Higgins JPT, Green S, editors. Cochrane handbook for systematic reviews of interventions version 5.1.0 (updated March 2011). The Cochrane Collaboration, 2011. http://handbook.cochrane.org; with permission.)

completion of a research study (see **Fig. 4**, **Table 3**). The review team is responsible for assessing selective outcome reporting. Pertinent stakeholders who influence publication bias are membes of the research team, research sponsors, editors, peer-reviewers, publishing companies, and possibly others. Strategies for identifying and dealing with meta-biases have to be described a priori in the protocol.[38]

Confidence in cumulative estimate The GRADE approach has been developed for grading the confidence in the estimate of effect.[55] This approach applies a series of factors (with their consequences) that can reduce or increase the quality of evidence.

Table 3
Biases of the Cochrane risk of bias tool for randomized trials and publication bias

Type of Bias	Description of Bias	Phase of the Research Study	Relevant Domains in the Cochrane Risk of Bias Tool for Randomized Trials[56]
Selection bias	Refers to systematic error in the way that participants are selected. This error can lead to systematic differences between the study groups that are compared and can ultimately affect the results of a research study	Selection bias covers the period from the start of randomization to the start of the intervention	• Sequence generation and allocation concealment
Performance bias	Refers to systematic error in the care provided and/or in the exposure to factors other than those of the intervention being studied. This error can lead to systematic differences between the study groups that are compared and can ultimately affect the results of a research study	Performance bias covers the period from the start of the intervention to the start of measuring outcomes	• Blinding of participants and personnel • Other potential threats to validity
Detection bias	Refers to systematic error in the way outcomes are measured and analyzed. This error can lead to systematic differences between the study groups that are compared and can ultimately affect the results of a research study	Detection bias covers the period from the start of measuring outcomes to the completion of all data analyses	• Blinding of outcome assessment • Other potential threats to validity
Attrition bias	Refers to systematic error in dealing with incomplete outcomes. This error can lead to systematic differences between the study groups that are compared and can ultimately affect the results of a research study	Attrition bias covers the period from the start of randomization to the completion of the analyzing of data phase	• Incomplete outcome data

(continued on next page)

Table 3
(continued)

Type of Bias	Description of Bias	Phase of the Research Study	Relevant Domains in the Cochrane Risk of Bias Tool for Randomized Trials[56]
Reporting bias	Refers to systematic error in the reporting of some or all of the outcomes. This error can lead to systematic differences between the study groups that are compared and can ultimately affect the results of a research study	Reporting bias covers the period of writing the article	• Selective outcome reporting
Other biases	Refers to any type of systematic error that are only relevant in certain circumstances and that were not covered by the previous biases, such as study design–specific biases, conflicts of interest, fraud, and so forth. This error can lead to systematic differences between the study groups that are compared and can ultimately affect the results of a research study	"Other biases" cover all phases of a research study except those covered by publication bias	
Publication bias	GRADE defines publication bias as "a systematic under-estimation or an over-estimation of the underlying beneficial or harmful effect due to the selective publication of studies"[55]	Publication bias covers the period after the completion of the report of a research study to the publication or nonpublication of data of this study	

Data from Refs.[55–57]

GRADE factors that can reduce the quality of the evidence are (1) limitations in study design or execution (risk of bias), (2) inconsistency of results, (3) indirectness of evidence, (4) imprecision, and (5) publication bias.[55] GRADE factors that can increase the quality of the evidence are (1) large magnitude of effect, (2) all plausible confounding would reduce the demonstrated effect or increase the effect if no effect was observed, (3) dose-response gradient.[55] One of the great merits of the GRADE approach is the transparent, explicit, and therefore reproducible explanation of the ratings of the quality judgements. The GRADE approach has been developed for conducting systematic reviews and guidelines. However, unlike guideline developers, review investigators should not provide recommendations based on the GRADE quality ratings, because a series of other factors need to be weighed by a guideline panel for such advice.[55] Before adopting the GRADE approach, investigators should assess whether their systematic review qualifies under the criteria for using GRADE.[58]

Phase 3. Undertaking the Systematic Review Process

Fig. 5 presents the 8 key action steps of undertaking the systematic review process of phase 3.[9,59] In this phase, the reviewers apply the methods described in the protocol

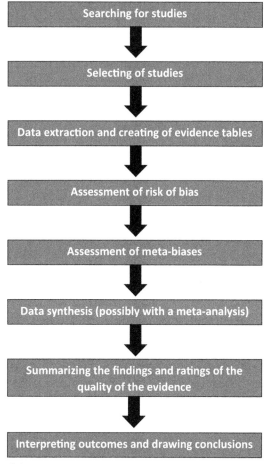

Fig. 5. The 8 steps of the systematic review process during Phase 3. (*Adapted from* Liberati A, Altman DG, Tetzlaff J, et al. The PRISMA statement for reporting systematic reviews and meta-analyses of studies that evaluate health care interventions: explanation and elaboration. PLoS Med 2009;6:e1000100; and Chandler J, Churchill R, Higgins J, et al. The methodological standards for the conduct of new Cochrane intervention reviews (Version 2.3 02 December 2013). Available at: http://editorial-unit.cochrane.org/sites/editorial-unit.cochrane.org/files/uploads/MECIR_conduct_standards%202.3%2002122013_0.pdf. Accessed August 19, 2016; with permission.)

in order to produce outcomes on the review questions, analyze them, and draw conclusions. Complete adherence to the protocol is not always possible because of unanticipated problems such as reporting issues in the eligible studies or the use of unexpected outcome measures or time points for measuring outcomes. A carefully prepared protocol can help to reduce such changes and the associated biases. Guidance on methodological standards can be found in the Methodological Expectations of Cochrane Intervention Reviews (MECIR) project.[59] These MECIR standards have been developed by the Cochrane Collaboration for the conduct of new Cochrane intervention reviews.

Phase 4. Reporting of the Systematic Review

As is necessary for all research studies, systematic reviews and meta-analyses also need to be reported in full and transparently to permit methods, results, and inferential reproducibility and to assess the validity of its findings.[60] The PRISMA statement is considered the reference standard for reporting systematic reviews and meta-analyses of studies that evaluate health care interventions.[13,39] For reviews that address other health questions, this statement may need to be modified.[39] To adequately comply with the PRISMA statement, review investigators should carefully address the 27 reporting items of the PRISMA 2009 checklist and scrutinize its guiding document.[13,39] The MECIR standard can also provide helpful guidance for transparent reporting.[59]

Ideally, the methods sections of a protocol and the review are similar; however, a complete overlap is not realistic. The methods of a protocol represent the planned methodology, and are generally more broad spectrum and could therefore possibly also include methods that will not be implemented. The methods section of the final review should only report the methods that were used. In a separate section, all differences between the planned methods of the protocol and those used in the final systematic review should be completely reported as well as the type, timing, and the rationale for these modifications. The consequences of these changes on outcomes should also be explained.[61] Reviewers should avoid making changes that could affect the outcomes of the review, because this could introduce reviewer's bias.[45]

APPLYING THE FINDINGS OF A SYSTEMATIC REVIEW TO INDIVIDUAL PATIENTS

Before applying a therapy to a patient, clinicians should first assess whether guidelines on this treatment are available. When such documents are not available, clinicians should consult systematic reviews. However, before applying the results of systematic reviews to individual patients, clinicians should ask some important questions[58,62]:

1. Are the patients in the systematic review similar to the patient under consideration?[62]
2. Did the systematic review consider all patient-important outcomes (ie, the values and preferences among patients) and what is the confidence in these parameters?[58] In general, little information is available in the literature on typical values and preferences or their variability among patients. This uncertainty can downgrade the confidence in the validity of these values and preferences.
3. Did the systematic review directly compare the interventions and measure the outcomes in which the clinician is interested?[62]
4. Are the outcomes based on subgroups in the systematic review credible?[63] Subgroup analyses should be interpreted with caution, because they are not based on randomized comparisons.[22,64]

5. Are the benefits (assess the effect size and the precision) of the treatment presented in the systematic review worth the potential risks?[58]
6. What is the confidence in the quality of the evidence in the systematic review on all important outcomes?[58] The GRADE approach assesses a series of factors to score the quality of the evidence.[58]
7. What is the quality of the systematic review? This is an important issue, because many systematic reviews and meta-analyses are not carefully done.[4] Specific tools are available to assess the quality of the systematic review[34,35] and the risk of bias.[44]
8. What are the costs of the intervention?[58]
9. What are potential barriers and facilitators to the implementation of the intervention?[65]

SUMMARY

Preparing and conducting systematic reviews and meta-analyses is a complex process that requires many judgements and the input from a wide variety of stakeholders.[45] This article presents an introduction on how to develop, conduct, and report on these research studies. This article also explains why clinicians should seek systematic reviews when they search for evidence to address their research questions. Systematic reviews are important for both medical and veterinary clinicians.[66] However, before applying the findings of systematic reviews and meta-analyses to particular patients, clinicians should weigh a variety of issues in these reviews, such as (1) the pertinent patient population, (2) whether all patient-important outcomes were assessed, (3) the balance between desirable and undesirable outcomes, (4) the magnitude and the quality of the evidence, (5) the costs of the intervention, and (6) the quality of the review. The quality of the review is particularly important, because a recent study[4] showed that most systematic reviews address unimportant questions and are poorly conducted and reported.

REFERENCES

1. Guyatt GH, Sackett DL, Sinclair JC, et al. Users' guides to the medical literature. IX. A method for grading health care recommendations. JAMA 1995;274:1800–4.
2. Systematic review from Wikipedia, the free encyclopedia. Available at: https://en.wikipedia.org/wiki/Systematic_review. Accessed May 20, 2016.
3. Smith R. The Cochrane Collaboration at 20. BMJ 2013;347:f7383.
4. Ioannidis JP. The mass production of redundant, misleading, and conflicted systematic reviews and meta-analyses. Milbank Q 2016;94(3):485–514.
5. Sargeant JM, O'Connor AM. Introduction to systematic reviews in animal agriculture and veterinary medicine. Zoonoses Public Health 2014;61(Suppl 1):3–9.
6. VetSRev-database of veterinary systematic reviews. Centre for Evidence-based Veterinary Medicine. The University of Nottingham. Available at: http://webapps.nottingham.ac.uk/refbase/. Accessed May 20, 2016.
7. Borenstein M, Hedges LV, Higgins JPT, et al. Preface. In: Borenstein M, Hedges LV, Higgins JPT, et al, editors. Introduction to meta-analysis. Chichester (United Kingdom): John Wiley; 2009. p. XXi–XXViii.
8. Mulrow CD. The medical review article: state of the science. Ann Intern Med 1987;106:485–8.
9. Deeks JJ, Frampton GK, Glanville JM, et al, European Food Safety Authority. Application of systematic review methodology to food and feed safety assessments to support decision making. EFSA J 2010;8(6):1637.

10. Petticrew M. Systematic reviews from astronomy to zoology: myths and misconceptions. BMJ 2001;322(7278):98–101.
11. Cook DJ, Mulrow CD, Haynes RB. Systematic reviews: synthesis of best evidence for clinical decisions. Ann Intern Med 1997;126(5):376–80.
12. Green S, Higgins JPT, Alderson P, et al. Introduction. Chapter 1. In: Higgins JPT, Green S, editors. Cochrane handbook for systematic reviews of interventions version 5.1.0. The Cochrane Collaboration; 2011. Available at: www.cochrane-handbook.org. Accessed May 20, 2016.
13. Moher D, Liberati A, Tetzlaff J, et al, PRISMA Group. Preferred reporting items for systematic reviews and meta-analyses: the PRISMA statement. PLoS Med 2009; 6:e1000097.
14. Cochrane Qualitative and Implementation Methods Group. Available at: http://methods.cochrane.org/qi/. Accessed September 16, 2016.
15. Cochrane Screening and Diagnostic Test Methods Group (SDTM). Available at: http://methods.cochrane.org/sdt/. Accessed September 16, 2016.
16. Centre for Reviews and Dissemination (CRD). Systematic reviews. CRD's guidance for undertaking reviews in health care. Available at: https://www.york.ac.uk/media/crd/Systematic_Reviews.pdf. Accessed November 6, 2016.
17. Higgins JPT, Green S, editors. Cochrane handbook for systematic reviews of interventions version 5.1.0. The Cochrane Collaboration; 2011. Available at: www.cochrane-handbook.org. Accessed May 20, 2016.
18. The Joanna Briggs Institute Reviewers' Manual 2014. The systematic review of prevalence and incidence data. Available at: http://joannabriggs.org/sumari.htm. Accessed September 25, 2015.
19. Becker LA, Oxman AD. Overviews of reviews. Chapter 22. In: Higgins JPT, Green S, editors. Cochrane handbook for systematic reviews of interventions version 5.1.0. The Cochrane Collaboration; 2011. Available at: www.cochrane-handbook.org. Accessed May 20, 2016.
20. Schünemann HJ, Moja L. Reviews: Rapid! Rapid! Rapid! ...and systematic. Syst Rev 2015;4:4.
21. Borenstein M, Hedges LV, Higgins JPT, et al. How a meta-analysis works. Chapter 1. In: Borenstein M, Hedges LV, Higgins JPT, et al, editors. Introduction to meta-analysis. Chichester (United Kingdom): John Wiley; 2009. p. 3–8.
22. Deeks JJ, Higgins JPT, Altman DG. Analysing data and undertaking meta-analyses. Chapter 9. In: Higgins JPT, Green S, editors. Cochrane handbook for systematic reviews of interventions version 5.1.0. The Cochrane Collaboration; 2011. Available at: www.cochrane-handbook.org. Accessed May 20, 2016.
23. Walker E, Hernandez AV, Kattan MW. Meta-analysis: Its strengths and limitations [review]. Cleve Clin J Med 2008;75(6):431–9.
24. Borenstein M, Hedges LV, Higgins JPT, et al. Factors that affect precision. Chapter 8. In: Borenstein M, Hedges LV, Higgins JPT, et al, editors. Introduction to meta-analysis. Chichester (United Kingdom): John Wiley; 2009. p. 51–6.
25. Borenstein M, Hedges LV, Higgins JPT, et al. Identifying and quantifying heterogeneity. Chapter 16. In: Borenstein M, Hedges LV, Higgins JPT, et al, editors. Introduction to meta-analysis. Chichester (United Kingdom): John Wiley; 2009. p. 107–26.
26. Higgins JPT, Thompson SG. Quantifying heterogeneity in a meta-analysis. Stat Med 2002;21:1539–58.
27. Higgins JPT, Thompson SG, Deeks JJ, et al. Measuring inconsistency in meta-analyses. BMJ 2003;327:557–60.
28. Higgins JP. Commentary: heterogeneity in meta-analysis should be expected and appropriately quantified. Int J Epidemiol 2008;37(5):1158–60.

29. Borenstein M, Hedges LV, Higgins JPT, et al. When does it make sense to perform a meta-analysis?. Chapter 40. In: Borenstein M, Hedges LV, Higgins JPT, et al, editors. Introduction to meta-analysis. Chichester (United Kingdom): John Wiley; 2009. p. 357–64.

30. Sing Chawla D. Retraction watch. We have an epidemic of deeply flawed meta-analyses, says John Ioannidis. Available at: http://retractionwatch.com/2016/09/13/we-have-an-epidemic-of-deeply-flawed-meta-analyses-says-john-ioannidis/. Accessed October 29, 2016.

31. Critical Appraisal Skills Programme (CASP). Making sense of evidence. Available at: http://media.wix.com/ugd/dded87_a02ff2e3445f4952992d5a96ca562576.pdf. Accessed October 29, 2016.

32. GATE CAT for systematic reviews: Intervention studies. Available at: https://www.fmhs.auckland.ac.nz/en/soph/about/our-departments/epidemiology-and-biostatistics/research/epiq/evidence-based-practice-and-cats.html. Accessed September 29, 2016.

33. Risk of bias in systematic reviews (ROBIS). ROBIS tool and the ROBIS guidance document. Available at: http://www.robis-tool.info/. Accessed August 13, 2016.

34. Shea BJ, Grimshaw JM, Wells GA, et al. Development of AMSTAR: a measurement tool to assess the methodological quality of systematic reviews. BMC Med Res Methodol 2007;7:10.

35. Shea BJ, Hamel C, Wells GA, et al. AMSTAR is a reliable and valid measurement tool to assess the methodological quality of systematic reviews. J Clin Epidemiol 2009;62(10):1013–20.

36. SIGN critical appraisal: notes and checklists. Methodology checklist 1: Systematic reviews and meta-analyses. Available at: http://www.sign.ac.uk/methodology/checklists.html. Accessed October 29, 2016.

37. Moher D, Shamseer L, Clarke M, et al. Preferred reporting items for systematic review and meta-analysis protocols (PRISMA-P) 2015 statement. Syst Rev 2015;4(1):1.

38. Shamseer L, Moher D, Clarke M, et al, The PRISMA-P Group. Preferred reporting items for systematic review and meta-analysis protocols (PRISMA-P) 2015: elaboration and explanation. BMJ 2015;349:g7647.

39. Liberati A, Altman DG, Tetzlaff J, et al. The PRISMA statement for reporting systematic reviews and meta-analyses of studies that evaluate health care interventions: explanation and elaboration. PLoS Med 2009;6:e1000100.

40. Chalmers I, Glasziou P. Avoidable waste in the production and reporting of research evidence. Lancet 2009;374(9683):86–9.

41. Cowan K, Oliver S. The James Lind Alliance guidebook, 2013. Version 5. Available at: www.JLAguidebook.org. Accessed September 29, 2015.

42. O'Connor D, Green S, Higgins JPT. Defining the review question and developing criteria for including studies. Chapter 5. In: Higgins JPT, Green S, editors. Cochrane handbook for systematic reviews of interventions version 5.1.0. The Cochrane Collaboration; 2011. Available at: www.cochrane-handbook.org. Accessed May 20, 2016.

43. Thompson MT, Van den Bruel A. Asking an answerable clinical question. Chapter 3. In: Thompson MT, Van den Bruel A, editors. Diagnostic tests toolkit. Chichester (United Kingdom): Wiley-Blackwell; 2012. p. 16–7.

44. Whiting P, Savović J, Higgins JP, et al. ROBIS group. ROBIS: A new tool to assess risk of bias in systematic reviews was developed. J Clin Epidemiol 2016;69: 225–34.

45. Green S, Higgins JPT. Preparing a Cochrane Review. Chapter 2. In: Higgins JPT, Green S, editors. Cochrane handbook for systematic reviews of interventions version 5.1.0. The Cochrane Collaboration; 2011. Available at: www.cochrane-handbook.org. Accessed May 20, 2016.

46. Light RJ, Pillemer DB. Summing up: the science of reviewing research. Cambridge (MA): Harvard University Press; 1984.

47. PROSPERO: Centre for Reviews and Dissemination. UK: University of York. Available at: http://www.crd.york.ac.uk/PROSPERO/. Accessed May 20, 2016.

48. Enabling Open Scholarship (EOS). Available at: http://www.openscholarship.org/upload/docs/application/pdf/2009-09/open_access_institutional_repositories.pdf. Accessed August 14, 2016.

49. The Directory of Open Access Repositories (Open DOAR). Available at: http://www.opendoar.org/. Accessed August 14, 2016.

50. Registry of Open Access Repositories (ROAR). Available at: http://roar.eprints.org/. Accessed August 14, 2016.

51. Cochrane database of systematic reviews. Available at: http://www.cochranelibrary.com/cochrane-database-of-systematic-reviews/. Accessed September 16, 2016.

52. Systematic Reviews. A journal published by BioMed Central. Available at: http://www.systematicreviewsjournal.com/. Accessed May 20, 2016.

53. CABI veterinary science database. Available at: http://www.cabi.org/publishing-products/online-information-resources/veterinary-science-database/. Accessed November 20, 2016.

54. Lefebvre C, Manheimer E, Glanville J. Searching for studies. Chapter 6. In: Higgins JPT, Green S, editors. Cochrane handbook for systematic reviews of interventions version 5.1.0. The Cochrane Collaboration; 2011. Available at: www.cochrane-handbook.org. Accessed September 25, 2016.

55. Schünemann H, Brozek J, Gyatt G, et al, editors. GRADE handbook. Handbook for grading the quality of evidence and the strength of recommendations using the GRADE approach. Available at: http://gdt.guidelinedevelopment.org/app/handbook/handbook.html. Accessed November 6, 2016.

56. Higgins JPT, Altman DG, Sterne JAC. Assessing risk of bias in included studies. Chapter 8. In: Higgins JPT, Green S, editors. Cochrane handbook for systematic reviews of interventions version 5.1.0. The Cochrane Collaboration; 2011. Available at: www.cochrane-handbook.org. Accessed November 6, 2016.

57. Meursinge Reynders R, Ladu L, Ronchi L, et al. Insertion torque recordings for the diagnosis of contact between orthodontic mini-implants and dental roots: protocol for a systematic review. Syst Rev 2015;4(1):39.

58. Schünemann H, Gyatt G, Oxman A. Criteria for applying or using GRADE. Available at: http://www.gradeworkinggroup.org/docs/Criteria_for_using_GRADE_2016-04-05.pdf. Accessed August 14, 2016.

59. Chandler J, Churchill R, Higgins J, et al. The methodological standards for the conduct of new Cochrane intervention reviews (version 2.3 02 December 2013). Available at: http://editorial-unit.cochrane.org/sites/editorial-unit.cochrane.org/files/uploads/MECIR_conduct_standards%202.3%2002122013_0.pdf. Accessed August 19, 2016.

60. Goodman SN, Fanelli D, Ioannidis JP. What does research reproducibility mean? Sci Transl Med 2016;8(341):341ps12.

61. Higgins JPT, Green S. Guide to the contents of a Cochrane protocol and review. Chapter 4. In: Cochrane handbook for systematic reviews of interventions version

5.1.0. The Cochrane Collaboration; 2011. Available at: www.cochrane-handbook. org. Accessed May 20, 2016.

62. Murad MH, Montori VM, Ioannidis JP, et al. How to read a systematic review and meta-analysis and apply the results to patient care: users' guides to the medical literature. JAMA 2014;312(2):171–9.

63. Guyatt G, Jaeschke R, Prasad K, et al. Summarizing the evidence. Chapter 14. In: Guyatt G, Rennie D, Meade MO, et al, editors. Users' guides to the medical literature. New York: McGraw-Hill Medical; 2008. p. 547–59.

64. Oxman AD, Guyatt GH. A consumer's guide to subgroup analyses. Ann Intern Med 1992;116(1):78–84.

65. Legaré F. Assessing barriers and facilitators to knowledge use. Chapter 3.4. In: Straus SE, Tetroe J, Graham ID, editors. Knowledge translation in health care: moving from evidence to practice. Chichester (United Kingdom): Wiley-Blackwell; 2009. p. 83–93.

66. Baltzell P. The role of systematic or critical reviews for interventions in veterinary medicine [MSc thesis]. Ames (IA): Iowa State University; 2015.

How to Report Exotic Animal Research

Nicola Di Girolamo, DMV, MSc(EBHC), PhD, DECZM(Herpetology)[a,b,*],
Alexandra L. Winter, BVSc, DACVS[c]

KEYWORDS

- Reporting • Bias • Methodology • Clinical epidemiology • Evidence-based medicine
- Randomized controlled trials • Medical writing • Statistics

KEY POINTS

- Reporting the results of primary research is a key step in knowledge creation; inadequate reporting may limit readers' ability to recognize the risk of bias.
- The EQUATOR (Enhancing the Quality and Transparency of Health Research) network provides an online database of current guidelines that have been developed and endorsed as a means to assist investigators in reporting research transparently and accurately.
- It is important that, during research planning stages, investigators ensure that the proposed study design is appropriate, and is likely to yield useful data.
- Defining the primary outcome is key, and this must be explicitly reported in the published article and accompanied by a sample size estimation.
- Study design elements, including details of randomization, allocation concealment, and blinding of participants (owners) are methodological issues that should always be reported.

Reporting the results of primary research is a key step in knowledge creation. Inadequate reporting greatly limits the ability of readers to clearly evaluate the relevance and reliability of the results. Reporting deficiencies include omission of key information (ie, selective reporting), incorrect study design, and misinterpretation of results, all of which contribute to research waste. One of the main problems of poor reporting is that it makes it impossible for readers to understand what was done by researchers. For example, when primary researchers only mention the term "random" without further explanation, readers have 2 options to interpret this limited description: (1) the investigators adequately generated a random sequence but failed to report it; or (2) the investigators did not perform adequate randomization. An important step to

Disclosure: The authors have nothing to disclose.
[a] Tai Wai Small Animal & Exotic Hospital, 75 Chik Shun Street, Tai Wai, Shatin, Hong Kong;
[b] EBMVet, Via Sigismondo Trecchi 20, Cremona, Italy; [c] American Veterinary Medical Association, 1931 N. Meacham Road, Suite 100, Schaumburg, IL 60173, USA
* Corresponding author. EBMVet, Via Sigismondo Trecchi 20, Cremona, Italy.
E-mail address: nicoladiggi@gmail.com

advance exotic animal practice is improved quality of research reporting. At present, almost all randomized controlled trials (RCTs) in veterinary medicine lack adequate reporting of key methodological elements (ie, primary outcome, power calculation, random sequence generation, allocation concealment, intention to treat); they also do not comply with current recommendations for statistical reporting (ie, effect measures with confidence intervals).[1] This article summarizes the most important methodological points to consider when reporting research results.

IMPROVING THE REPORTING OF RESEARCH: THE USE OF REPORTING GUIDELINES

At present, several guidelines have been produced to assist investigators in reporting research. The EQUATOR (Enhancing the Quality and Transparency of Health Research) network provides an up-to-date, comprehensive, searchable database of reporting guidelines as well as links to other resources relevant to research reporting on its website: http://www.equator-network.org. These guidelines are basically a checklist of items that are considered essential to report. Most new or updated guidelines are accompanied by an explanation and elaboration article that provides background and context, as well as detailed information for researchers on each item. Although these reporting guidelines are explicitly not intended to allow journal editors, reviewers, and others to assess the quality of a study, when adhered to, improved reporting is expected. The most applicable and useful of current reporting guidelines for exotic animal research are CONSORT 2010 (Consolidated Standards of Reporting Trials), for the reporting of RCTs; STARD (Standards for Reporting of Diagnostic Accuracy), for the reporting of studies of diagnostic accuracy; STROBE (Strengthening the Reporting of Observational studies in Epidemiology), for the reporting of observational studies; CARE (Case Reports), for the reporting of case reports; and TRIPOD (Transparent Reporting of a multivariable prediction model for Individual Prognosis Or Diagnosis), for prognostic studies. With improved quality of published exotic animal research, this should in turn allow systematic reviews to be published with use of the PRISMA (Preferred Reporting Items for Systematic reviews and Meta-Analyses) guideline, and PRISMA-P (Preferred Reporting Items for Systematic Review and Meta-Analysis Protocols), for systematic reviews and meta-analysis protocols. Such reporting guidelines do not cover only the methods section but the entire article, from the abstract to the conflict-of-interest disclosure.

TITLE

The objective of the title is to summarize the content of the article, trigger readers' curiosity, and facilitate indexing. Titles may be descriptive, noting the conducted research methods (ie, indicative title), or state key study findings (ie, declarative title). It has been suggested that declarative titles may attract clinicians,[2] and many journals do not allow this title style because of concerns that they are misleading[3]; however, a recent RCT found no evidence that declarative titles influence readers' perceptions of study conclusions.[4] Furthermore, use of new article level metrics (eg, Altmetrics) indicates that articles with declarative titles are among the most shared.[5] In order to help ensure that a study is appropriately indexed and easily identified, investigators should describe the type of study in the title. For RCTs, the word randomized should be inserted in the title[6]; for example, "Effect of Pimobendan in Dogs with Preclinical Myxomatous Mitral Valve Disease and Cardiomegaly: the EPIC Study – A Randomized Clinical Trial."[7] For diagnostic accuracy studies the title should include at least 1 measure of accuracy (eg, sensitivity, specificity, predictive values, area under the curve).[8] For observational studies, a commonly used term (eg, case control, cohort, cross-sectional) should be included.[9]

ABSTRACT

Abstracts should be clear, transparent, and sufficiently detailed to convey the main elements of the study, including the question, primary outcome measure, study design, and main conclusions.[6] Abstracts may influence whether busy clinicians will read the full article, and, if a study is not open access, practitioners may need to make clinical decisions from abstracts only. Consider also that, with new technologies and means of accessing information, the abstract content alone may serve as the basis for creative methods of dissemination (eg, infographics [#visualabstract], video abstracts) designed to increase engagement. Although individual journals may impose style guidelines, the core reporting guidelines, such as CONSORT 2010, also provide specific instructions for abstracts (eg, CONSORT for abstracts).[10] Main items required for abstracts of RCTs are reported in **Table 1**. Investigators are encouraged to work with journal editors to comply with style requirements while avoiding the omission of essential study design elements (eg, for RCTs, avoid only reporting the final number of participants randomized and analyzed; also report the number originally allocated and randomized).

INTRODUCTION

The introduction assists the reader in understanding the context of the research, including what is the current scientific knowledge on the topic and why the topic deserves

Table 1
Items to include when reporting a randomized trial in a journal or conference abstract

Item	Description
Title	Identification of the study as randomized
Investigators	Contact details for the corresponding author
Trial design	Description of the trial design (eg, parallel, cluster, noninferiority)
Methods	
Participants	Eligibility criteria for participants and the settings where the data were collected
Interventions	Interventions intended for each group
Objective	Specific objective or hypothesis
Outcome	Clearly defined primary outcome
Randomization	How participants were allocated to interventions
Blinding (masking)	Whether or not participants, care givers, and those assessing the outcomes were blinded to group assignment
Results	
Numbers randomized	Number of participants randomized to each group
Recruitment	Trial status
Numbers analyzed	Number of participants analyzed in each group
Outcome	For the primary outcome, a result for each group and the estimated effect size and its precision
Harms	Important adverse events
Conclusions	General interpretation of the results
Trial registration	Registration number and name of trial register if applicable
Funding	Source of funding

From Hopewell S, Clarke M, Moher D, Wager E, Middleton P, Altman DG, et al. (2008) CONSORT for Reporting Randomized Controlled Trials in Journal and Conference Abstracts: Explanation and Elaboration. PLoS Med 5(1): e20. Available at: https://doi.org/10.1371/journal.pmed.0050020.

further investigation. Ideally, investigators should assess the status of current scientific knowledge by means of a thorough literature search, a systematic review; and either performing a systematic search or referring to a recent systematic review on the topic (See Laura Pavlech's article "Information Resources for the Exotic Animal Practitioner" & Reint Meursinge Reynders's article "An Introduction to Systematic Reviews and Meta-Analyses for Exotic Animal Practitioners," in this issue). In the absence of such evidence it is still advisable to consult with a medical librarian at the outset to ensure an appropriate and thorough literature search. The final paragraph of the introduction presents the specific objectives, hypotheses, or both of the research.

METHODS

The Methods section provides a detailed report of the what and the how of the described research process. However, in order to maximize reader comprehension and to permit repeatability of research, several methodological aspects need to be transparently reported (**Table 2**). Again, by clearly defining the type of study design, investigators can then refer to the appropriate reporting guideline and supporting materials for guidance. Even where aspects of trial design may have been suboptimal, use of the appropriate reporting guideline helps avoid selective reporting that can bias readers.

Study Design

The appropriate design of the study is the first thing to choose once a research question is posed, and it should be reported accordingly. In the veterinary literature, there is frequent difficulty in meeting these basic criteria. It is important that, during the research planning stage, investigators pay careful attention to developing a study that best adheres to the ideal study design for the research question posed. A table that summarizes the most important study designs and their characteristics is included (**Table 3**). For RCTs, the number of arms (eg, parallel, multiarm), eventual multiple treatments per arm (eg, crossover, factorial), the number of institutions (ie, single institution, multicenter), and the conceptual framework (ie, superiority, noninferiority) should be reported in this section.[6] Tools are being developed that can assist investigators in selecting the correct reporting guideline for their research[11]; initial investigation suggests that this tool can help investigators to select the correct guideline for their study type.

Primary and Secondary Outcomes

Studies that assess the effectiveness of an intervention (either randomized or not), or the risk associated with an exposure, evaluate response variables (eg, mortality, quality of life, disease occurrence rate), or outcomes, between different groups.[6,9] Typically, investigators measure many outcomes (eg, laboratory results, mortality, recovery time) during a study. However, this frequently contributes to inappropriate reporting because of multiplicity of analyses. For example, when researchers use many variations of treatment arms, subgroups, and time points or conduct many analyses (ie, data driven approach), it is common to report the results of spurious statistically significant findings.[12,13] In order to avoid this shortcoming, outcomes need to be prespecified during the research planning stage. A primary outcome must be explicitly reported in the published article. That primary outcome is then the basis for a priori sample size estimation. Many studies have more than 1 primary outcome; potential harms of an intervention should be considered a primary outcome. Secondary outcomes need to be reported, and clearly indicated as such; the sample size calculation should always be tailored to the primary outcome. Any change of

Table 2
Methodological details to include when reporting a randomized trial, or a diagnostic accuracy study

Section/Topic	Items to Report	Item No. in the Reporting Guideline Checklist CONSORT 2010	STARD 2015
Trial design	Description of trial design (eg, parallel, factorial) including allocation ratio	3a	—
	Important changes to methods after trial commencement (eg, eligibility criteria), with reasons	3b	—
	Whether data collection was planned before the index test and reference standard were performed (prospective study) or after (retrospective study)	—	5
Participants	Eligibility criteria for participants	4a	6
	On what basis potentially eligible participants were identified (eg, symptoms/signs, results from previous tests, inclusion in registry)	—	7
	Settings and locations where the data were collected	4b	8
	Whether participants formed a consecutive, random, or convenience series	—	9
Interventions	The interventions for each group with sufficient details to allow replication, including how and when they were administered	5	—
Test methods	Index test, in sufficient detail to allow replication	—	10a
	Reference standard, in sufficient detail to allow replication	—	10b
	Rationale for choosing the reference standard (if alternatives exist)	—	11
	Definition of and rationale for test positivity cutoffs or result categories of the index test, distinguishing prespecified from exploratory	—	12a
	Definition of and rationale for test positivity cutoffs or result categories of the reference standard, distinguishing prespecified from exploratory	—	12b
Outcomes	Any changes to trial outcomes after the trial commenced, with reasons	6b	—
Sample size	How sample size was determined	7a	18
	When applicable, explanation of any interim analyses and stopping guidelines	7b	—
Random sequence generation	Method used to generate the random allocation sequence	8a	—
	Type of randomization; details of any restriction (eg, blocking and block size)	8b	—
Allocation concealment mechanism	Mechanism used to implement the random allocation sequence (eg, sequentially numbered containers), describing any steps taken to conceal the sequence until interventions were assigned	9	—

(continued on next page)

		Item No. in the Reporting Guideline Checklist	
		CONSORT	STARD
Section/Topic	**Items to Report**	**2010**	**2015**
Implementation	Who generated the random allocation sequence, who enrolled participants, and who assigned participants to interventions	10	—
Blinding	Blinding to intervention or to results of index/reference test	11a	13a, 13b
	If relevant, description of the similarity of interventions	11b	—
Statistical methods	Statistical methods used to compare groups for primary and secondary outcomes or for comparing measures of diagnostic accuracy	12a	14
	Methods for additional analyses; eg, subgroup analyses, adjusted analyses, and analyses of variability in diagnostic accuracy, distinguishing prespecified from exploratory	12b	17
	How indeterminate index test or reference standard results were handled	—	15
	How missing data on the index test and reference standard were handled	—	16

Table 2
(*continued*)

Data from Moher D, Hopewell S, Schulz KF, et al. CONSORT 2010 explanation and elaboration: updated guidelines for reporting parallel group randomised trials. J Clin Epidemiol 2010;63(8):e1–37; and Bossuyt PM, Reitsma JB, Bruns DE, et al. STARD 2015: an updated list of essential items for reporting diagnostic accuracy studies. BMJ 2015;351:h5527.

outcomes between the time of study conception and publication that was not pre-specified (eg, switching outcomes) is considered scientific misconduct.[14]

Power Calculation

The number of participants enrolled in a study should be tailored to the research question.[15] Veterinary trials frequently enroll a limited number of patients compared with human trials,[1] which limits the power of the studies, increasing the chance of false-negative findings (type II statistical errors).[16] However, inclusion of too many animals results in unnecessary expense and time, and is also not ethical once the superiority of an intervention or a diagnostic technique has been established. Furthermore, with an increased number of patients, there is increasing risk of finding statistical significance without clinical significance.[17] On this basis, published studies, in particular intervention studies, must report a power calculation that justifies the sample size. The power calculation should have been performed *a priori*, during the stage of trial development, instead of adjusted after trial completion. Post-hoc power calculations should not be reported, because they produce invalid estimates.[18] An appropriate power calculation reported for an interventional trial should include (1) the estimated outcomes in each group (ie, the clinically important difference between the groups), (2) the type I error probability (usually 5%), (3) the statistical power (or the type II error probability; usually 80%–90%), and (4), the expected standard deviation of the measurements when continuous outcomes are used.[13,19] At present, only 16.7% to 22% of veterinary RCTs report a power calculation, versus 98.3% of the RCTs in human medicine.[1,15]

Table 3
Clinical questions, with appropriate study designs and relevant reporting guidelines

Clinical Question	Ideal Study Design	Brief Explanation	Reporting Guideline
Efficacy or effectiveness of an intervention (medical/surgical)	RCT	Patients are randomized to 2 or more treatment groups. The results (as measured by prespecified outcomes) are compared between those groups	CONSORT 2010
Accuracy of a diagnostic technique	Diagnostic accuracy study	Consecutive or random patients receive an index test and a reference standard test. Results of the tests are compared providing at least sensitivity and specificity	STARD 2015
Cause (especially of a common disease)	Cohort study	Patients are divided into 2 or more groups based on preexisting characteristics (eg, exposure to a toxic, administration of a drug). The outcomes are compared between those groups, controlling for potential confounders	STROBE
Cause (especially of a common disease)	Cross-sectional study	In a group of patients, the presence of an exposure (eg, a toxin) and a disease are evaluated at the same time	STROBE
Cause (especially of a rare disease)	Case-control study	A group of patients with a disease is compared with a group of patients without the disease regarding exposure to some factor (eg, a toxin, a cancerogenic substance)	STROBE
Prognostic value of 1 or multiple factors	Prognostic study	The relationship between 1 or multiple factors and an outcome (eg, mortality) are evaluated	TRIPOD

Data from The EQUATOR network. Available at: www.equator-network.org.

Randomization Procedures

Randomization, when properly performed, avoids selection bias by balancing both known and unknown prognostic factors in the assignment of treatments.[20] Furthermore, random assignment permits the use of probability theory to express the likelihood that any difference in outcome between intervention groups merely reflects chance.[21] In addition, randomization may facilitate further blinding of investigators, participants, and evaluators to the treatment assigned.[22] Successful randomization in practice depends on adequate generation of an unpredictable allocation sequence and concealment of that sequence until treatment assignment occurs.[6]

Methods for generating a random sequence are reported in just one-fifth of veterinary randomized trials.[1] Often, randomization is only mentioned to describe the division of the subjects, typically: "[...] the ferrets were randomly allocated to 2 groups [...]." However, such text is inadequate, because it does not explain the type of randomization scheme (eg, simple, restricted, minimization), lacks a description of the instruments used to generate the random sequence (ie, use of computer software, a random number table, coins, cards, or all of these). As stated in the

CONSORT 2010 checklist: "readers cannot judge adequacy [of randomisation] from such terms as 'random allocation' 'randomization' or 'random' without further elaboration."[6] It could be hypothesized that investigators used the term random without generating a random sequence, and that the word random was just used to indicate that investigators did not liberally assign participants to a specific treatment arm. In order to properly report random sequence generation, 2 features are required[6]: (1) explanation of the method by which the random sequence is generated (eg, computer, coin tosses); alternatively, the statement that a statistician performed the sequence generation is acceptable. (2) Specific explanation of the type of randomization scheme (eg, simple randomization, permuted block [to avoid imbalances in allocation], stratification [to balance the distribution of certain baseline risk factors]) should be provided.

Although reporting on appropriate details of randomization is improving in human medicine,[23] reporting of randomization for veterinary trials did not improve significantly in the last decade.[1] One study observed that random sequence generation was reported in approximately half (48.9%; 95% confidence interval [CI], 37.8%–59.9%) of parallel controlled clinical trials in client-owned dogs and cats published from 2000 to 2005 in 12 veterinary journals.[24] In a similar subgroup (parallel manifest RCTs of clinical patients) of a more recent study, the random sequence generation was reported in 42.4% (95% CI, 25.9%–60.6%; 14 out of 33).[1] Veterinary investigators should be aware of this and improve on reporting of the randomization mechanism used.

Allocation Concealment

In an RCT, the randomization list should be concealed to prevent investigators being aware of which treatment group each participant is assigned to. This requirement is fundamental in order to permit readers to evaluate the risk of selection bias. One of the first adequate reports of allocation concealment was in the landmark streptomycin trial of 1948: "the details of the [allocation] series were unknown to any of the investigators or to the coordinator and were contained in a set of sealed envelopes, each bearing on the outside only the name of the hospital and a number."[25] In the early 1990s, only one-quarter of the RCTs published in 4 journals of obstetrics and gynecology contained information showing that steps had been taken to conceal assignment.[26] Reporting of allocation concealment in RCTs published in general medical journals improved in the last 15 years from 34.4% to 64.7%.[27] In leading veterinary journals, only one-tenth of the RCTs published in veterinary journals mentioned allocation concealment.[1] This finding is worrying because there is evidence that lack of allocation concealment is empirically associated with bias.[28] Trials in which concealment was either inadequate or unclear (did not report or incompletely reported a concealment approach) yielded larger estimates of treatment effects than trials in which investigators reported adequately concealed treatment allocation.[28] Because concealing treatment assignments up to the point of allocation is always possible regardless of the study topic,[26] it should be properly performed and reported.

BLINDING

In research, there is often the need to blind (ie, to make people unaware) investigators (personnel and outcome assessors) and/or participants for several reasons (**Table 4**). When reporting any type of study, it should be made clear to readers which individuals were blinded, and to what. The use of terminology such as single, double, and triple blinding should be avoided because such terms can be variably interpreted and fail

Table 4
Potential benefits of blinding of various individuals during randomized trials and applicability to veterinary trials

Category Blinded	Potential Benefits	Applicable in Veterinary Trials?
Participants: owners/caregiver	Less likely to have biased psychological or physical responses to intervention	Unclear
	More likely to comply with trial regimens	Yes
	Less likely to seek additional adjunct interventions	Yes
	Less likely to leave trial without providing outcome data, leading to lost to follow-up	Yes
Trial investigators	Less likely to transfer their inclinations or attitudes to participants	Unclear
	Less likely to differentially administer cointerventions	Yes
	Less likely to differentially adjust dose	Yes
	Less likely to differentially withdraw participants	Yes
	Less likely to differentially encourage or discourage participants (ie, owners) to continue trial	Yes
Outcome assessors	Less likely to have biases affect their outcome assessments, especially with subjective outcomes of interest	Yes

Modified from Schulz KF, Grimes DA. Blinding in randomised trials: hiding who got what. Lancet 2002;359:696–700.

to explicitly explain blinding procedures.[29] The following categories of blinding should be clearly reported:

Blinding of Participants/Owners

In animal trials, blinding of participants corresponds with blinding of owners/care-givers. Most actions carried out by human participants not blinded to a treatment that may bias a trial (ie, do not fulfill trial regimen, search for new interventions, or leave the trial) may be performed by owners/caregivers. However, although in human trials participants enrolled in a group that received a new treatment might bring favorable expectations or increased apprehension, in veterinary trials it has generally been perceived that owner perceptions are less likely to influence outcomes, although this may not actually be the case.

Blinding of Personnel

It should be clear whether trial personnel, including those that provide the intervention or take care of the animals during the trials (eg, veterinarians, nurses, technicians) are aware of the intervention provided. Trial personnel may have a biased perception of the effectiveness of the interventions and may interact with owners suggesting that they exit the trial, may administer multiple interventions to 1 treatment group, or may provide additional care in 1 treatment group, among other potential forms of bias.

Blinding of Outcome Assessors

The outcome assessors are the investigators who evaluate by means of objective or subjective means the results of a study. Blinding of outcome assessors is potentially indicated in every study design. In randomized trials, blinding of outcome assessors means that they are not aware of whether or not the participants that they are assessing received the treatment. Blinding of outcome assessors is fundamental in RCTs, because knowledge of the treatment group could dramatically influence the assessor.[29] In diagnostic accuracy studies, outcome assessors should be blinded to the results of other tests performed on study participants. Knowledge of the results of other tests could influence the assessor.

RESULTS
Participant Flow

It is highly recommended in all study designs to depict the flow of participants with a flow diagram (**Fig. 1**).[6,8] Information required to complete a flow diagram for a RCT, for example, includes the number of participants evaluated for potential enrollment into the trial and the number excluded at this stage because they either did not meet the inclusion criteria or declined to participate. For each intervention group it also requires the numbers of participants which were randomly assigned, received treatment as allocated, completed treatment as allocated, and were included in the main analysis, with numbers and reasons for exclusions at each step.[30] Investigators should exercise care when constructing the flow diagram, and solicit input from methodologists or statisticians as needed. In a recent study evaluating compliance with CONSORT, the level of compliance with all elements of the flow diagram was lacking.[31] Crucial elements such as number of subjects lost because of attrition or numbers of patients included in intention-to-treat analyses were not clearly reported, such that results might easily be misleading to readers.

Main Results: Use of Effect Size Estimation Methods

A statistically significant result does not provide information on the magnitude of the effect and thus does not necessarily mean that the effect is robust.[32] Current CONSORT 2010 guidelines suggest that, "For each outcome, study results should be reported as a summary of the outcome in each group [...] together with the contrast between the groups, known as the effect size.." Although almost every RCT published in selected medical journals provided point estimates with measures of uncertainty (ie, 95% CI), veterinary studies mostly provided a measure of statistical significance (ie, P values) without such measures.[1] Over-reliance on P values when reporting and interpreting results of an RCT or other research study may be inappropriate and misleading.[33,34] Furthermore, unadjusted estimates and confounder-adjusted estimates (especially in observational studies) need to be reported, making clear which confounders were adjusted for and why they were included.[9] Veterinary investigators should work more closely with statisticians and improve the quality of published evidence by including point estimates and measures of uncertainty (See Michelle Giuffrida's article "Basic statistics for the exotic animal practitioner," in this issue). In small studies, as is often the case in exotic animal medicine, it is advisable to provide the entire data set of individual results.

Diagnostic accuracy studies

For diagnostic accuracy studies with binary categorical outcomes (eg, disease present/absent, test positive/negative), it is of fundamental importance to report the cross-tabulation of the index test results compared with the results of the reference standard test in a 2×2 table. Sensitivity, specificity, positive predictive value, and negative predictive value are all critical data to report in order to ascertain the accuracy of the index test. For diagnostic accuracy studies with numerical outcomes

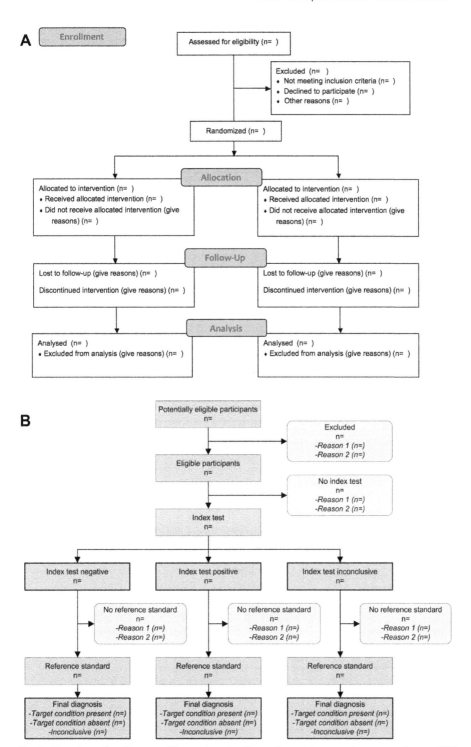

Fig. 1. Templates for diagrams illustrating the flow of participants when reporting an RCT (*A*), and a diagnostic accuracy study (*B*); according to CONSORT 2010[6] and STARD 2015[8] recommendations. n= the number of participants.

(eg, new mean values for measuring blood pressure in ferrets), the mean difference, with 95% CI and limits of agreement, should be reported.[35]

Other Results: Subgroup and Sensitivity Analyses

Subgroup analyses (ie, stratification by 1 characteristic of study participants) and sensitivity analyses (ie, methods to determine the robustness of an assessment by examining the extent to which results are affected by changes in methods, models, values of unmeasured variables, or assumptions)[36] may be crucial in the determination of the ability to generalize results. Such analyses should be clearly reported and labeled as such in every study. It should be transparently indicated whether these analyses were planned *a priori* or not.

DISCUSSION

The discussion reports the results of the study in the context of existing evidence.[6,8,9] The investigators should cautiously interpret the results considering the objectives, limitations, multiplicity of analyses, results from similar studies, and other relevant evidence. In brief, the investigators should (1) summarize the results considering the study objectives; (2) discuss the limitations of the study, addressing sources of potential bias (both direction and magnitude), imprecision, and multiplicity of analyses; and (3) discuss the ability to generalize (external validity) the results (ie, how much the results of the study are applicable to clinical populations). Again, referring to the appropriate reporting guideline checklist helps investigators to remember to include all relevant details.

Box 1
Selected examples of poor reporting

Nonreporting or delayed reporting

Studies are not published because of negative or unexpected results (even if preliminary results have been presented)

Selective reporting

Published article(s) do not include all results, with "cherry-picking" of
- Outcomes (eg, only statistically significant findings)
- Analyses (eg, subgroups)

Incomplete reporting

Lack of complete and transparent reporting of methods that in turn limits reproducibility

Lack of reporting of all results such that data cannot included in future metaanalyses

Lack of reporting of adverse effects or harms of interventions or diagnostic tests

Misleading reporting

Deliberate or inadvertent misinterpretation of study methods, results, or both (eg, reporting a study as randomized when it is not; using "spin" to present negative results in a positive manner)

Unacknowledged inconsistency between information sources

Study protocol details differ between publication and trial registry/database

Adapted from Simera I, Kirtley S, Altman DG. Reporting clinical research: guidance to encourage accurate and transparent research reporting. Maturitas 2012;72:84–7.

SUMMARY

This article discusses aspects of research reporting. Other than purely literary reporting, there is a multitude of other types of reporting deficiencies that increase research waste (**Box 1**). Awareness of such problems is the first step toward improvement.

REFERENCES

1. Di Girolamo N, Meursinge Reynders R. Deficiencies of effectiveness of intervention studies in veterinary medicine: a cross-sectional survey of ten leading veterinary and medical journals. PeerJ 2016;4:e1649.
2. Haynes RB. More informative titles. ACP J Club 1994;121(1):A10.
3. Aronson J. When I use a word … declarative titles. QJM 2010;103:207–9.
4. Wager E, Altman DG, Simera I, et al. Do declarative titles affect readers' perceptions of research findings? A randomized trial. Res Integrity Peer Rev 2016;1(11).
5. Di Girolamo N, Reynders RM. Health care articles with simple and declarative titles were more likely to be in the Altmetric Top 100. J Clin Epidemiol 2016. [Epub ahead of print].
6. Moher D, Hopewell S, Schulz KF, et al. CONSORT 2010 explanation and elaboration: updated guidelines for reporting parallel group randomised trials. J Clin Epidemiol 2010;63(8):e1–37.
7. Boswood A, Häggström J, Gordon SG, et al. Effect of pimobendan in dogs with preclinical myxomatous mitral valve disease and cardiomegaly: the EPIC Study–a randomized clinical trial. J Vet Intern Med 2016;30(6):1765–79.
8. Bossuyt PM, Reitsma JB, Bruns DE, et al. STARD 2015: an updated list of essential items for reporting diagnostic accuracy studies. BMJ 2015;351:h5527.
9. Vandenbroucke JP, von Elm E, Altman DG, et al. Strengthening the Reporting of Observational Studies in Epidemiology (STROBE): explanation and elaboration. PLoS Med 2007;4(10):e297.
10. Available at: https://www.ncbi.nlm.nih.gov/pmc/articles/PMC2211558/.
11. Shanahan D, de Sousa IL, Marshall D. Improving author adherence to reporting guidelines. Conference on Open Access Scholarly Publishing (COASP) 2016. Poster. Arlington (VA), September 20–21, 2016.
12. Messerli FH. Chocolate consumption, cognitive function, and Nobel laureates. N Engl J Med 2012;367(16):1562–4.
13. Giuffrida MA. Defining the primary research question in veterinary clinical studies. J Am Vet Med Assoc 2016;249:547–51.
14. Goldacre B, Drysdale H, Powell-Smith A, et al. The COMPare trials project. 2016. Available at: www.COMPare-trials.org. Accessed November 19, 2016.
15. Giuffrida MA. Type II error and statistical power in reports of small animal clinical trials. J Am Vet Med Assoc 2014;244:1075–80.
16. Freiman JA, Chalmers TC, Smith H Jr, et al. The importance of beta, the type II error and sample size in the design and interpretation of the randomized control trial. Survey of 71 "negative" trials. N Engl J Med 1978;299:690–4.
17. Kim J, Bang H. Three common misuses of P values. Dent Hypotheses 2016;7(3):73–80.
18. Goodman SN, Berlin J. The use of predicted confidence intervals when planning experiments and the misuse of power when interpreting results. Ann Intern Med 1994;121:200–6.
19. Campbell MJ, Julious SA, Altman DG. Estimating sample sizes for binary, ordered categorical, and continuous outcomes in two group comparisons. BMJ 1995;311:1145–8.

20. Schulz KF. Randomised controlled trials. Clin Obstet Gynecol 1998;41:245–56.
21. Greenland S. Randomisation, statistics, and causal inference. Epidemiology 1990;1:421–9.
22. Armitage P. The role of randomisation in clinical trials. Stat Med 1982;1:345–52.
23. Hopewell S, Dutton S, Yu LM, et al. The quality of reports of randomised trials in 2000 and 2006: comparative study of articles indexed in PubMed. BMJ 2010;340: c723.
24. Brown DC. Sources and handling of losses to follow-up in parallel-group randomized controlled clinical trials in dogs and cats: 63 trials (2000–2005). Am J Vet Res 2007;68:694–8.
25. Medical Research Council. Streptomycin treatment of pulmonary tuberculosis: a medical research council investigation. BMJ 1948;2:769–82.
26. Schulz KF, Chalmers I, Grimes DA, et al. Assessing the quality of randomization from reports of controlled trials published in obstetrics and gynecology journals. JAMA 1994;272(2):125–8.
27. To MJ, Jones J, Emara M, et al. Are reports of randomized controlled trials improving over time? A systematic review of 284 articles published in high-impact general and specialized medical journals. PLoS One 2013;8(12):e84779.
28. Schulz KF, Chalmers I, Hayes RJ, et al. Empirical evidence of bias. Dimensions of methodological quality associated with estimates of treatment effects in controlled trials. JAMA 1995;273:408–12.
29. Schulz KF, Grimes DA. Blinding in randomised trials: hiding who got what. Lancet 2002;359:696–700.
30. Hopewell S, Hirst A, Collins GS, et al. Reporting of participant flow diagrams in published reports of randomized trials. Trials 2011;12:253.
31. Godwin OP, Dyson B, Lee PS, et al. Compliance to the CONSORT statement on participant flow diagrams in infectious disease randomized clinical trials. J Pharma Care Health Sys 2015;2:130.
32. Landis SC, Amara SG, Asadullah K, et al. A call for transparent reporting to optimize the predictive value of preclinical research. Nature 2012;490:187–91.
33. Rothman KJ. A show of confidence. N Engl J Med 1978;299:1362–3.
34. Sterne JA, Davey Smith G. Sifting the evidence–what's wrong with significance tests? BMJ 2001;322:226–31.
35. Bland JM, Altman DG. Statistical methods for assessing agreement between two methods of clinical measurement. Lancet 1986;1:307–10.
36. Schneeweiss S. Sensitivity analysis and external adjustment for unmeasured confounders in epidemiologic database studies of therapeutics. Pharmacoepidemiol Drug Saf 2006;15:291–303.

Moving?

Make sure your subscription moves with you!

To notify us of your new address, find your **Clinics Account Number** (located on your mailing label above your name), and contact customer service at:

Email: journalscustomerservice-usa@elsevier.com

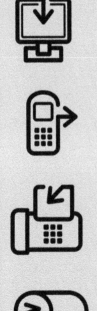

800-654-2452 (subscribers in the U.S. & Canada)
314-447-8871 (subscribers outside of the U.S. & Canada)

Fax number: 314-447-8029

Elsevier Health Sciences Division
Subscription Customer Service
3251 Riverport Lane
Maryland Heights, MO 63043

*To ensure uninterrupted delivery of your subscription, please notify us at least 4 weeks in advance of move.

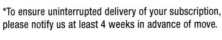
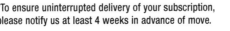

Printed and bound by CPI Group (UK) Ltd, Croydon, CR0 4YY

07/10/2024

01040501-0010